Dermatology

IN

PRACTICE

Dermatology

IN

PRACTICE

Anthony du Vivier

MD, FRCP

Department of Dermatology
King's College Hospital
London, UK

M Mosby-Wolfe

London Baltimore Bogotá Boston Buenos Aires Caracas Carlsbad, CA Chicago Madrid Mexico City Milan Naples, FL New York Philadelphia St. Louis Sydney Tokyo Toronto Wiesbaden

Typesetting by M to N Typesetters, London
Text and captions set in Plantin; figures set in Univers
Produced by Mandarin Offset
Printed in Hong Kong, 1990
Reprinted in Hong Kong, 1992, 1993, 1995.

Catalogue records for this book are available from the
US Library of Congress and British Library.

ISBN 0-397-44698-5

Publisher:	Fiona Foley
Series design:	Sue Michniewicz
Design:	Judith Gauge
Illustration:	Marion Tasker
Editorial assistants:	Justine Lisa King
	Nicola Bowen
Index:	Anne McCarthy
Production:	Seamus Murphy

PREFACE

This book has been written with the family practitioner specifically in mind. Most small textbooks of dermatology are designed for undergraduates, are fairly comprehensive at a superficial level and include disorders which a physician might only come across once or twice in a lifetime. It is tempting to include these rarer disorders because major advances have been made in understanding them, for example bullous pemphigoid and dermatitis herpetiformis. These discoveries have brought dermatology out of the dark ages of brilliant description, which so mystified and infuriated our colleagues, into a renaissance of science which rivals advances in medicine as a whole. The aetiology of common disorders such as eczema and psoriasis regrettably remains depressingly mysterious.

However, I have concentrated on those skin disorders which I see most days or at least once every few weeks, so that by inference the general practitioner should come across them regularly. I tell myself that I would be disappointed if a practitioner could not diagnose and manage them. I have tried to cover them in more detail than usual and have drawn attention to common errors and misconceptions.

I have included rarer disorders, but in a manner which allows only for diagnosis. I have left details of their aetiology and management to larger, more comprehensive tomes. I hope by this means to have satisfied the appetites of the undergraduate and permitted the physician to identify the disorder, prior to referral for investigation.

I have given much emphasis to physical signs because I believe diagnosis presents greater difficulty in dermatology than in any other speciality. This is not because the disorders are inherently difficult, but because time spent in a skin department as an undergraduate is either non-existent or understandably brief in view of the demands of the big four clinical attachments. The introductory chapter on terminology is thus particularly important because it is the vocabulary of dermatology, which must be understood in order to make a diagnosis.

The second major problem in dermatological practice is therapeutics. Most patients will have received an antifungal, an antibacterial and a combined steroid/anti-infective preparation before reaching the specialist, which gives the impression of a rather hit and miss approach. I have therefore spent time detailing how I manage common skin conditions.

I have been fortunate in my publishers, who gave me carte blanche to illustrate adequately my more comprehensive 'Atlas of Clinical Dermatology' and have allowed me to bring a liberal supply of illustrations to this book. I am hopeful that the text will be clear enough to bring some understanding of my speciality but the illustrations and their captions have been chosen to tell an accompanying story. I have also included some brief visual aids to highlight what I consider to be vital clues to diagnosis and fundamental points of management. In summary, I hope to have provided a manual for general practice which illustrates how to diagnose and treat the top twenty common skin diseases. An alternative title to the book might have been 'Bread and Butter Dermatology'.

Anthony du Vivier
London.

ACKNOWLEDGEMENTS

This book is dedicated to my lovely wife and favourite family practitioner, Judith Brett, and to her colleague and our good friend the late Tom Kelly; to the monks at Ampleforth College in Yorkshire, who profoundly influenced me; to the physicians at St. Bartholomew's Hospital, Dowling Munro and the late Peter Borrie, who introduced me to dermatology, and the late Sir Ronald Bodley Scott and Gordon Hamilton Fairley, who made it possible for me to pursue a career in medicine. I am also grateful to Richard Stoughton in the United States, who told me more about the science of the subject, and to my close colleagues, Andrew Pembroke and Jeremy Gilkes, who put me right when I get it wrong.

I would like to thank the following for providing illustrative material: Dr Y.M. Clayton, St John's Hospital for Diseases of the Skin (Figs 10.11, 12.12, 12.16); Dr Frank Dann, Honolulu (Fig. 10.16); Dr P.H. McKee, St Thomas's Hospital (Figs 1.34, 3.3, 3.4, 5.3, 6.7, 7.4, 21.6); Miss G. Midgley, St John's Hospital for Diseases of the Skin (Figs 12.12, 12.13); St Bartholomew's Hospital (Figs 11.20, 13.1); Institute of Dermatology, UMDS, Guy's & St Thomas's Hospitals (Figs 9.8, 10.5, 10.14, 14.3, 14.11, 14.12, 14.13, 17.18, 22.2, 22.8); St Mary's Hospital Medical School (Figs 6.9, 12.3, 22.3, 23.17, 23.18).

The rest of the photographs have been taken by Mr Barry Pyke and his excellent Department of Medical Photography and Illustrations at King's College Hospital. I am most grateful for their skill and help.

I have attempted to acknowledge the original source of all colour photographs other than those from our own collection but apologise if any attributions have been omitted.

CONTENTS

1 THE DERMATOLOGICAL DIAGNOSIS

INTRODUCTION

The 'spot diagnosis' is a delusion, a belief strongly adhered to by medical students despite its obvious deficiencies. It is always impressive to see an experienced dermatologist arrive instantly at a diagnosis but, just as Sherlock Holmes astounded Dr Watson with observations regarding his life history at their first encounter in the Pathology Department at St. Bartholomew's Hospital, it is a matter of a series of rapid observations resulting in correct deduction. It is not enough to 'glance' at an eruption and expect to make a diagnosis. Dermatology, like any other branch of medicine, is a science and diagnosis results from detailed history taking, thorough examination and accurate observation. It is essential that this should take place in consulting rooms with plenty of natural sunlight affording good illumination. A British winter's evening is an anathema for examining the skin.

The teaching of dermatology varies. Some medical schools have excellent training programmes but others (including, surprisingly, some of those in the US) do not teach dermatology at a student level at all; sometimes the course is optional. This is regrettable, because approximately twenty per cent of consultations in family practice relate to the skin. Even in good centres, students will not have enough exposure to the diagnosis and management of skin disorders, for understandably their time is limited. It is therefore an excellent idea to spend a few sessions as a postgraduate in family practice with the local dermatologist. The problem with dermatology is that all is and has been revealed from the start. The conditions have therefore been classified many years ago in ancient languages which are no longer learnt at school. This nomenclature gives rise to confusion. Also, because every disorder is visible, an explanation is expected, whereas disorders of the liver, for example, are only slowly being coded as the needle biopsy reveals a vast array of pathology. However, the aetiology of each skin disorder is gradually being elucidated and major advances are being made in therapy, so that the field is rapidly expanding and has already given rise to specialists within the speciality.

HISTORY

Taking the history (Fig. 1.1) of a skin disorder is usually a less prolonged affair than in general medicine. Indeed sometimes it is more productive to examine the skin early in the consultation to get some idea of the problem and then to proceed to ask the relevant questions. These enquiries include:

How long has it been present? Some eruptions begin acutely, for example drug eruptions, whereas others are more insidious, such as pityriasis versicolor.

How does it behave? Some disorders are liable to relapse and remission, for example urticaria, which may not be present on the day of the consultation. However, a history of red itchy swelling appearing anywhere on the skin, which disappears without trace within twenty-four hours, is characteristic. Factors

THE HISTORY	
general questions:	how long has it been present? how does it behave? how did it start? what did it look like initially? is it anywhere else? what affects it? from where do you come? have you been abroad recently and if so where?
assess symptoms:	does it itch? is it painful? is it sore? does it burn?
ascertain:	past history of skin and related disorders family history associated symptoms past medical history previous and current drug therapy occupation social history effect of the disease on the patient

▲ **Fig. 1.1** *Taking the history.*

relating to the relapses may be important, for example exposure to bright sunlight may precipitate recurrent attacks of herpes simplex.

How did it start? In pityriasis rosea, a patch appears and remains solitary for several days after which a large number of smaller patches appear all over the torso. This single lesion is known as the herald patch and is an important clue to diagnosis.

What did it look like initially? Some patients are very observant and can record the progress of their condition accurately. For example, in impetigo, they note that it starts as blisters which quickly break and form crusts. Their descriptions may be very helpful if the rash has temporarily disappeared, as happens with urticaria and herpes simplex. Often however, if it has disappeared, it is wise to suggest that the patient returns immediately when it recurs and has access to an 'SOS appointment' so that the eruption can be seen at its height.

Is it anywhere else? Patients may complain about something they consider important but disregard a long-standing skin condition elsewhere. Thus an acute weeping eczema on the face may clearly be the prime problem to the patient but the cause of it may be an ointment being used to treat chronic varicose eczema on the leg, which is thought to be totally unrelated by the patient. Therefore all the skin should be examined to avoid this happening.

What affects it? The patient's view is sometimes invaluable. The patient may suspect the sun, the cat, something at work, 'nerves' or some tablets as the cause of the skin complaint, and often the patient is correct.

From where do you come? A knowledge of diseases endemic in various parts of the world is useful: a Vietnamese may have erythema nodosum secondary to tuberculosis, a Philippino may have leprosy and a West Indian may have sarcoidosis.

Have you been abroad recently and if so where? Foreign travel exposes patients to diseases which are uncommon in their country of origin. For example, the insect which bit the patient may have been infected with the protozoan, *Leishmania* sp., which causes leishmaniasis, and Baghdad boil (cutaneous leishmaniasis) can occur in less exotic places, such as the Mediterranean.

Symptoms

Does it itch? Some disorders always itch, for example scabies, and the very intensity of the complaint may suggest the diagnosis. The rash of secondary syphilis on the other hand virtually never itches. Psoriasis and pityriasis rosea are quixotic and may or may not itch.

Is it painful? Few dermatological disorders are acutely painful but the classic example is that of herpes zoster. Pain dominates the history (you do not need to ask) and the suspicion is confirmed when the unilateral vesicular eruption is revealed on examination.

Is it sore? An eruption such as eczema or psoriasis may become sore when it dries out and cracks, particularly in cold climatic conditions.

Does it burn? Few skin disorders burn and patients thus afflicted volunteer the symptom. The rash of erythropoietic protoporphyria burns and the localization of the symptoms to light-exposed skin might suggest the diagnosis. More often than not, burning is a psychosomatic symptom which affects the mouth, genitalia or face.

Associated symptoms

The skin disorder may follow a prior illness. Thus a fever and sore throat due to a *Streptococcus* frequently precede guttate psoriasis, erythema nodosum and Henoch–Schönlein purpura. The rash, however, may result from a drug given to treat an illness, for example the unfortunate prescription of ampicillin for a sore throat in a young adult with unsuspected infectious mononucleosis; or the skin rash may be one of the presenting features of a systemic disease, such as sarcoidosis or lupus erythematosus.

Past history of skin and related disorders

A past history of skin and related disorders is often relevant. It is stated in text books that children with atopic eczema always recover. Although this is true in the majority of cases, the fact that the skin looks normal in these individuals does not mean that the propensity for the disease has disappeared. The skin of someone who has had eczema is potentially able to react in that manner again given the right circumstances. This is particularly relevant to young women who have had eczema as children. They begin to develop it again on the hands, either as a result of an occupation such as hairdressing or when looking after small children. Alternatively, a patient may develop late onset eczema and the clue to its cause may be other symptoms of atopy such as hay fever or asthma in childhood.

Family history

Many common skin diseases are inherited including psoriasis, ichthyosis and eczema. In the case of eczema, the family history of a related disorder, such as asthma, hay fever or urticaria, may be present even if eczema is not. Sometimes the patient denies a family history at the initial consultation but this is usually simply because no one has ever mentioned a skin disorder to them previously and subsequent questioning at a family reunion may provide information that the patient was unaware of.

Past medical history

A previous illness may help to explain the present complaint. Thus a difficult and protracted labour may be responsible for a diffuse loss of hair three months later (telogen effluvium). A chronic illness, such as diabetes mellitus, might make the patient more prone to a chronic candidal paronychia.

Previous and current drug therapy

Clearly a systemic agent may be the cause of a skin disorder, such as a phenothiazine, a diuretic or a tetracycline for a phototoxic eruption or an antibiotic for a morbilliform rash. Drugs such as systemic steroids are immunosuppressive and make a patient more prone to infections with commensals, such as pityriasis versicolor. Family practitioners are very good at listing the oral agents which a patient is taking in their letters of referral to the specialist, but sometimes topical remedies are forgotten. These are important because the therapy prescribed may have been correct and yet ineffective in a particular patient. It is not known why this is nor why, for example, some patients with psoriasis will respond to tar and others will not or why one patient with acne will respond to tetracyclines and another will not. However, there is no point in represcribing the drug.

Alternatively, the prescribed therapy may actually be making the disease worse and patients will often note this. This may be because the condition has been misdiagnosed, for example when tinea or rosacea are diagnosed as eczema and treated with steroids. Alternatively, a complication may have occurred in a steroid-responsive dermatosis, so that the steroid is no longer appropriate, as when molluscum contagiosum is superimposed upon eczema. Equally the patient may have become sensitized to the prescribed agent. This occurs particularly when varicose eczema is treated with agents containing topical antibiotics, such as neomycin. Another possibility is that the patient may have developed an irritant reaction to a drug, such as dithranol used in the treatment of psoriasis. Finally, alcohol is a drug which is often forgotten. In sufficient quantity it tends to exacerbate psoriasis, discoid eczema and rosacea.

Occupation

Just as coal miners are prone to pneumoconiosis, so certain occupations predispose to skin disease. Percival Pott established the link between carcinoma of the skin of the scrotum and previous exposure to soot in men who had cleaned chimneys as children. Dubreuilh pin-pointed the relationship of malignant melanoma on the face of workers in the vineyards of Bordeaux to exposure to ultraviolet light. In modern times, a sclerodermatous condition, with systemic involvement including angiosarcoma of the liver, has occurred in industrial workers exposed to vinyl-chloride. Exposure to contact allergens at work is often suspected because the patient gets better at the weekend or when away on holiday. Dermatitis secondary to chromate has become common in builders working with cement. Probably the most common occupational skin diseases seen in dermatology are primary irritant dermatitis and chronic candidal paronychia in housewives, nurses and barmaids, caused by the frequent exposure of the hands to water.

Social history

The situation at home is of great importance. Other members of the household may be itching which may suggest a diagnosis of scabies. The family cat and its cohabitants may be the source of the insect bites. Psychological factors are as critical in skin disorders as they are in other branches of medicine. The unhappiness of a marriage or relationship, guilt (religious or otherwise), success or failure at work, or difficult children, all take their toll and it is difficult to manage any chronic skin disease without a knowledge of these problems. It may be that the whole eruption is caused by the patient (dermatitis artefacta) or that the failure to recover is because the patient does not wish to get better, preferring instead to continue to evoke sympathy and attention because of the condition. Sometimes patients simply overreact to a minor skin condition, the presence of which is the final straw in a life style that has got completely out of control.

Effect of the disease on the patient

The patient is likely to be anxious regarding the nature of the disorder. Infectivity and malignant disease are the commonest fears so that informed reassurance to the contrary, if appropriate, may be of enormous help to the patient. Sometimes the concern may amount to a phobia, for example regarding herpes simplex in the 1970s and now acquired immune deficiency syndrome (AIDS) in the 1980s, and further psychological help will be required.

The functional effects may be important. An eruption on the feet may make it difficult to walk and one on the hands difficult to work. The appearances of the condition on exposed parts may make the patient feel leprous and ostracized. Extraordinary variations in patients' reactions occur. Some will put up with a considerable degree of psoriasis and yet others will be disgusted and aggrieved by minimal disease. All these factors have to be considered when deciding how aggressively to treat a disorder.

THE EXAMINATION

Ideally the whole patient should be examined. This is not usually necessary for warts, but it is for most conditions. A basal cell carcinoma of the face may be accompanied by other solar-induced malignancies elsewhere, such as a malignant melanoma on the back, an area which the patient cannot easily see; an eruption on one hand may be explained by spread of tinea from the toe nails and feet; and a condition of both hands which is unresponsive to therapy may be due to psoriasis found on the elbows and in the scalp.

It is sensible to examine the skin in an orderly manner, starting at the hands, so as not to miss the burrows of scabies, and then proceeding up the arms, face, trunk and so on. The hair, nails and mouth should not be forgotten.

It is important also to palpate the lesions. Disorders involving primarily the dermis, such as sarcoidosis or lymphoma, can be distinguished from those affecting the epidermis, such as eczema, because they are firmly palpable. Finally, patients are reassured by a thorough general medical examination and they are relieved that the doctor is prepared to feel their skin. It helps to dispel the fear that their condition made them 'untouchable'.

VOCABULARY

Just as râles, rhonchi and bronchial breathing are physical signs which once elicited contribute to a pulmonary diagnosis, so there is a vocabulary which must be grasped to establish the nature of a skin disorder. The main lesions may be defined as follows:

Primary lesions

Macule: a flat lesion less than 1cm in diameter (Figs 1.2 & 1.3).

Papule: a raised lesion less than 0.5cm in diameter (Figs 1.4 & 1.5).

Nodule: a papule greater than 0.5cm in diameter (Fig. 1.6).

Patch: a flat lesion greater than 1cm in diameter (Fig. 1.7).

Plaque: a slightly raised lesion greater than 1cm in diameter (Fig. 1.8).

Pustule: a raised lesion less than 0.5cm in diameter containing yellow fluid which may be infected or sterile (Fig. 1.9).

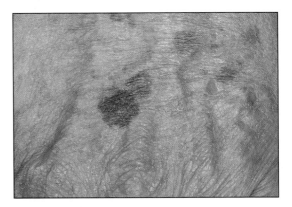

▲ **Fig. 1.2** *Macules. Flat lesions less than 1cm in diameter. These pigmented macules are solar lentigines.*

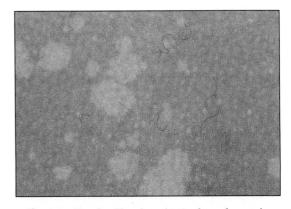

▲ **Fig. 1.3** *Macules. These hypopigmented macules vary in size and have enlarged by confluence. They are due to pityriasis versicolor.*

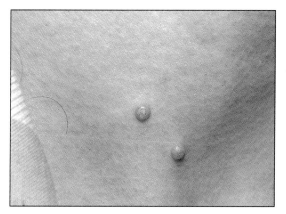

▲**Fig. 1.4** *Papules. Raised lesions less than 0.5 cm in diameter. These are flesh coloured with central dimpling of the surface and are due to molluscum contagiosum.*

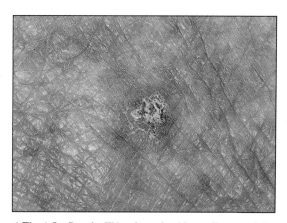

▲**Fig. 1.5** *Papule. This red papule with an adherent scale is a solar keratosis. Note the surrounding lentigines from solar damage.*

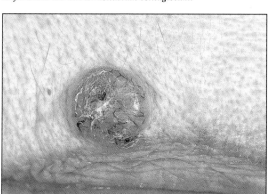

▲**Fig. 1.6** *Nodule. A raised lesion greater than 0.5 cm in diameter, in this case a cystic basal cell carcinoma on the upper lip. Note the telangiectasia.*

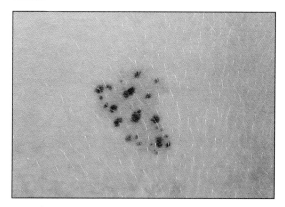

▲**Fig. 1.7** *Patch. Flat lesion greater than 1 cm in diameter, in this case a congenital melanocytic naevus known as naevus spilus.*

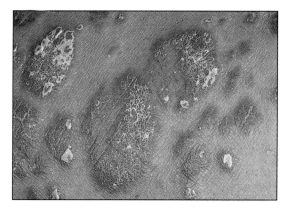

▲**Fig. 1.8** *Plaque. Slightly raised lesion greater than 1 cm in diameter. These plaques due to psoriasis are a deep-red colour, are well defined and have a thick white scale.*

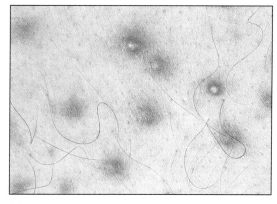

▲**Fig. 1.9** *Pustule. Raised lesion less than 0.5 cm in diameter containing yellow fluid which may be infected or sterile. These sterile pustules are associated with papules and are due to acne vulgaris.*

Vesicle: a raised lesion less than 0.5cm in diameter containing clear fluid (Figs. 1.10 & 1.11).

Bulla (blister): a vesicle which is greater than 0.5cm in diameter (Fig. 1.12).

Wheal: a transient red swelling of the skin, often with central pallor (Fig. 1.13). Wheals can be of various shapes and sizes.

Telangiectasia: dilatation of capillaries (see Fig. 1.6).

Secondary lesions

Crust: a dried exudate which may have been serous, purulent (Fig. 1.14) or haemorrhagic.

Excoriation: a shallow haemorrhagic excavation resulting from scratching. It may be linear (Fig. 1.15) or discrete (punctate).

Lichenification: a thickening of the skin with exaggeration of the skin creases (Fig. 1.16).

Necrosis: death of skin tissue; it is usually black in colour (Fig. 1.17).

Scar: the final stage of any healing process which involves the deeper dermis, resulting in a white smooth firm shiny lesion (Fig. 1.18).

Erosion: partial break in the epidermis.

Ulcer: full thickness loss of the epidermis (Fig.1.19).

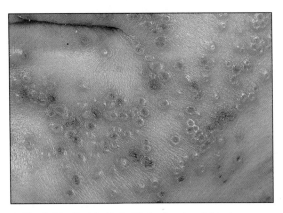

▲ **Fig. 1.10** *Vesicle. Raised lesion less than 0.5cm in diameter containing clear fluid. These vesicles, some of which are becoming brown as they dry, are due to herpes simplex in a patient with eczema (eczema herpeticum).*

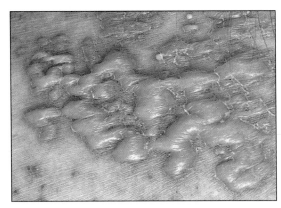

▲ **Fig. 1.11** *Vesicle. The clear fluid may become turbid as in herpes zoster.*

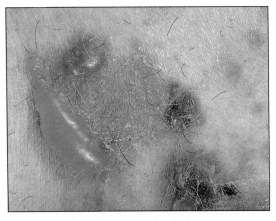

▲ **Fig. 1.12** *Bulla. A vesicle greater than 0.5cm in diameter. These are tense blisters due to bullous pemphigoid. Haemorrhagic scabs occur as they dry.*

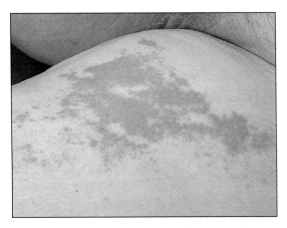

▲ **Fig. 1.13** *Wheals. Transient red swellings of the skin which are of various shapes and sizes and occur in urticaria.*

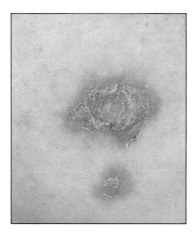

◀**Fig. 1.14**
*Crust. Dried
exudate, which
may have been
serous, purulent or
haemorrhagic.
These yellow
crusts are due to
impetigo.*

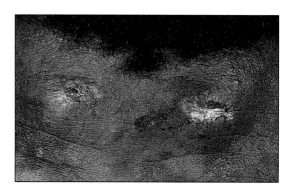

▲**Fig. 1.15**   *Excoriation. A shallow haemorrhagic excavation
resulting from scratching. These linear excoriations were
artefactual.*

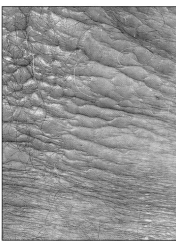

◀**Fig. 1.16**
*Lichenification.
Thickening of the
skin with
exaggeration of the
skin creases due to
continual rubbing.*

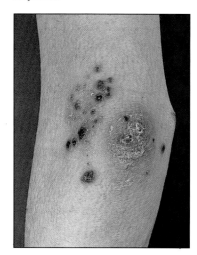

◀**Fig. 1.17**
*Necrosis. Death of
skin tissues, in this
case secondary to
allergic vasculitis.*

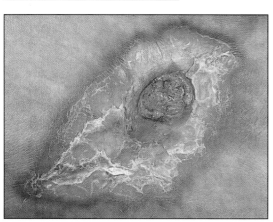

▲**Fig. 1.18**   *Scar. Permanent destruction of the skin
secondary to healing of a disorder which involves the deeper
dermis. Here there is a well-defined waxy yellow-red plaque
with a red-brown margin and an area of ulceration due to
necrobiosis lipoidica diabeticorum.*

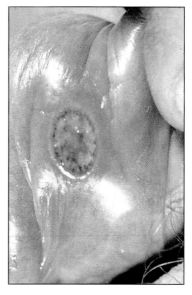

◀**Fig. 1.19**
*Ulcer. A full-
thickness break in
the epidermis.
This lesion is a
syphilitic chancre.*

Atrophy: a thinning and transparency of the skin due to diminution of either the epidermis or the dermis, or both (Fig. 1.20).

Sclerosis: a circumscribed or diffuse hardening or induration of the skin due to dermal or subcutaneous oedema, cellular infiltration or collagen proliferation (Fig. 1.21).

An eruption may be either essentially monomorphic, for example molluscum contagiosum, or consist of various forms (polymorphic), for example acne, where comedones, papules, pustules, cysts and scars may be found (Fig. 1.22). The lesion may evolve through various stages, for example from macules, vesicles, pustules and crusts sometimes to post-inflammatory pigmentation as in herpes simplex.

Certain other characteristics of the lesions must be observed as described below.

MORPHOLOGY OF THE LESIONS

Colour

A wealth of colours occurs in skin disorders, which is critical for diagnosis. Thus eczema is pink, psoriasis is red and pityriasis versicolor is frequently brown; the papules of lichen planus are purple, of scabies, red, of xanthomata, yellow or orange (Fig. 1.23), and of the blue naevus, blue. The pigments and colours of a malignant melanoma are varied whereas those of a

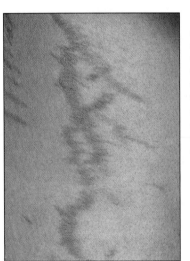

◄**Fig. 1.20**
*Atrophy.
Diminution of
epithelial cells or
connective tissue,
or both, resulting
in a thinned and
transparent
epidermis or
depression in the
dermis, or both as
in these striae.*

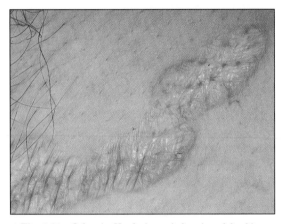

▲**Fig. 1.21** *Sclerosis. Hardening or induration of the skin. In lichen sclerosus et atrophicus, the white areas are sclerotic and the wrinkled areas are atrophic.*

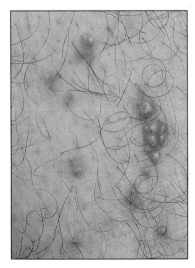

◄**Fig. 1.23**
*Colour. Yellow
papules occur in
xanthomata due to
hyperlipidaemia.*

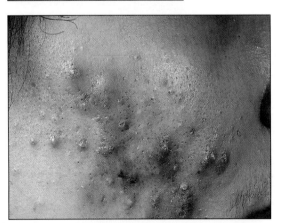

▲**Fig. 1.22** *Polymorphic eruptions. Blackheads, papules, pustules, nodules and scarring are present in this example of acne vulgaris.*

solar lentigo are quite uniform (see Fig. 1.2). Purpura (Fig. 1.24) is distinguished from erythema (Fig. 1.25) because the latter is red and blanches with pressure whereas the former is purple and does not.

Scale

The skin is shed imperceptibly all the time. This becomes visible as scales if at least part of the disorder affects the epidermis. In eczema there is fluid in and around the epidermal cells producing a disordered epithelium. In psoriasis the basal cells are mitotically active and a hyperproliferative epidermis results. These disorders are scaly and because they are red are known as erythematosquamous diseases. The scale is fine in eczema (Fig. 1.26) and thick and silvery in psoriasis (see Fig. 1.8). In pityriasis versicolor, where there is colonization of the outermost layer of the epidermis by a fungus, the scale may be barely perceptible until the macules are scraped with a blunt scalpel. The scale may be either tenacious, as in a solar keratosis (a pre-malignant disorder of the epidermis; see Fig. 1.5), or easily scraped off revealing minute bleeding points, as in psoriasis. The scale may be either uniformly spread across the lesion, as in eczema, or more marked peripherally, as in pityriasis rosea. On the other hand, if the primary pathology is in the dermis, as in lichen planus or granuloma annulare (Fig. 1.27), no scaling is produced at all.

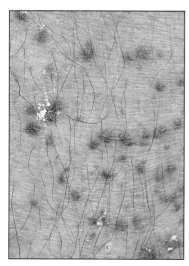

◀**Fig. 1.24** *Colour. Purple papules are present in allergic vasculitis.*

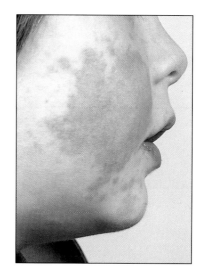

◀**Fig. 1.25** *Colour. A blotchy redness (erythema) is present in this child with fifth disease due to a parvovirus.*

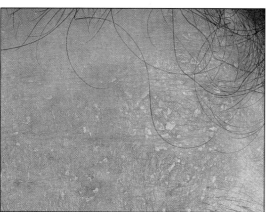

▲ **Fig. 1.26** *Scale. Seborrhoeic eczema: the scale is fine on a background of erythema and is known as an erythematosquamous disorder.*

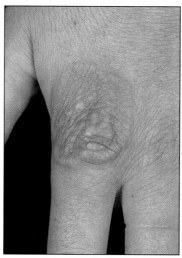

◀**Fig. 1.27** *Pattern. Granuloma annulare: the lesion is annular, spreading peripherally and regressing centrally.*

Shape

Lesions may be round or discoid as in nummular eczema, oval as in pityriasis rosea or all manner of shapes and sizes as in psoriasis (see Fig. 1.8). Lesions of lichen planus are polygonal.

Pattern

Lesions may be arranged in a particular pattern which may be linear (some epidermal naevi, artefacts, phyto-photodermatitis and the Koebner phenomenon), grouped (insect bites and herpes simplex), reticular or net-like (oral lichen planus) or annular (Figs 1.27 & 1.28). The latter may be round, arciform, polycyclic (Fig. 1.29) or iris- (target-) like (Fig. 1.30).

Surface

The lesion may be rough, as in a seborrhoeic wart (Fig. 1.31), or smooth, as in a dermal melanocytic naevus (a mole).

Consistency

The lesion may be firm as in a dermatofibroma, soft as in a dermal mole, hard as in a secondary deposit or tethered as in scleroderma.

Margin

The lesion may be discrete as in psoriasis or indistinct as in many forms of eczema. There may be more activity peripherally with a tendency to central

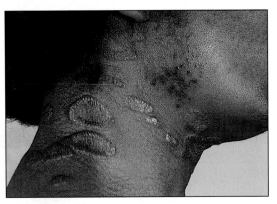

▲**Fig. 1.28** *Pattern. Sarcoidosis: the lesions are annular in arrangement and raised with no scaling indicating that the pathology is in the dermis or deeper.*

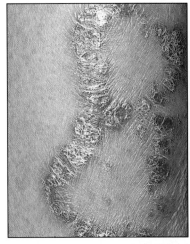

◀**Fig. 1.29** *Pattern. Psoriasis: the lesion is arranged into more than one ring and is thus polycyclic. It is a deep-red colour with a thick white scale and is another erythemato-squamous disorder.*

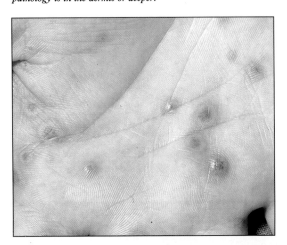

▲**Fig. 1.30** *Pattern. Erythema multiforme: iris or target lesions consisting of a pink macule with a purple central papule are present.*

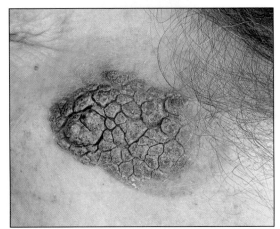

▲**Fig. 1.31** *Surface. Seborrhoeic wart: the surface of this plaque is rough and split (fissured). The lesion is well defined and pigmented.*

healing, as in tinea. The margin may be raised and rolled as in basal cell carcinoma (Fig. 1.32) or irregular and notched as in a malignant melanoma.

DISTRIBUTION OF THE LESIONS

The importance of the morphology of the skin lesions has been emphasized. Consideration of the distribution of these lesions is the next critical step in diagnosis.

The distribution of some skin eruptions is often explicable. Herpes zoster is a viral infection usually involving a single cutaneous nerve. The eruption is therefore unilateral and corresponds to the dermatome affected (Fig. 1.33). The finding of vesicles surrounded by erythema confirms the diagnosis. The superficial fungus which causes pityriasis versicolor is lipophilic and is dependent upon active sebaceous glands. It therefore only occurs after puberty, predominantly on the trunk where the sebaceous glands are most active. In contrast psoriasis, for totally obscure reasons, principally affects the scalp, elbows, knees and buttocks. It is possible that visible areas, such as the face, are often spared from psoriasis because of constant ultraviolet exposure. Lichen planus has a predilection for the fronts of the wrists, ankles, umbilicus, lumbar area and genitalia. Its diagnosis may be confirmed by finding oral lesions. This distribution is also not understood.

THE ANATOMY OF THE SKIN

The dermatological diagnosis is incomplete without an understanding of the anatomy of the skin. It is composed of an epidermis, a dermis and certain appendages (Fig. 1.34).

The epidermis has four layers. The lowest is the basal cell layer. Above this is the spinous or Malpighian layer, which is sometimes called the prickle cell layer because the desmosomes that attach one epidermal cell to another are clearly visible. If the desmosomes

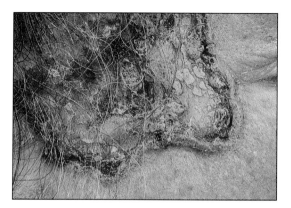

▲**Fig. 1.32** *Margin. Basal cell carcinoma: the margin is raised, pearly in colour and rolled.*

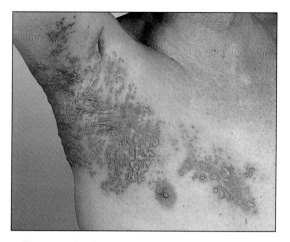

▲**Fig. 1.33** *Distribution. Herpes zoster: the eruption is unilateral in the distribution of a cutaneous nerve (T2) and in the early stages consists of vesicles surrounded by erythema (see Fig. 1.11).*

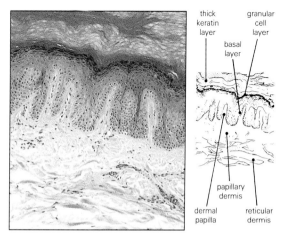

▲**Fig. 1.34** *Skin anatomy. Palmar skin illustrates the thick dead keratin layer, the viable epidermis and the dermis.*

11

are damaged as in the autoimmune disease, pemphigus, or in a genetic abnormality such as Hailey–Hailey disease or Darier's disease, the epidermal cells become separated (acantholysis) and intraepidermal blistering results. The granular layer succeeds the prickle layer. It contains keratohyalin granules, which are precursors of keratin and certain lipids that are discharged into the intercellular space and are probably responsible for intercellular cohesion. Keratin (a protein) makes up the final outermost layer which is the stratum corneum in which the keratinocytes have become flat anucleated corneocytes (squames). In the palms and soles a non-stainable layer (known therefore as the stratum lucidum) exists between the granular and horny layer.

There are four cell types in the epidermis. The keratinocyte in the basal layer is mitotically active. It moves outwards to form the keratin of the stratum corneum, a process that takes 28 days. The keratinocyte may be stimulated to further mitosis by trauma and its control mechanism is abnormal in psoriasis. It has a large dark staining nucleus with one or more nucleoli; its cytoplasm contains ribosomes, mitochondria and tonofilaments. Tonofilaments consist of keratin polypeptides which insert into desmosomes and reduce the mechanical stresses within the epidermis by distributing them evenly between the cells.

Melanocytes are situated in the basal cell layer of the epidermis and are responsible for producing the pigment, melanin. They occur in a ratio of approximately 1:5 with basal cells. Since they do not stain with haematoxylin and eosin, they appear as clear cells in routine sections. Caucasians have the same number of melanocytes as Negroes but have less and smaller melanosomes (pigment-containing electron-dense granules produced within the melanocyte during the process of melanogenesis). Melanosomes are present in the dendrites of melanocytes and are ingested by neighbouring keratinocytes. These melanin granules partially surround the nucleus of the keratinocyte and protect it from ultraviolet light. Each melanocyte serves several keratinocytes.

The Langerhan cell is a dendritic cell of mesenchymal origin which is situated in the suprabasal layer but which is not visible with haematoxylin and eosin stains, though it can be stained with monoclonal antibodies to antigenic components on its surface. Under an electron microscope rather characteristic tennis racquet shaped granules are visible in the cytoplasm. The Langerhan cell is involved in immune function and is responsible for the processing of allergens and their presentation to lymphocytes.

The Merckel cell is present throughout the skin. Like the Langerhan cell, it cannot be visualized with conventional stains but can be distinguished ultrastructurally. It subserves sensory function and is most abundant in areas of maximum sensitivity.

The junction of the epidermis with the dermis consists of undulating projections of epidermis into the dermis which are known as rete ridges and conversely of loops in between them which are known as dermal papillae. A basement membrane separates the epidermis from the dermis and is visible under the light microscope when stained pink with periodic acid–Schiff (PAS). It consists of several layers distinguishable by electron microscopy. A basal cell plasma membrane is attached to the epidermis by hemidesmosomes and underneath this is an electron-lucid zone (lamina lucida) and underneath that an electron-dense basal lamina. A network of anchoring fibrils and fine fibrils connect this to the dermis. These layers are abnormal in inherited disorders such as epidermolysis bullosa and in immunological disorders such as bullous pemphigoid. Blistering of the skin results.

The dermis nourishes and supports the epidermis. The most abundant cell in the dermis is the fibroblast which synthesizes three dermal proteins: collagen, which provides structural support, and elastin and reticulin, which contribute to the elasticity and tensile strength of the dermis. They are all located in an amorphous material known as the ground substance. There are many subtypes of collagen, abnormalities of which may lead to one of the varieties of the Ehlers–Danlos syndrome. Similar abnormalities of elastic tissue gives rise to conditions such as pseudoxanthoma elasticum. The collagen bundles in the deeper (reticular) dermis are coarser than those in the superficial (papillary) dermis and may also be distinguished by special stains. The other cells of the dermis are mast cells, macrophages and lymphocytes.

Arteries and veins in the subcutaneous fat give rise to two horizontal vascular plexuses linked by ascending intercommunicating vessels. These are clearly visible physiologically in many adolescents (cutis marmorata) and are permanently dilated in erythema ab igne. These vascular channels have an enormous reserve capacity for vasodilatation, particularly during exercise when it is necessary to lose heat rapidly. In pathological states such as erythroderma this vasodilatation may result in high output cardiac failure. Lymphatics are also present in the dermis and peripheral sensory nerves and sympathetic autonomic nerves supply the vasculature and hair follicles.

There are three main skin appendages. The pilo-sebaceous unit consists of a hair follicle (which is an invagination of the epidermis) one or more sebaceous glands, and the arrector pili muscle. The sebaceous gland secretes sebum a substance resulting from the disintegration of the glandular cells of the sebaceous glands. Their activity is increased with puberty and is abnormal in acne vulgaris.

Eccrine sweat glands occur throughout the skin and are concerned with thermoregulation. The gland itself is a coiled structure found in the reticular dermis, and excretory ducts spiral through the papillary dermis and epidermis to the surface. The apocrine gland is located principally in the axilla and pubic area. Although it has a highly important function in animals with regard to scent, its significance in humans is unknown. However the breakdown products of apocrine secretions by bacterial flora are responsible for body odour. The duct of the apocrine gland enters the pilosebaceous follicle just above the sebaceous gland.

Specialized structures of the skin (hair and nail) are dealt with in the respective chapters devoted to their abnormalities.

TOOLS OF THE TRADE

Dermatology in common with family practice is one of the last bastions of clinical medicine, and 'high tech' — although undoubtedly now a feature — is unnecessary most of the time. Dermatologists probably request fewer laboratory tests than many specialists in other disciplines. However, a dermatologist does need:

- **An ordinary microscope** for the examination of skin scrapings fixed in potash for fungi and for the identification of the acarus, nits and pediculi.
- **Various basic surgical instruments:** such as a curette, scissors, needle holder, forceps and scalpel. Curettage of warts and pyogenic granuloma, and excision of dermatofibroma and benign moles are all procedures that any medical practitioner can perform, provided that the specimens are sent for histological examination. The various surgical techniques are better demonstrated in outpatient departments than described here. Diagnostic incisional skin biopsy is best performed by the dermatologist, as the choice of which part of a skin eruption to biopsy requires experience to obtain a satisfactory pathological specimen. It may also be

useful to process the specimen for immunofluorescence, electron microscopy, cell markers or microbiology in addition to routine pathology. Malignant tumours should be referred because their management is often complicated.

- **A cautery machine,** which is essential for simple minor surgical procedures such as cautery of skin tags and spider naevi or after a curettage.
- **A Wood's light,** which is an ultraviolet lamp emitting radiation with a wavelength of 360nm. This is a useful diagnostic tool; under its rays, erythrasma, a corynebacterial infection of the skin, fluoresces a coral-pink colour and certain ringworm infections of the scalp hairs fluoresce green.

THE DERMATOLOGIST AND COLLEAGUES

The family practitioner is the closest associate. It is extremely helpful if the skin department has a 'hot line', so that arrangements can easily be made by the practitioner for a patient to be seen that day. Acute eruptions, distressed patients and suspicious pigmented moles should be seen immediately.

In the hospital, the dermatologist is a frequent visitor to every ward, usually because of drug eruptions, and thus comes into contact with all specialists. However, certain specialists prescribe drugs which cause eruptions more often than others, for example rheumatologists; and disorders of certain organs (for example the liver) have a high frequency of cutaneous complications. Some specialities have a particularly close liaison with the dermatologist. For example, pathologists and dermatologists need to meet regularly to review the previous week's dermatopathology as it is extremely difficult for either speciality to work constructively without regular dialogue. Most pathology departments also have facilities for immunofluorescence, which is now an essential investigative technique in the diagnosis of disorders such as bullous pemphigoid and dermatitis herpetiformis.

Although most dermatologists look at their own skin specimens for the diagnosis of fungal disorders, the microbiology department is indispensible for culturing specimens. The microbiologist is also an important colleague as he or she can give advice regarding appropriate antimicrobial therapy in patients with infective or infected skin diseases. The virologist, in addition to culturing specimens, will often examine directly under the electron microscope specimens taken from vesicles and give an immediate answer. This is particularly important in distinguishing serious disorders such as primary herpes simplex, Kaposi's varicelliform eruption, generalized herpes zoster and, formerly, smallpox from each other.

Most dermatologists work closely with a plastic surgeon and a radiotherapist, and have combined clinics for the management of malignant disease of the skin. A liaison with a good general physician is very helpful with regard to the sick patient, for it is a rare dermatologist who can keep up with all the developments in general medicine, when matters are proceeding so quickly in dermatology itself. A liaison psychiatrist in the skin department is invaluable. A significant number of dermatological patients have affective disorders and whereas they might be un-willing to see a psychiatrist in a department of psychological medicine, they find the venue of the skin department acceptable.

Paramedical staff are essential. Many nurses regret-tably go through their training with little or no exposure to the management of skin diseases. As a result, they may be puzzled by the presence of a healthy person with a skin rash in a hospital bed. However, the nurse who understands the use of dithranol in psoriasis and topical corticosteroids in eczema, the application of dressings and the treatment of leg ulcers is invaluable in a day-care and inpatient

setting. My own view is that nurse practitioners have a greater part to play in dermatology. They could treat warts with liquid nitrogen and be invaluable in advising and counselling patients with acne, skin cancer and eczema (including the parents of children with eczema) amongst other things. Other paramedical staff include physiotherapists for the supervision of ultraviolet B therapy and photochemotherapy and dietitians. Although dietary measures have only been proven to be highly effective in the management of dermatitis herpetiformis (with the elimination of gluten), eczema and urticaria are sometimes treated by dietary manipulation. The elimination of dairy products in small children with eczema can, however, be hazardous without the help of a dietitian.

The photographic department is very important for recording lesions, such as malignant melanomas, and for monitoring progress which otherwise would be difficult to recall. Polaroid cameras offer an ideal opportunity for patients or their doctors to do this.

Most skin departments have the help of a cosmetic expert to teach patients to disguise disfiguring dis-orders such as port-wine stains.

Finally, the pharmacist is a key member of the team for many old-fashioned preparations are still in use which have to be prepared in the pharmacy; for example, dithranol in Lassar's paste, ung. cocois co., and menthol and phenol in aqueous cream.

2 GLUCOCORTICOSTEROIDS

INTRODUCTION

Steroids completed the dawn of dermatological therapeutics which had been heralded by antibiotics. They revolutionized the treatment of many skin disorders during the 1950s and 60s and they are so fundamental to the treatment of eczema that they merit description in this early chapter.

Their story parallels that of any major therapeutic advance. After the initial euphoria dermatologists issued warnings about overuse and the media publicized the problems. In some ways, dermatologists may have overplayed their hand, for the side-effects of steroids are certainly easy to record photographically and can be well described during lectures. The time has come for a rehabilitation of these drugs. It is still all too common to find practitioners scarcely using them at all and patients refusing to use them. The side-effects are related to either misdiagnosis or overtreatment and in experienced hands should rarely occur. Their benefits far outweigh their potential side-effects and they remain the most important treatment for eczema, which is the most common skin disease. The recent deregulation of hydrocortisone, such that it is now available over the counter without prescription, goes some way towards redressing the balance and calming the fears of doctors and general public alike.

In 1949 Hench and his colleagues demonstrated the effectiveness of cortisone acetate in the treatment of rheumatoid arthritis and following this dermatologists experimented with the drug topically. Cortisone is inactive topically but Sulzberger demonstrated in 1952 that compound F (which turned out to be identical to cortisol produced from the adrenal cortex and is now known as hydrocortisone) was effective in inflammatory disorders such as eczema. Hydrocortisone is simply cortisone with a –OH group at the C11 position. Cortisone is converted to hydrocortisone when it is given systemically but not when it is applied topically, which explains why it does not work topically.

Biochemists were subsequently able to increase the anti-inflammatory properties of systemic steroids. Thus a double bond at the C1–2 position increases the effect of hydrocortisone and produces the synthetic steroid prednisolone. Subsequently it was shown that a fluorine atom at the C9 position considerably increased the anti-inflammatory action of the steroid molecule but also increased the mineralocorticoid activity. The latter could be minimized by various additions (Fig. 2.1) which included a –OH group at the 16-alpha position (triamcinolone), a methyl group at the 16-alpha position (dexamethasone), or a methyl group at the 16-beta position (betamethasone). All these measures enhanced the therapeutics of severe skin disorders where systemic steroids were indicated, but these drugs were not particularly active topically.

The breakthrough in topical steroids came when it was appreciated that bioavailability could be improved by esterification of the steroid molecule, which made it lipophilic and suited the special conditions of the skin. Thus an acetonide at the C16–17 position of

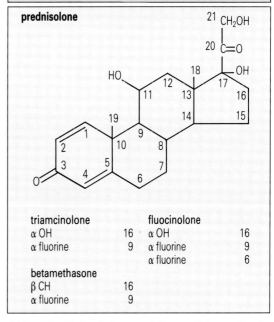

Fig. 2.1 *Hydroxylation or methylation and fluorination of prednisolone produces triamcinolone, betamethasone and fluocinolone which are powerful systemically but not topically.*

triamcinolone transforms a relatively inactive topical steroid into a potent topical steroid, triamcinolone acetonide (Adcortyl, Ledercort, UK; Aristocort, Kenalog, US). An additional fluorine atom at the C6 position of the steroid molecule and a 16-alpha and 17-alpha acetonide ester (Fig. 2.2) produced fluocinolone acetonide (Synalar, UK and US) in 1958 and

dermatology was on the move. This was quickly followed by betamethasone valerate (Betnovate, UK; Valisone, US) which is simply betamethasone with a valerate ester at the C17 position (Fig. 2.2).

A major landmark in the investigation of topical steroids was the discovery by Dr Richard Stoughton and his colleague Dr A.W. MacKenzie that a blanching or vasoconstriction (Fig. 2.3) occurred on the skin a few hours after the application of a steroid. This proved to be a superb screening system for new steroids in that it became clear that the degree of vasoconstriction produced by a steroid paralleled the likely potency of the drug in a clinical situation. (Dermatologists then went through a period of wrapping their patients up in polythene or plastic suits and bags to increase the penetration of their steroids into the skin and thus enhance their potency. Vasoconstriction tests had demonstrated that this would increase the potency of a steroid a hundred-fold.) The test system eventually led to the development in 1974 of clobetasol propionate (Dermovate, UK; Temovate, US) which has a chlorine atom in the C21 position and propionate ester in the C17 position. This is the strongest steroid available to date, and in many instances it has made the need for plastic occlusion obsolete.

As might be expected, the more powerful the steroid is, the more likely it is to produce side-effects. Thus, all topical steroids are absorbed and so clobetasol propionate is potentially able to produce Cushing's syndrome if misused, but class III steroids such as

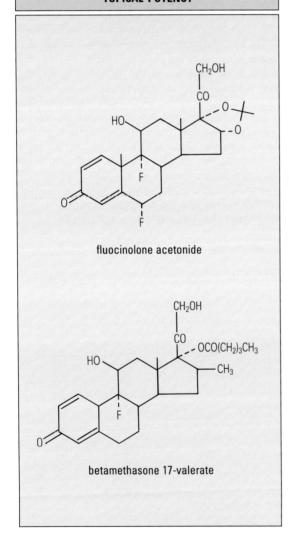

ESTERIFICATION INCREASES TOPICAL POTENCY

fluocinolone acetonide

betamethasone 17-valerate

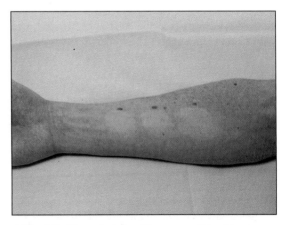

▲ **Fig. 2.2** *Esterification of the C16 and C17 positions greatly enhances topical efficacy and results in fluocinolone acetonide (Synalar) and betamethasone valerate (Betnovate, UK; Valisone, US).*

▲ **Fig. 2.3** *Vasoconstriction. Three areas of blanching are visible 6 hours after applications of potent topical steroids. In general the greater the degree of blanching produced, the greater the potency of the steroid.*

betamethasone valerate and fluocinolone acetonide have rarely ever been recorded as doing so. Similarly, local side-effects are potentially more likely with the potent steroids. Attempts are being made to disassociate potential side-effects from potency, but so far this has been unsuccessful. An interesting drug developed in the 1970s was clobetasone butyrate (Eumovate, UK), which had a keto group rather than a –OH group at the C11 position, thus simulating cortisone acetate, coupled with a chlorine atom at the C21 and the butyrate at the C17 position. It seems to have no systemic toxicity at all, but on the other hand is only a moderately potent steroid.

Considerable progress has been made not only in enhancing the intrinsic activity of the steroid but also in improving the drug delivery system. It has been shown that ointment vehicles are more effective than creams in penetrating the stratum corneum, and various modifications have been made to improve the vehicles to which the active steroids are added. Propylene glycol enhances penetration, although in some patients there is the disadvantage that there is a transitory stinging associated with the drug. Keratolytics such as salicylic acid or urea also improve penetration.

Many dermatologists had a tendency to request pharmacists to dilute commercially available steroid preparations, but this was unsatisfactory because the mixing of a vehicle such as white soft paraffin with the proprietary vehicle may destabilize the steroid. To meet this need, ready diluted steroids are now available, which is helpful in eczema because it is a principle of the treatment to start with a powerful steroid to gain control and then continue with a weaker one for maintenance.

MODE OF ACTION OF STEROIDS

Steroids penetrate cell membranes easily and attach to receptors in the cytoplasm. The receptor–steroid complex interacts with DNA resulting in modified RNA and protein synthesis. These modified proteins are responsible for the important immunosuppressive and anti-inflammatory effects, among others, of steroids.

(1) **Anti-inflammatory.** Steroids decrease inflammation whether produced by bacteria, chemical or physical injury, ultraviolet light or immunological events. Macrocortin, one of the modified proteins, interferes with prostaglandin synthesis. Vasodilatation, leakage from capillaries, margination of white cells and chemotaxis are inhibited, which is of importance with eczema.

(2) **Immunosuppression.** Steroids suppress lymphocyte activity and block the access of lymphokines to target cells. They will therefore reduce the effects of a contact allergic dermatitis and may well have important lympholytic effects in disorders such as lichen planus where there is a heavy infiltrate of lymphocytes in the skin. They will, of course, allow infections to spread as a result of this immunosuppression.

(3) **Antimitotic.** Topical steroids are known to interfere temporarily with epidermal DNA synthesis and it is probably this action which is important in the treatment of psoriasis, a disorder of epidermal hyperproliferation. It possibly also explains the rebound deterioration of psoriasis on stopping therapy. This inhibition of cell division is responsible for the side-effect of epidermal atrophy.

(4) **Vasoconstriction.** This phenomenon has provided an extremely useful test system for ranking topical steroids. Hydrocortisone barely vasoconstricts at all, but fluocinolone acetate produces a degree of vasoconstriction which is 100 times as marked as that produced by hydrocortisone. Betamethasone valerate is 360 and clobetasol propionate 1640 times as potent a vasoconstrictor as hydrocortisone. The significance of vasoconstriction from a therapeutic point of view is not known but it is quite probable that the worsening of rosacea is due to a rebound vasodilatation.

(5) **Mineralocorticoid activity.** Sodium retention and potassium depletion are not a problem with currently available topical steroids but initially when the anti-inflammatory effects of hydrocortisone were increased by placing a fluorine atom at the C9 position (fludrocortisone), oedema secondary to sodium retention occurred secondary to mineralocorticoid effects and therefore proved unacceptable.

(6) **Glucocorticosteroid activity.** All the effects of systemic steroids which result in Cushing's syndrome are possible with percutaneous absorption of topical steroids, but they rarely occur nowadays unless large amounts (greater than 50g per week) of class IV steroids (or class III steroids under polythene occlusion) are used over many weeks or months.

(7) **Antimetabolic effects.** Systemic steroids cause muscle wasting but again this is rarely seen with topical steroids. However topical steroids do affect collagen producing the well-known side-effects of dermal atrophy, ecchymoses and striae (see Fig. 1.20).

STEROID CLASSIFICATION

Based on vasoconstrictor studies and clinical trials, steroids may be simply grouped into four classes (Fig. 2.4). Familiarity with these classes greatly increases the therapeutic effectiveness of the practitioner. Certain diseases will only respond to the strongest class of steroid whereas others will to milder ones. Certain sites are more penetrable (face and flexures) than others (palms and soles) so the class of steroid must be chosen accordingly.

Class I

These are the weakest steroids: indeed 0.5% hydrocortisone is virtually ineffective and is not worth prescribing. One per cent hydrocortisone is now available over the counter as it has been available on prescription for 35 years and has a very safe 'track record' indeed. Local side-effects, such as atrophy, striae or ecchymoses, are so rare that they are unlikely to be seen by either the specialist or the family practitioner; the same applies to systemic side-effects. Clearly it should not be used for infections but it is the treatment of choice for eczema on the face. It is often not effective for eczema elsewhere on the body and it has no effect whatever in psoriasis or lichen planus. Hydrocortisone is available in a 2.5% formulation which increases its potency slightly. There are some slightly stronger steroids than these, which include dexamethasone sodium phosphate (Decadron, UK and US), flumethasone pivalate (Locasalen, US; not available in the UK), flucortolone caproate (Ultralan, UK), and fluprednidene acetate (Decaderm, UK).

Class II

These are moderately potent steroids, examples of which are: fluocinolone acetonide 1:10, clobetasone butyrate, flucortolone pivalate 0.1% with flucortolone hexanoate 0.1% (Ultradil, UK) (and these two drugs at 0.25% — Ultralanum, UK), and flurandrenolone 0.0125% (Haelan). Hydrocortisone 1% combined with urea which increases penetration (Alphaderm, Calmurid HC) is also available.

These agents are useful in the management of eczema, particularly atopic eczema in children on areas other than the face. They are also useful for seborrhoeic eczema in intertriginous areas.

CLASSES OF TOPICAL STEROIDS			
Class	Potency	Steroid	UK trade name (US name)
I	mild	hydrocortisone 0.5–2.5%	Efcortelan Hydrocortistab
II	moderate	clobetasone butyrate 0.05% fluandrenolone 0.0125% fluocinolone acetonide 0.0025% hydrocortisone with urea	Eumovate Haelan Synalar 1:10 (Synalar) Alphaderm (Alphaderm) Calmurid
III	potent	beclomethasone dipropionate 0.025% betamethasone dipropionate 0.05% betamethasone valerate 0.1% fluocinolone acetonide 0.025% fluocinonide 0.05% hydrocortisone 17 butyrate 0.1% triamcinolone acetonide 0.1%	Propaderm Diprosone (Diprosone) Betnovate (Valisone) Synalar (Synalar) Metosyn (Lidex) Locoid (Locoid) Adcortyl (Trymex)
IV	very potent	clobetasol propionate diflucortolone valerate halcinonide 0.1%	Dermovate (Temovate) Nerisone Halciderm (Halog)

◀**Fig. 2.4**
Classification of topical steroids. Classes are based on vasoconstrictor studies and clinical trials.

Class III

These are potent steroids and include betamethasone valerate, fluocinolone acetonide, beclomethasone dipropionate (Propaderm, UK) and fluocinonide (Metosyn, UK; Lidex, US). Virtually all of these steroids are characterized by a fluorine atom at the C9 position. The exception to this is hydrocortisone 17 butyrate (Locoid, UK and US) which sounds deceptively non-potent because of the inclusion of hydrocortisone in its title; however, the butyrate ester greatly enhances its intrinsic activity and it is a potent steroid.

Potent steroids are indicated for the more resistant eczemas such as seborrhoeic eczema on the trunk, eczema of the hands and feet, discoid eczema and lichenified atopic eczema.

Class IV

These are the most potent available topical steroids and include clobetasol propionate, diflucortolone valerate 0.3% (Nerisone Forte, UK) and halcinonide 0.1% (Halciderm, UK; Halog, US).

These drugs have been an important therapeutic advance in the treatment of lichen planus since this disease only partially responds to class III steroids and plastic occlusion is usually necessary to enhance the effect. They are highly effective in lichen simplex and are useful in localized plaques of discoid lupus erythematosus. They are more effective than class III steroids in psoriasis but are not the treatment of choice and should only be reserved for limited disease. They are to be avoided in eczema, except when the disease is on the palms and soles. These are potent drugs and practitioners should be wary of long-term usage.

STEROID COMBINATIONS

(1) Antibiotics and antibacterials. Combination with an antibacterial is indicated if there is clinical evidence of secondary sepsis. This is a common occurrence in eczema and often a systemic antibiotic is required as well. Neomycin, gentamycin, gramicidin, bacitracin and fucidin are all available in combination. They should be used with great care in varicose eczema because contact sensitivity to antibiotics is commonplace in this area. Combination with tetracycline is occasionally not acceptable to the patient, because of the yellow colour of the preparation. This discolour-

ation applies also to hydroxyquinolines, which are also occasional sensitizers and have a weak effect against both bacteria and fungi.

(2) Anti-*Candida* agents. There is no indication for such combinations if the primary cause is *Candida*, but *Candida* may be a secondary invader particularly of eczema in intertriginous areas and in the napkin area in children, when it is reasonable to combine nystatin or an imidazole with hydrocortisone; combination with more potent steroids (for example Mycolog, US) is probably not.

(3) Broad spectrum antifungals. The imidazoles are effective not only against *Candida* but also against ringworm. Combinations are sometimes useful in general practice whilst awaiting the results of mycology from a suspected case of tinea in the groin but they are quite unnecessary if the diagnosis is confirmed.

(4) Anti-*Candida* and antibiotic combinations. The only indication for these drugs is in an eczematous intertrigo where there is the fear of secondary invasion by bacteria and *Candida*. Some dermatologists do use these preparations combined with hydrocortisone, particularly for napkin eruptions and intertriginous eczema, but if there is no overt evidence of such secondary infection hydrocortisone on its own will be just as effective.

It is unnecessary to combine more potent steroids with these combination drugs. Tri-Adcortyl (UK), which contains triamcinolone acetonide, nystatin, neomycin and gramicidin, is frequently mistaken for a panacea and prescribed for any eruption in the groin. Unfortunately it is often prescribed for ringworm, for which it has no effect whatsoever, except to make the condition worse. It has the further disadvantage that it contains ethylenediamine which is a potent sensitizer, and also that it stains clothing yellow. Similarly Trimovate (UK) — clobetasone butyrate with nystatin and tetracycline — stains yellow and is rarely required. The worst combination is Dermovate NN ointment (UK) for there is no skin disorder which requires a class IV steroid and an antibiotic (neomycin) and an anti-*Candida* agent (nystatin). It is perfectly reasonable to combine an antibacterial such as neomycin with Dermovate for the treatment, for example, of septic discoid eczema, but this combination does not exist. Dermovate NN should never be used in the groin.

(5) Salicylic acid is added to some steroids, for example flumethasone pivalate, betamethasone dipropionate (Diprosalic, UK only) to improve penetration. Urea and propylene glycol are similarly added.

OTHER DELIVERY SYSTEMS

(1) **Intralesional steroids.** These are useful as they bypass the process of percutaneous absorption. They are indicated (Fig. 2.5) in granuloma annulare, keloids, hypertrophic lichen planus and nodular prurigo. They should be injected either into the lesion or subcutaneously, but not intradermally, otherwise atrophy will result.

(2) **Tape impregnated with steroid.** A tape impregnated with flurandrenolone can be applied to localized lesions and left on for 12–24 hours to give a continual release of steroid. It has similar indications as intralesional steroids.

COMMON INDICATIONS FOR STEROIDS AND THE CHOICE OF STRENGTH

Indications for steroids are given throughout the book and are summarized in Figs 2.5–2.7. The choice of steroid depends upon:

(1) **The disease.** It is clear that some diseases respond better than others to weaker steroids, and this applies to eczema in particular. Lichen planus on the other hand only responds to the most powerful class IV steroids. Psoriasis will respond to Class III and IV steroids but not to class I or II. Systemic steroids (Fig. 2.7) are helpful in the acute situation particularly for eczema and drug eruptions and they are used over a

period of 3 or 4 weeks. Disorders such as bullous pemphigoid require much more long-term systemic therapy. Systemic steroids have been completely abandoned in the treatment of psoriasis because of unacceptable chronic side-effects and because of the hazard of pustular psoriasis, which is occasionally lethal.

(2) **The site.** The effective penetration of any drug through the skin depends upon the site. The thicker the stratum corneum, the less the drug can penetrate. The face is the easiest to penetrate and therefore is most vulnerable. The palms and soles are the thickest areas of skin and therefore skin disorders involving these areas are most difficult to treat. A helpful guide to thickness of the stratum corneum in increasing thickness is: (1) face; (2) flexures; (3) body and limbs; (4) palms, soles and scalp. Thus, as a general rule facial eczema should respond to class I steroids, flexural to class II, truncal eczema to class III and

COMMON INDICATIONS FOR TOPICAL STEROIDS
eczema
pityriasis rosea
lichen planus
some forms of psoriasis
alopecia areata
vitiligo

▲ **Fig. 2.6** *Common indications for topical steroids.*

COMMON INDICATIONS FOR INTRALESIONAL STEROIDS (TRIAMCINOLONE)
keloids
granuloma annulare
alopecia areata
hypertrophic lichen planus
nodular prurigo

▲ **Fig. 2.5** *Common indications for intralesional steroids (triamcinolone).*

COMMON INDICATIONS FOR SYSTEMIC STEROIDS
pemphigus, pemphigoid
vasculitis including lupus erythematosus
severe drug reactions
severe lichen planus
acute eczema

▲ **Fig. 2.7** *Common indications for systemic steroids.*

palmar to class IV. Flexural areas (groin, axillae, elbows) and intertriginous sites (under breasts and folds of fat, under the foreskin) are particularly amenable to percutaneous absorption of drugs, and hence to side-effects if class III or IV steroids are used, because of the increased temperature and humidity similar to that produced by polythene occlusion.
(3) Secondary sepsis. Eczema is particularly liable to be complicated by bacterial sepsis and occasionally by *Candida*, especially in intertriginous sites, and a combination preparation may be required.

SIDE-EFFECTS

Side-effects have been much emphasized but most are completely avoidable if the correct diagnosis is made and correct strengths and amounts of steroids are prescribed.
(1) Perioral dermatitis and rosacea. The problems of perioral dermatitis (chapter 17) and the exacerbation of rosacea (chapter 17) with steroids is either iatrogenic or due to misuse of a steroid by the patient. There is no indication for the use of topical steroids in rosacea or acne. Nor should potent topical steroids be used for seborrhoeic eczema of the face.
(2) Infections. Infections treated with powerful immunosuppressants such as steroids will obviously get worse, and the steroids themselves cannot be blamed for this. It is fundamental that the correct diagnosis must be made. If tinea is present but not suspected and a steroid is prescribed, the inflammatory

response and hence physical signs will be masked resulting in tinea incognito (chapter 12). Warts (especially plane warts), mollusca contagiosa and herpes simplex (especially associated with eczema) are occasionally misdiagnosed and inappropriately treated. Scabies is often misdiagnosed as eczema and allowed to spread.
(3) Adrenal suppression. Adrenal suppression is quite unnecessary. It was seen to a limited extent during the late 1970s, when class IV steroids were used without supervision and were applied in large quantities. This is rarely seen today. Infants are a special case, in that they appear to absorb more steroid because of their greater surface area to body size, and class III and IV steroids are contraindicated under the age of 18 months. Adrenal suppression only occurs nowadays if patients have access to repeat prescriptions of class IV steroids without supervision. A short synacthen stimulation test should be performed if there is a suspicion of adrenal insufficiency.
(4) Local side-effects. These are often avoidable. They comprise telangiectasia (dilated capillaries), epidermal, dermal and subcutaneous atrophy (Fig. 2.8), striae and purpura, and are due to the effects of the steroids on cell division and on the supporting structures in the skin. Telangiectasia occurs most commonly on the face. Atrophy and striae occur in the flexures when class III or IV steroids are either used excessively by the patient for psoriasis or eczema in the groin or are prescribed for tinea cruris. Atrophy and bruising (purpura) occur most commonly on the backs of the hands and forearms (Fig. 2.9) when class III or IV steroids are used incorrectly by the patient.

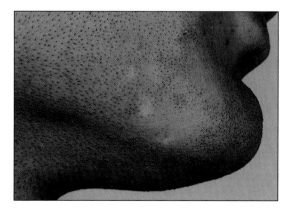

▲**Fig. 2.8** *Steroid atrophy and loss of pigmentation. This man has alopecia areata, which has been treated with injections of triamcinolone, and three areas of dermal atrophy and loss of pigmentation have resulted.*

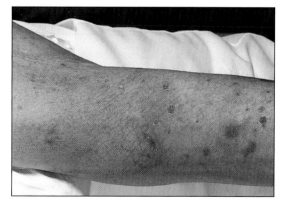

▲**Fig. 2.9** *Steroid atrophy and purpura. Purpura, atrophy and abnormal visibility of the vasculature are the visible side-effects of a class IV topical steroid. Psoriasis is often better treated with other means.*

Patients do vary considerably in the amounts that they apply and the frequency of their application. It is very important to instruct the patient to apply these drugs sparingly and to limit their applications to the site of the disease.

(5) Folliculitis. A septic folliculitis does occur in the treatment of eczema, in particular on the limbs with class III or IV steroids, and it is not always avoidable but it does respond well to antibiotics. Painful pustules surrounded by erythema are present. A sterile folliculitis (Fig. 2.10) comparable to the pustules of acne may also result.

(6) Glaucoma. Glaucoma sometimes occurs with long-term treatment of eczema around the eyes.

(7) Allergic reactions. Allergic reactions to topical steroids are uncommon, except to antibiotics in the steroid combinations used in the treatment of varicose eczema. However, certain steroids contain chlorocresol and parabens (preservatives in creams) which occasionally sensitize, and a few still contain lanolin and fragrances, which are also sensitizers.

SUMMARY

A summary of how to avoid common problems with steroids is given in Figure 2.11. An important consideration is patients who request regular repeat prescriptions. They often need re-evaluation. If they have psoriasis, it may be that the steroid is not the treatment of choice and that they need referral to hospital for consideration of dithranol, tar, ultraviolet light or some other mode of therapy. Patients with eczema who are using steroids in large quantity are often either using them as emollients or have widespread excoriations without much eczema, in which case bandages are much more effective than topical steroids.

AVOIDING COMMON PROBLEMS IN STEROID USE

make the correct diagnosis

beware of the face
    never prescribe a steroid for acne or rosacea
    never prescribe a steroid stronger than class I for eczema of the face

do not treat infections with steroids. Infections will flourish

do not treat infants with class III or adults with class IV steroids long-term: adrenal suppression may result

beware of class III or IV steroids in flexural areas: local side-effects are common

avoid prescribing more than 50g at a time of class III or IV steroids

re-evaluate patients who require regular repeat prescriptions: they may need referral

---

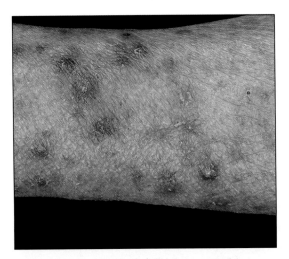

▲**Fig. 2.10** *Steroid folliculitis. This lady was applying a class III steroid inappropriately daily to treat her dry skin. Pustules surrounded by erythema (folliculitis) and some purpura have resulted.*

▲**Fig. 2.11** *Avoiding common problems in steroid use.*

If the steroid is not working, it is always worthwhile considering whether the diagnosis is correct (Fig. 2.12). If it is incorrect the patient will often observe that the disorder seems to be getting worse, and this is particularly so for infections such as tinea.

If the diagnosis is correct, it may be that the steroid is either not strong enough for the disease, for example hydrocortisone is ineffective in discoid eczema or lichen planus, or is not effective for the site involved, for example hydrocortisone will work perfectly for seborrhoeic eczema on the face but is ineffective for seborrhoeic eczema on the trunk. Alternatively, if the cause of eczema has not been identified, patch testing may be required to identify a possible contact allergen.

The appropriate choices of steroid class for different sites and diseases are summarized in Figure 2.13.

WHAT TO DO IF THE STEROID IS NOT WORKING

reconsider the diagnosis
the true diagnosis may be:
    acne
    rosacea
    infection
    contact allergy

re-evaluate the steroid
it may not be strong enough for:
    the site
    the disease
secondary infection may be present

▲ **Fig. 2.12** *What to do if the steroid is not effective.*

CHOICE OF STEROID CLASS BY DISEASE AND SITE

Class	Disease/Site
I	eczema on the face
II	atopic eczema elsewhere especially children and in the flexures
III	lichenified atopic eczema discoid eczema pityriasis rosea seborrhoeic eczema of the trunk varicose eczema psoriasis
IV	lichen simplex discoid eczema eczema and psoriasis of the palms and soles lichen planus vitiligo alopecia areata discoid lupus erythematosus

▲ **Fig. 2.13** *Choice of steroid class by disease and site.*

3 ECZEMA

INTRODUCTION

The skin probably has only a limited number of ways in which it can react. As a result the commonest pattern, which is eczema, is not a homogeneous disorder and does not constitute a diagnosis in itself but is, rather like anaemia, a set of symptoms and physical signs which require classification to determine its origin (Fig. 3.1). The terms 'eczema' and its relative 'dermatitis' are unsatisfactory. Some use the terms synonymously, but others prefer to reserve dermatitis for a disorder with an exogenous or external cause (contact dermatitis), and eczema for an endogenous disease. However, this is also unsatisfactory because what is now called endogenous disease may in due course be shown to have an exogenous explanation. Moreover, the term 'dermatitis' is also used as a prefix for quite separate and unrelated diseases, such as dermatitis artefacta and dermatitis herpetiformis, which only confuses matters further.

Eczema has various stages (Fig. 3.2) which depend on the degree of inflammation in the skin. These stages are known as acute, subacute or chronic and one or all of these stages may be present in a patient at any one time. The stages can be more easily understood by considering the pathology (Figs 3.3 & 3.4). The blood vessels are dilated (seen clinically as erythema) and are surrounded by inflammatory cells which migrate into the epidermis resulting in a varying amount of oedema, both between the epidermal cells (known as spongiosis) and within them. The epidermal cells consequently malfunction, so that the epithelium is thickened (acanthosis) with excess production of keratin (hyperkeratosis) and scaling.

TYPES OF ECZEMA
atopic eczema
seborrhoeic eczema
discoid (nummular) eczema
pompholyx (hand and foot eczema)
juvenile plantar dermatosis
lichen simplex
lichen striatus
varicose eczema (Chapter 16)
contact dermatitis (Chapter 4)

◀ **Fig. 3.1** *Types of eczema.*

THE STAGES OF ECZEMA	
stage	feature
acute	weeping, papules, vesicles and bullae
subacute	glistening of serum, redness, scaling and crusting
chronic	dryness, redness, scaling and fissuring

▲ **Fig. 3.2** *Stages of eczema.*

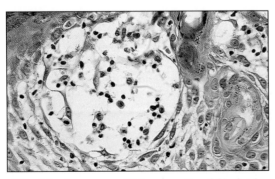

▲ **Fig. 3.3** *Acute eczema. High power section of skin showing intercellular oedema (spongiosis) with vesicle formation. H & E stain.*

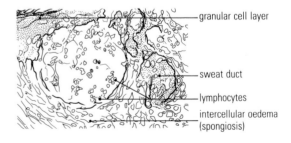

granular cell layer

sweat duct

lymphocytes

intercellular oedema (spongiosis)

Clinically, the oedema produces red papules which may become papulovesicles or bullae (Fig. 3.5) with a serous exudation (acute or wet eczema) if the oedema is considerable. In less acute cases (subacute eczema) there is a glistening of serum and crusting (Fig. 3.6). In chronic or dry eczema, the acanthosis and hyper-

keratosis predominate so that the skin is red, dry, scaly, slightly thickened (Fig. 3.7) and with a tendency to crack and fissure. The papules, particularly in pigmented races, are often centred around hair follicles and the appearance is known as *follicular eczema* (Fig. 3.8).

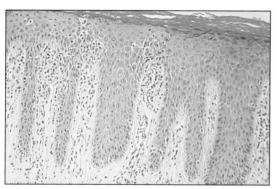

▲ **Fig. 3.4** *Chronic eczema. Section of skin showing hyperkeratosis, marked acanthosis with prolongation of the epidermal ridges and spongiosis. Within the dermis there is a*

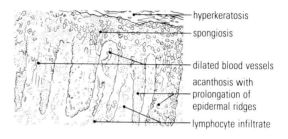

lymphocytic infiltrate surrounding dilated blood vessels. H & E stain.

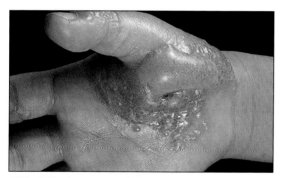

▲ **Fig. 3.5** *Acute eczema. Vesicles, which weep and may become confluent and bullous, dominate the clinical picture as in this patient with an acute pompholyx.*

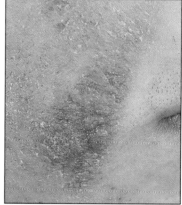

◀ **Fig. 3.6** *Subacute eczema. There is glistening of serum, redness, scaling and crusting. Secondary infection frequently supervenes.*

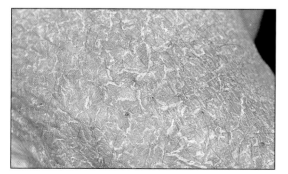

▲ **Fig. 3.7** *Chronic eczema. The skin is dry, pink and scaly with a tendency to painful splitting (fissuring) of the skin.*

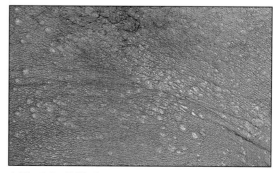

▲ **Fig. 3.8** *Follicular eczema. In coloured races in particular, the papular response in eczema is centred around the hair follicles.*

Eczema is intensely pruritic in all forms except seborrhoeic eczema. As a result, patients scratch and rub the skin which leads to excoriation and lichenification (Fig. 3.9) and in pigmented skins to lichenoid papules (Fig. 3.10). The epidermal barrier is disordered in eczema. This predisposes to infection which is encouraged by scratching. Post-inflammatory hypo- and hyperpigmentation (see Fig. 3.9) are frequent consequences of eczema, which in coloured races may constitute a problem because it takes time for the proper pigmentation to be restored.

ATOPIC ECZEMA

Definition
A chronic self-limiting inflammatory disorder, mainly of childhood, punctuated by relapses and remissions, usually genetically determined and associated with other atopic disorders.

Diagnostic features
- Onset at three months of age.
- Face and flexures.
- Dryness, redness and scaling.
- Sometimes weeping.
- Excoriation and lichenification.
- Symmetry.

Aetiology
The mystery surrounding the aetiology of atopic eczema constitutes one of the most serious omissions in our knowledge of skin diseases today. It predominantly affects children, and parents find this ignorance very difficult to accept. Almost all believe it to be an allergy, and certainly there are a number of immunological abnormalities to be found, but the nature of the allergen, if it exists, completely eludes us. It is more likely to be a disorder of the immune system with an unexplained deficiency or immaturity of the cell-mediated arm of the system, as evidenced by reduced numbers of suppressor T cells, permitting an increase in humoral activity, as evidenced by increased IgE levels.

A number of observations may be made about the disease:

(1) **The atopic state.** Asthma, hay fever and urticaria are commonly associated with atopic eczema, either in the patient or his immediate family. These disorders are inherited as autosomal dominants with incomplete penetrance.

(2) **White dermographism.** After stroking normal skin, erythema and oedema (wheal and flare) occurs, but only a white line occurs on atopic skin which also appears generally pale. The significance of this abnormal tendency to vasoconstriction is not explained, but some believe that there is an impaired ß-adrenergic response leading to excessive α-adrenergic stimulation, perhaps comparable to a similar mechanism in asthma.

(3) **Skin prick tests.** These are frequently positive, especially to the house-dust mite, pollens, cat and dog hair, and food allergens. Consequently, some have suggested that measures such as a withdrawal of the patient to a house-dust free environment and special diets may be of benefit, but unfortunately these do not lead to improvement or resolution of the eczema in most instances.

(4) **IgE (Immunoglobulin E).** The levels of IgE are raised in some but disconcertingly not all patients, which may indicate there is heterogeneity within the disease. There is some evidence in those who do have raised IgE levels that these levels reflect the activity of the disease. Radioallergosorbent testing (RAST),

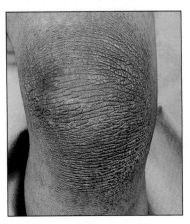

◀**Fig. 3.9** *Lichenification. The skin is thickened and the creases prominent. Hyperpigmentation is common in coloured races. This child has atopic eczema.*

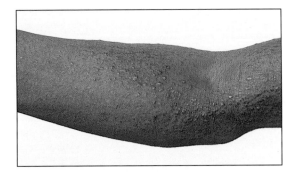

▲**Fig. 3.10** *Lichenoid eczema. A papular pattern of eczema may occur in dark skins. The papules are flat-topped and thus lichenoid.*

used to determine which specific antigens the IgE is synthesized against, corresponds to the results of the skin prick tests. Food challenges based on positive tests are unreliable in that correlation between positive RAST and positive food challenges only occurs in a third of cases. Negative RAST, however, does correspond with negative food challenges.

(5) Reduced delayed hypersensitivity. Patients with atopic eczema probably have a decreased incidence of sensitivity to contact allergens, for example in North America to the common plant allergen poison oak (*Rhus diversiloba*), so that skin patch tests are rarely helpful. Skin test responses to candidal and streptococcal antigens and *in vitro* lymphocyte transformation responses to these and other mitogens are reduced.

(6) Increased susceptibility to virus infections. Atopic patients have abnormalities of cellular immunity such that they have reduced numbers of E-rosette forming T cells, T cells with receptors for IgG and suppressor T cells. They therefore have a reduced ability to produce a cell-mediated response and are more susceptible to wart, vaccinia, herpes simplex and molluscum contagiosum viruses.

(7) Increased susceptibility to bacterial sepsis. Staphylococcal and streptococcal infections are common and many patients are densely colonized with *Staphylococcus aureus*, although overt infection may not be present. This may be an inherent defect or due to the disordered epidermal barrier function which occurs in all forms of eczema.

(8) Diet. A dietary abnormality is the most fashionable theory relating to the cause of atopic eczema, particularly amongst parents. In the early 1970s, it was suggested that there was a transient IgA deficiency in the gastrointestinal tract during infancy in these patients, which permitted access of foreign allergens. It was proposed that strict dietary avoidance of cow's milk by breast feeding alone might prevent the atopic state, but this has not been shown to be the case. It may be however that maternal diet needs to be controlled during the whole of pregnancy in patients with a strong atopic family history.

In a small number of children, exclusion of milk products and other foods, particularly of a citrus nature, is followed by improvement and is therefore worthy of a therapeutic trial. However, it is very difficult to assess the response of eczema to dietary exclusion, because it is a disease so liable to fluctuation in activity. Certainly, dietary manipulation gives none of the satisfaction of reproducibility of response as seen with gluten withdrawal in dermatitis herpetiformis, for example.

(9) Inherent dryness (xerosis). Virtually all patients with atopic eczema have a constitutionally dry skin which remains with them all their lives. This dryness differs from ichthyosis and is probably part of eczema itself. Any xerosis is very susceptible to climatic change and it is noticeable that eczema is much worse for most patients during the winter months, when there is a chill factor and the relative humidity is low. Xerotic skin is also extremely susceptible to substances which irritate the skin, such as wool, water and detergents.

Clinical features

Atopic eczema is common, affecting over one per cent of children in the UK. It occurs in all races. It usually begins at about three months of age. Occasionally, it can appear for the first time in adult life, but often such patients are simply unaware that they had the disease as an infant until they subsequently question their parents. The condition often starts on the face (Fig. 3.11) and spreads to the trunk and limbs. The flexures (Fig. 3.12) are especially affected, and in

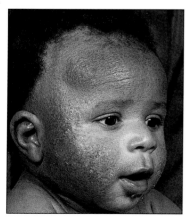

◄**Fig. 3.11**
Atopic eczema. The disorder usually starts on the face, classically at 3 months. The eczema is subacute on his cheeks and lichenified and chronic on his forehead.

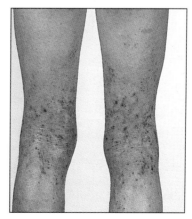

◄**Fig. 3.12**
Atopic eczema. The eruption is symmetrical, usually affecting the flexures. Scratching results in excoriations and lichenification.

particular the eyelids, neck, elbows, wrists, posterior gluteal folds, knees and ankles. It is strikingly symmetrical. The physical signs are of an ill-defined redness and fine scaling, together with serous exudation, vesiculation and crusting in the more acute states. The skin is generally dry or xerotic.

Atopic eczema is very itchy and excoriations and lichenification result from scratching and rubbing. The degree of scratching varies but in some cases excoriations, with consequent pigmentary abnormalities and occasionally scarring, may dominate the physical signs, overshadowing the eczematous changes when the condition is sometimes known as *Besnier's prurigo* (Fig. 3.13). Post-inflammatory hypo- or hyperpigmentation is common in coloured skins.

The eczema waxes and wanes in intensity, sometimes without obvious reason and at other times as a result of climatic changes, secondary infection or emotional and physical illness. It constitutes therefore a fluctuating disease and remedies have to be tailored to each individual's needs.

Atopic eczema is often complicated by infection (Fig. 3.14).

Bacterial sepsis

Eczema, particularly in its acute or subacute stages, frequently becomes secondarily infected. The eczema is either studded with yellow pustules, oozing yellow purulent material (Fig. 3.15), or covered with yellow crusts, when it is described as impetiginized eczema.

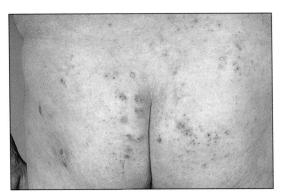

▲**Fig. 3.13** *Besnier's prurigo. Sometimes excoriations dominate the clinical picture with very little evidence of active eczema.*

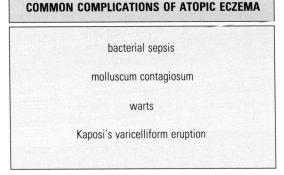

COMMON COMPLICATIONS OF ATOPIC ECZEMA

bacterial sepsis

molluscum contagiosum

warts

Kaposi's varicelliform eruption

▲**Fig. 3.14** *Common complications of atopic eczema.*

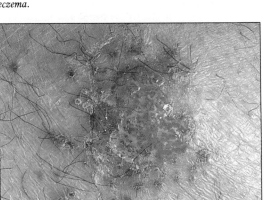

▲**Fig. 3.15** *Septic eczema. The epidermis is disrupted in eczema and secondary bacterial sepsis, manifest as a yellow purulent exudate with crusting, may occur.*

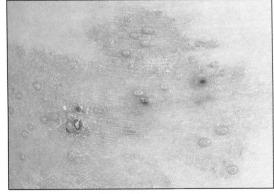

▲**Fig. 3.16** *Eczema and mollusca contagiosa. Atopics are prone to certain viruses. Flesh-coloured papules of mollusca are present.*

Molluscum contagiosum and warts

The atopic patient appears to be more prone to these viruses. Warts are readily diagnosed, but molluscum contagiosum (Fig. 3.16) is frequently not recognized by the patient and sometimes not by the practitioner, so that the patient applies topical steroids to the infection, mistaking it for eczema, and as a result the virus flourishes unrestrained.

Kaposi's varicelliform eruption

This is an important, serious, secondary infection of atopic eczema with either vaccinia or herpes simplex which can occur even in patients whose eczema is in remission. It was customary never to vaccinate

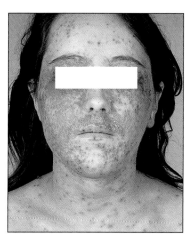

◀ **Fig. 3.17** *Kaposi's varicelliform eruption. Atopics are prone to infections with herpes simplex. Discrete vesicles, which become scabbed, are present.*

eczematous subjects against smallpox for this reason, but since smallpox has been eradicated and vaccination against it is no longer necessary, vaccinia should theoretically never be a cause again. However, herpes simplex infections are quite common. The virus colonizes eczematous and non-eczematous skin, and leads to a widespread eruption (Fig. 3.17) of discrete, tense vesicles (see Fig. 1.10) surrounded by erythema, coupled with a viraemia. The patient therefore may be extremely ill with other organ involvement including the central nervous system. The use of acyclovir is mandatory and usually life-saving. An atopic subject should be advised to avoid contact with individuals with an active herpes simplex infection.

Differential diagnosis

(1) Infancy — seborrhoeic eczema. The distinction between this and atopic eczema is not always straightforward but a number of pointers are given in Figure 3.18.

(2) Childhood. It should present no problem with differential diagnosis.

(3) Adult life. In a patient who has never had eczema previously there are two important considerations. (i) *Contact dermatitis*: if a patient denies a past or family history of eczema, it is always worth considering contact dermatitis, particularly to metal, which may affect similar sites, for example the neck (necklace or its clasp), forearms and elbows (metal strap of handbag), and wrists (watchstrap or bracelet). Patch tests would be positive to nickel in contact dermatitis but negative in atopic eczema. (ii) *Scabies*: there is usually no past or family history of atopic eczema, but there may be a history of someone else itching. The quality of the itch is different to eczema in that it is more severe, especially at night. The finding of burrows and the identification of the acarus under the microscope will clinch the diagnosis.

Prognosis

Most children's eczema improves during childhood and probably more than half are completely free of the disease by the age of thirteen. There may be some relapse during adolescence or early adult life but the majority recover by the age of thirty. There are, however, a few who suffer from it for virtually all their lives. It is difficult to predict in an individual case the prognosis, but severe disease in infancy and the involvement of the fronts of the elbows and knees often augur a poorer prognosis. The reaction of the child and its parents to the disease may prolong the healing stage.

DIFFERENTIAL DIAGNOSIS OF INFANTILE ATOPIC FROM SEBORRHOEIC ECZEMA

	Atopic eczema	Seborrhoeic eczema
onset (age)	3 months	6 weeks
duration	chronic	approximately 6 weeks
itch	yes	no
family history of atopy	yes	no
distribution	face and limb flexures	scalp, face, axillae and napkin area

▲ **Fig. 3.18** *Differential diagnosis of infantile atopic from seborrhoeic eczema.*

Management of atopic eczema:

Introduction

The cause of atopic eczema is unknown, so that whilst there is no cure it should be stressed that for the vast majority the condition resolves with time. Many children are better by the age of two or three years.

Since there is no specific remedy and the disease has a variety of forms and complications, treatment is not straightforward. The dryness, the eczema itself, the degree of scratching, the presence or absence of infection and extraneous psychological and social factors (Fig. 3.19), all need to be assessed.

Management of the xerosis

Attention to improving the dryness every day is critical. It is well worthwhile getting into a routine of using lubricants first thing in the morning and at bath time. An explanation of the simple physics of the adverse effects of low temperature and low relative humidity on the skin during the winter months is important. The lubrication needs to be increased during these times. Irritants such as woollen clothing (cotton is much better), soaps and 'bubble baths' should be prohibited. It is important to dry the skin properly after a bath. The most useful emollients are as follows.

Soap substitutes

Emulsifying ointment is the one most frequently used. It consists of 30 parts emulsifying wax, 20 parts liquid paraffin and white soft paraffin made up to 100 parts. The ointment must be soft, so that if it has been kept in the pharmacist's refrigerator before dispensing, it should be put into a warm place, such as the airing cupboard, to soften. It is used in exactly

---

POINTS TO CONSIDER IN MANAGING ECZEMA

treat the dryness — use emollients
assess the eczema
    choose the correct steroid for the site and
      activity of the disease
    remember tar
is infection present?
are there psychological, social and dietary factors?
how much scratching is there?
    consider medicated bandages
    prescribe antihistamines

▲ **Fig. 3.19** *Points to consider in managing eczema.*

---

the same manner as a soap. It will lather slightly and so wash the skin, but much more important, it is a marvellous hydrator of the skin. If the mother also suffers from eczema, it will be helpful for her hands whilst bathing the child.

Bath additives

There are many bath additives available commercially, most of them based on liquid paraffin. Equally, emulsifying ointment itself may be stirred in hot water in a jug and then added to the bath. The point of all these preparations is to increase further the lubrication of the skin.

General purpose emollients

Again, there are many emollients commercially available. Individuals vary in their acceptance of them, but usually one or two are found to be satisfactory. Lanolin, liquid paraffin and urea are common ingredients. Aqueous cream in the UK and Aquaphor in the US are very popular. These moisturizers should be used liberally and the child should be allowed to have a pot by the bedside and encouraged to apply it at any time, especially when awaking at night.

Vehicles

A vehicle is an inert carrier of the active ingredient. For the treatment of eczema 'creams' in general are not satisfactory vehicles because they tend to have a drying effect. 'Ointments' are far better. It is often impressive how the cream form of a particular steroid may be totally ineffective and yet a switch to the ointment form of that same steroid transforms the response.

Management of the eczema

Emollients only help the xerosis and have no effect on the eczema itself. Topical steroids and tar are the most effective agents for the eczema.

Topical glucocorticosteroids

An understanding of topical steroids is fundamental to the management of eczema, and reassurance of the patient and the parents depends upon this. They are highly efficacious anti-inflammatory agents if used sensibly. Their use is considered in detail in Chapter 2. In summary, the choice of steroid depends on the site and stage of the eczema.

(1) The site. Hydrocortisone is the only steroid which is permitted on the face; 0.5% is usually ineffective, so in practice 1.0 or 2.5% is needed. However, for the body and limbs, hydrocortisone is often too mild and a more powerful steroid is required, either a moderately potent (class II) or a potent one (class III). Frequently it is helpful to use a potent one first, in order to gain control, before returning to the less powerful one. The most potent steroids (class IV) are rarely required in atopic eczema.

(2) The stage. The type of eczema is important. The dry, red, scaly variety responds to the above measures. Chronic lichenified eczema will not respond to hydrocortisone, except on the face, nor to a moderate steroid, and in these cases powerful steroids are indicated. The very thickness of the skin is such that the weaker steroids cannot penetrate in sufficient quantity to be effective. Where excoriation predominates, bandages and sedatives are required, otherwise patients will use large quantities of topical steroids, hoping for an effect which will not materialize. If the eczema continues to deteriorate, despite the correct strength of steroid, sepsis may be present.

Persuading patients to use topical steroids
The fear of side-effects from topical steroids has got quite out of hand. It is true that there was a time when they were being misprescribed in the UK without any thought to diagnosis, so that acne, rosacea and infections were being inappropriately treated. Also, vast amounts were being used, often of very potent steroids, for eczema and psoriasis and thus local and occasionally systemic side-effects occurred. Today, side-effects of topical steroids are much less common, but an almost pathological loathing for them has developed despite the fact that they represent the single most effective remedy for controlling the disease if used sensibly. The result of this prejudice is that many patients do not get properly cared for at all. The pendulum must swing back to a sensible mean. Fortunately, the regulatory bodies have led the way, both in the US and in the UK, by permitting over-the-counter sale of 1% hydrocortisone, which demonstrates their confidence in its safety.

It is important to show concern about the use of the steroids, but in a reassuring way. It is useful to make the patient or parent bring the tube that has been previously prescribed, this being the only way of determining how much steroid is being used. It is helpful to instruct the patient to apply a very thin smear, only to the eczema and not to normal skin. There is strong evidence that the steroid remains active in the skin for twenty-four hours, so that once-daily applications are sufficient. Patients have completely different concepts of how much to apply. It is reasonable to point out that only the ointment in

contact with the skin is effective, and not that piled up high on top of it. There is also a tendency to use the steroids as lubricants, and by proper instruction in the use of emollients it is often possible to reduce the amount of steroid being applied. If more than 30g is being used every week, the patient should be seen by a specialist and other measures considered, including hospitalization. Systemic steroids are rarely required for atopic eczema and their prescription should be a specialist's decision.

Tar
Tar was the mainstay of treatment before the advent of hydrocortisone in 1952. The mode of action of tar is quite unknown but it is well worth considering in eczema, especially in the modern climate of prejudice against topical steroids. There are various ways of prescribing tar:

(1) Proprietary medicaments. A 10% coal tar solution, or 5% coal tar extract and allantoin, is useful as ointment.

(2) Extempore formulations. Twenty per cent coal tar solution in emulsifying ointment is an excellent soap substitute and the child can have it beside the bed to apply to the eczema at night if he wakes.

(3) Combined preparations. Proprietary preparations of tar and hydrocortisone are available, and extempore formulations may be made with class II or III steroids, such as 3% coal tar in clobetasone butyrate or in betamethasone 17-valerate ointment.

(4) Bandages impregnated with tar. Bandages containing tar or ichthammol (a form of tar) are invaluable in Besnier's prurigo.

Management of infection
Bacterial sepsis
For all minor degrees of sepsis there are various proprietary medicaments which combine an antibacterial agent, usually neomycin, fucidic acid, tetracycline or a quinolone, with the appropriate strength of steroid. Sensitization to these antibacterial agents is uncommon in atopic eczema and they can be used without concern.

Although steroid–antibiotic combinations are often recommended, treatment with a topical steroid alone may still be effective, probably because the drug restores the barrier function and limits bacterial activity. However, in more severe sepsis, where there is frank pus and yellow crusts, combined preparations and systemic antibiotics are required. Erythromycin has been the drug of choice, since penicillin resistance is fairly common, but erythromycin resistance is increasing and flucloxacillin (floxacillin) may be required.

Molluscum contagiosum and warts

If a child has one of these infections, it is important to tell the mother not to put the steroid anywhere near it otherwise the virus will spread. In fact, it is best to treat them with liquid nitrogen as quickly as possible, so that the eczema can be attended to.

Kaposi's varicelliform eruption

The management of this condition has been revolutionized by the use of acyclovir 200mg orally, five times daily for five days, and acyclovir 5% cream applied topically five times daily to the lesions. Acyclovir is usually given orally but if there is any systemic complication, it should be given intravenously.

Management of excoriated eczema

Acute episodes of scratching of the skin leading to multiple excoriations may be precipitated by an emotional crisis or a physical illness. Topical steroids do not work well on their own in this situation but the *use of occlusive bandages on the limbs is extremely helpful*, a weak or moderately potent topical steroid being applied first. The occlusion of the bandage will increase the potency of the steroid, so that there is no need to use potent steroids.

The bandages either contain tar (coal tar and zinc paste bandages), ichthammol, zinc and calamine, or zinc, calamine and clioquinol. These bandages are left on for three days and just a few applications can make an enormous difference to the eczema. The practice nurse can apply them and instruct the mother so that she can apply them herself.

Other aspects of management

Antihistamines

Antihistamines are very useful adjuncts to therapy and are helpful at night to reduce nocturnal scratching. Their sedative effect is valuable and hence the new non-hypnotic antihistamines, such as terfenadine, are not so helpful. Phenothiazine antihistamines are preferable at night. During the day, chlorpheniramine or brompheniramine are less sedative and therefore more useful. Antihistamines are well tolerated by children and they may be given adult doses. Hydroxyzine hydrochloride has anxiolytic activity and is particularly useful in anxious adults.

Diet

If all other therapy fails and if the mother or patient is eager, it is reasonable to try milk and dairy product avoidance. However this should be done under the supervision of a dietitian, because it is possible to induce malnutrition in children through restriction of vital vitamins, protein and calcium. Elimination diets are extremely tedious and not very gratifying.

Hospitalization

Most patients recover in hospital, often without any particular change in management or diet. Recovery may be due to good nursing, removal from an allergic environment at home (house dust) or removal from psychological stress at home. It is to be avoided in children but is often of great help to adults.

Psychological aspects

All aspects of the art of the practice of medicine are required to treat atopic eczema. Explanation, reassurance, sympathy, interest and encouragement are vital, so that the patient and parents can build up a trust in the physician, particularly as the condition is chronic and given to exacerbations.

The management of the child with severe atopic eczema, however, can be one of the most difficult problems in dermatology. Despite a lengthy consultation, carefully explaining everything that is known about the aetiology, the parents are often dissatisfied and still end up asking what is the cause of the disease. If the consultation is a difficult one, it frequently indicates that all is not well between the parents. Often the child senses this and manipulates the parents who, for example, permit such malpractice as allowing the child to sleep in their bed at night, which further drives a wedge between them. Another sign of parental unhappiness is the mother who cannot control the child during the consultation and therefore cannot concentrate on the advice being given by the doctor. It indicates that she cannot cope and lacks attention from her husband. Thus the parents may need as much help if not more than the afflicted child.

The consultation for older individuals is usually easier because the parental influence is past and a dialogue is more forthcoming with the patient. Nevertheless more specialized psychological help is sometimes necessary.

SEBORRHOEIC ECZEMA OF INFANCY

Definition

A common self-limiting condition occurring within the first few weeks of life, affecting primarily the scalp, face, axillae and napkin area, which resolves within a few weeks.

Diagnostic features

- Onset at six weeks of age.
- Non-itchy and apparently not uncomfortable.
- Yellow scales on the scalp and in the eyebrows.
- Erythema, scaling and sometimes rawness under the neck, in the axillae and in the napkin area.
- Resolves within six weeks.

Aetiology

The cause of the disorder is quite unknown. It is a separate entity from adult seborrhoeic eczema and, although its distribution is similar, the infantile disease does not lead to the adult form. It was thus named because the scales which appear are rather yellow and greasy, particularly on the scalp, and the theory was that sebaceous gland activity was over-active in these infants. This has been confirmed; the glands are enlarged and sebum secretion is increased.

There is no familial tendency and the mother may have several children before having one who develops

seborrhoeic eczema, so that it does not seem to be due to a failure to care for the skin properly. Some authorities question whether there is a nutritional element to the disorder, but there is no positive evidence for this.

Clinical features

The eruption usually begins with yellow coarse scales in the scalp (Fig. 3.20), so-called 'cradle cap'. It spreads on the face, with yellow crusts around the eyebrows and ears particularly, and then under the neck, in the axillae (Fig. 3.21) and in some cases onto the body (Fig. 3.22). Sometimes the condition starts in the napkin area rather than on the face and in most cases the napkin area is usually involved at some stage. Secondary infection either with bacteria or with *Candida albicans* may occur, but this is often over-diagnosed.

Management

(1) Reassurance. The condition improves over the ensuing few weeks. This is true even if a quite florid eruption affects most of the skin. It should be pointed out to the mother that the infant is otherwise perfectly healthy and not distressed by the rash.

(2) Treatment of the cradle cap. Two per cent salicylic acid in aqueous cream is helpful for removing the crusts.

(3) Emollients, such as emulsifying ointment for bathing instead of soap, and aqueous cream as a moisturizer, may be used in the same way as for atopic eczema.

(4) Topical steroids. The condition does respond to mild topical steroids. One per cent hydrocortisone is the drug most commonly used, but occasionally class II steroids are required. Some dermatologists advocate combining the steroid with an antibacterial and an anticandidal agent, but this is not essential.

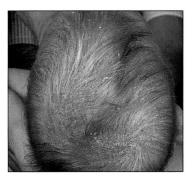

Fig. 3.20
Cradle cap. Yellow scales surrounded by erythema on the scalp are the commonest manifestation of seborrhoeic eczema in infancy.

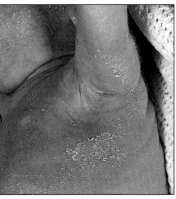

Fig. 3.21
Seborrhoeic eczema of infancy. The eczema is red and scaly and the face and axillae are involved. The condition resolves in infancy.

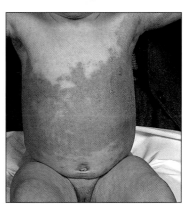

Fig. 3.22
Seborrhoeic eczema of infancy. The eruption may be extensive and involve the flexures and trunk.

ADULT SEBORRHOEIC ECZEMA

Definition
An eczematous process of varying degrees of severity with a propensity for the scalp, face, flexures and upper trunk.

Diagnostic features
- Dryness, redness and scaling.
- Scalp.
- Face: glabella, eyebrows, eyelids, ala nasi, moustache area, sideburns and ears.
- Torso: presternum and upper back.
- Flexures: axillae, groins and under breasts.

Aetiology
The cause is unknown but Sabouraud, in the last century, suspected that it was caused by the fungus, *Pityrosporum ovale*. This theory was subsequently discarded but it has recently been re-examined in the light of the new systemic antifungal agent ketoconazole, which is active against *P. ovale* and which clears the rash of seborrhoeic eczema, although it relapses on stopping treatment. Certainly, *P. ovale* is found among the scales of dandruff and in the associated skin eruption of seborrhoeic eczema, but it may also be found in unaffected skin. Thus this may be an epiphenomenon, for if it is the cause it is curious how the disorder responds to topical steroids, which theoretically should make an infection worse. Interestingly, seborrhoeic eczema is common in the acquired immunodeficiency syndrome (AIDS), possibly because immunosuppression encourages secondary infection with a commensal, such as *P. ovale*, and hence seborrhoeic eczema. On the other hand, the eczema may be a manifestation of the stress of having AIDS.

The term 'seborrhoeic' is a misnomer. The dry, yellow scales of the disease were thought to represent dried sebum, but in fact they are exfoliated cells of the stratum corneum. Although the eruption occurs on the face and the front and back of the chest, where there are a large number of sebaceous glands, it is also encountered in sites where there are few sebaceous glands, for example the groin and axillae.

The condition is much more common in Celts than in any other racial group. Minor varieties of it, particularly affecting the scalp and face, are extremely common. The more widespread and severe variety is much less common in Western societies than it used to be, possibly due to improved standards of nutrition and health. The disorder is commonest in young adults. It is probably one of the most common disorders of the skin, often seen in a very minor form when it is frequently associated with stress and anxiety. Many patients note that it disappears instantly on a relaxing holiday, particularly in the sun, but begins to return as soon as they arrive home. There is some scientific evidence too that it is related to stress, in that it was much more common during the last two World Wars. It is also more common in patients with Parkinson's disease for unknown reasons.

Clinical features
The essential morphological change is of an ill-defined roughness, redness and scaling of the skin to a varying degree. Although considered part of the same disease, it is possible to recognize three entities, based on the distribution of the eruption:

(1) Face and scalp. The distribution is as indicated under Diagnostic Features. One or all of the sites may be involved (Figs 1.26 & 3.23). The condition is symmetrical and often does not itch at all, unlike other forms of eczema. The scalp is most commonly involved, as either a dandruff, which is an exaggeration of the normal process of exfoliation of the cells of the stratum corneum, or coupled with an ill-defined erythema when it is classified as a true seborrhoeic eczema.

(2) Presternum and upper back. The condition is chronic and consists of fairly well-defined pink, scaly, annular patches over the sternum (Fig. 3.24), or in the interscapular area. Often both areas are involved.

(3) Flexural seborrhoeic eczema. This is the least common variety, the obese and middle-aged being more prone to it. It is a form of intertrigo involving the major flexures (Fig. 3.25). The eruption is symmetrical and is either pink with a fine scale or bright red, raw and sore.

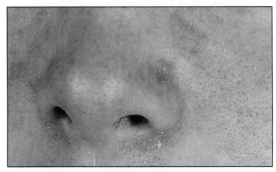

▲**Fig. 3.23** *Adult seborrhoeic eczema. The sides of the nose are dry, pink and scaly. The eyebrows, ears, cheeks and scalp are often involved.*

Differential diagnosis

(1) Face and scalp. There is usually little difficulty in this case. Although it is sometimes confused with psoriasis, the latter is much more difficult to treat and this in itself may suggest the diagnosis. Also the lesions of psoriasis are a deeper red colour than the pink of seborrhoeic eczema and the scales are thicker.

(2) Presternal and upper back. This is sometimes mistaken for pityriasis versicolor because the two diseases have a similar distribution, but the lesions of pityriasis versicolor are asymmetrical and brown or off-white, whereas those of seborrhoeic eczema are pink and symmetrical.

(3) Seborrhoeic intertrigo. Tinea infections are sometimes misdiagnosed as seborrhoeic intertrigo and it is always important to take scrapings for mycology of any eruption that occurs in a flexural area. However, the margin of the eruption is slightly raised and more scaly with a tendency to central healing in tinea as opposed to the more uniform appearance of eczema.

Management

Scalp

Mild seborrhoeic eczema of the scalp is commonly called dandruff. It responds well to frequent washing (often daily) with shampoos which contain tar, selenium sulphide or ketoconazole. The latter are effective against *P. ovale*. If erythema is present, topical steroids are indicated, usually class III, since the thickness of the scalp prevents adequate penetration of weaker steroids. Tar preparations may be of benefit. In severe cases, the disorder pityriasis amiantacea may develop, in which case ung. cocois co. should be used.

Face

Hydrocortisone, either as 1.0% or occasionally as 2.5%, is very effective for the face. It is reasonable to use creams because they are more cosmetically acceptable than ointments on the face. The patient should be warned not to put the steroid in the eye. More potent steroids are never indicated for eczema on the face as they cause a perioral or periorbital dermatitis (see Chapter 17). The disorder invariably returns although it ultimately goes into remission. It can be kept under control with 1% hydrocortisone cream bought over the counter. Side-effects are unusual. However, these patients sometimes have concomitant acne vulgaris and should be warned not to put the steroid onto this as it exacerbates acne. It may be necessary to treat the acne with systemic antibiotics.

Presternum and upper back

This variety is singularly difficult to treat. It does not respond to hydrocortisone, but does to the potent class III steroids, although it tends to relapse very quickly. Patients often have concomitant acne and may require oral antibiotic therapy. The condition may respond to ultraviolet light, but again it tends to return.

Seborrhoeic intertrigo

(1) Minor variants. The disorder can usually be controlled with class II topical steroids, because flexural areas are warm and moist allowing efficient penetration of the drug. Because there is sometimes secondary infection with bacteria and *Candida*, combined antibacterial, anticandidal and hydrocortisone preparations may be used. A proprietary formulation containing miconazole, which has antibacterial and anticandidal activity, and 1% hydrocortisone is useful.

(2) Major variants. This variety of seborrhoeic eczema may be quite inflamed and widespread, and often requires rest and occasionally hospitalization.

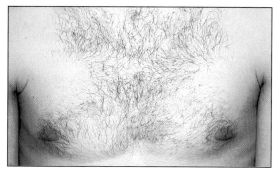

▲ **Fig. 3.24** *Adult seborrhoeic eczema. Pink scaly patches may occur on the front and back of the chest and be remarkably persistent.*

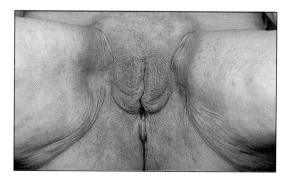

▲ **Fig. 3.25** *Intertriginous seborrhoeic eczema. There is erythema and scaling uniformly and symmetrically involving the genitalia and genitocrural folds.*

35

The principals of therapy are:

(a) *Soaks*: saline, aluminium acetate or potassium permanganate soaks are most commonly used. The groin can be soaked in a bidet or in a bowl, whereas more widespread disease requires soaking in bath water. Potassium permanganate crystals added to the water to produce a pink colour are excellent but it stains the nails and the patient should be warned to wear rubber gloves. Ten-minute soaks once or twice daily are sufficient after which the area should be patted dry with a paper towel or an old dispensable towel.

(b) *Topical steroids*: potent topical steroids are usually required and often need to be coupled with an antibiotic.

(c) *Systemic antibiotics*: erythromycin or flucloxacillin (floxacillin) are the antibiotics of choice, as in other forms of infected eczema.

DISCOID (NUMMULAR) ECZEMA

Definition

A morphological description of an eczema which constitutes a distinct disorder in older individuals, but may be an extension of atopic eczema in youth. It particularly affects the limbs.

Diagnostic features
- Itchy.
- Dry, red and scaly or exudative red and crusted.
- Well-defined discoid or coin-shaped.
- Limbs, principally.

Aetiology

There are two types of discoid eczema. In young adults it is probably an extension of the atopic

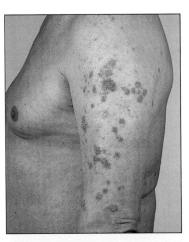

◄**Fig. 3.26** *Discoid eczema. Itchy round coin-shaped (nummular) lesions occur on the limbs. It occurs in young adults or the elderly and usually remits after a few months.*

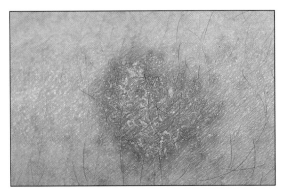

▲**Fig. 3.27** *Discoid eczema. The lesions are round and uniformly red and scaly.*

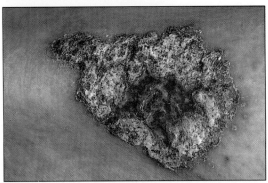

▲**Fig. 3.28** *Septic discoid eczema. The lesions often become purulent with yellow crusts.*

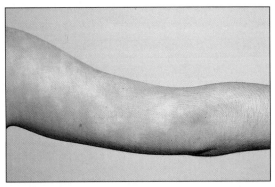

▲**Fig. 3.29** *Hypopigmented discoid eczema. In young adults who like the sun, the discoid eczema results in hypopigmented patches which are often mistaken for pityriasis versicolor.*

diathesis. In the elderly the cause is quite unknown despite its rather distinctive pattern. It is more common in males and runs a remitting and relapsing course but ultimately disappears. Some of the older patients abuse alcohol.

Clinical features
The condition is particularly itchy, the limbs (Fig. 3.26) being affected predominantly. The lesions are extremely well defined and therefore completely different from other forms of eczema. They are round, hence the term 'nummular' (from *nummus*, Latin for coin). The surface is dry, rough, red and covered with a fine scale (Fig. 3.27). If secondary sepsis has occurred there is weeping and crusting (Fig. 3.28). There is a variant in young adults who like the sun, which causes temporary loss of pigmentation (Fig. 3.29) and is sometimes confused with pityriasis versicolor, but this condition occurs predominantly on the trunk with less marked extension onto the limbs.

Management
(1) Emollients.
(2) Antihistamines.
(3) Potent topical steroids. The condition does not respond to low or moderate potency steroids, so that potent class III or often class IV steroids are required. Because secondary sepsis is common, a combination with a topical antibacterial agent is helpful.
(4) Hypopigmented variety. The patient is usually most concerned about the disturbance to the suntan which results in a rather off-white patchy effect on the limbs. Advice not to sunbathe, thus allowing the normal skin to return to its previous pale colour to blend in with the hypopigmented areas, is usually not greeted with any enthusiasm. The eczematous patches should be treated with steroids but the hypopigmented patches recover slowly and may take many months. This disorder does go into remission after a few years.

POMPHOLYX (DYSHIDROTIC ECZEMA)

Definition
A distinctive primary vesicular eruption of the sides of the fingers and toes and palms and soles associated with hyperhidrosis. It may become dry, fissured and chronic.

Diagnostic features
- Itchy.
- Vesicles and occasionally bullae present.
- Sides of the fingers and/or toes.
- Palms and soles.
- Becomes dry, cracked and painful.
- Occurs especially in the summer.
- Associated hyperhidrosis.

Aetiology
The cause of this common condition is quite unknown. It affects both sexes, is most frequent in young adults and early middle age and is usually precipitated by warm weather. Many of the patients have a tendency to sweat easily on the palms and soles, hence its alternative name, dyshidrotic eczema. Although this hyperhidrosis must be relevant, the theory that the bubbles (Fig. 3.30) represent beads of sweat no longer receives any scientific support. Some patients have an annual attack lasting three or four weeks every summer but others have a more chronic course. Some of them have an atopic background, but this is not a consistent finding. A few are positive to nickel and perfumes on patch testing, but avoidance of the allergen although improving the condition is not necessarily followed by cure. Many of the patients are under intense pressure and it is one of the skin disorders where personal circumstances are deemed to be particularly relevant.

Occasionally, a satisfactory explanation is forthcoming when the pompholyx on the hands represents a reaction to a cutaneous problem on the feet. However, this is often overdiagnosed because pompholyx is not restricted to the hands (cheiropompholyx) but frequently occurs on the feet (podopompholyx). Nevertheless, it is recognized that it may be precipitated by an acute tinea or contact dermatitis of the feet.

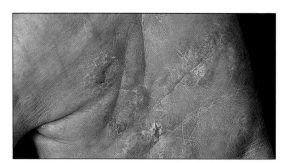

▲ **Fig. 3.30** *Pompholyx. Intensely itchy vesicles, which may become confluent and form bullae, occur on the palms and sides of the fingers, particularly in the summer.*

Clinical features

The patient complains of small 'bubbles' under the skin of the palms (see Fig. 3.30) and sides of the fingers. These are intensely itchy. They subsequently break, weep and then dry out. The skin becomes cracked and painful (Fig. 3.31). On examination, tiny vesicles are found on the palms and the palmar skin on the sides of the fingers. The feet may be similarly involved. The vesicles may coalesce and massive blisters may result (see Fig. 3.5) which incapacitate the patient to such an extent that they cannot use their hands and feet. The eruption is remarkably symmetrical. Secondary infection is common in the more acute cases and sometimes a lymphangitis and lymphadenopathy occur.

The more acute cases settle down rapidly with treatment. Others are more chronic and the vesicles keep recurring. The skin is more eczematous than in the very acute type. The condition ultimately goes into remission. There is a very common minor variant of pompholyx which is sometimes known as recurrent focal peeling or *keratolysis exfoliativa*, where small areas of focal desquamation occur on the palms. It rarely gives rise to any symptoms, although anxious patients sometimes request an explanation. There is no treatment for it.

Management

Acute vesiculo-bullous pompholyx

(1) **Rest.** The patient is often so incapacitated that he cannot work, and rest is indicated.

(2) **Soaks.** Saline, Burrow's solution (5% aluminium acetate) or potassium permanganate are all useful, the latter especially for the feet.

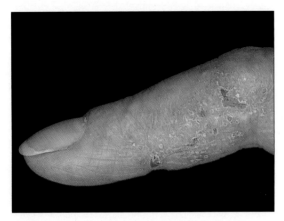

▲ **Fig. 3.31** *Pompholyx. The vesicles dry and the skin becomes fissured and painful.*

(3) **Antibiotics.** Secondary sepsis is often present and erythromycin is a useful choice.

(4) **Steroids.** (a) *Topical*: although potent steroids are traditionally prescribed, especially in combination with antibiotics, they are not particularly effective in acute cases. (b) *Systemic*: this is the treatment of choice, if there are no medical contraindications. Prednisolone (30mg) is prescribed and the dose is reduced by 5mg every fourth day. Systemic steroids usually lead to improvement within forty-eight hours.

Subacute and chronic pompholyx

(1) **Topical steroids.** Class III or IV steroids are indicated. They do dry up the vesicles and relieve the irritation. Weaker steroids are ineffective because they do not adequately penetrate the thick palmar skin. Care should be taken to prevent the steroids spreading onto the non-affected skin on the dorsal aspects of the hands. A combination with antibiotics is indicated if pustules or yellow crusts (sepsis) are present. Systemic steroids are sometimes necessary in chronic cases, but should be avoided as much as possible.

(2) **Emollients.** These are useful for the second stage when dryness and fissuring predominate.

(3) **Oral antihistamines.** They are useful as sedatives and antipruritics.

Investigations in pompholyx

Occasionally an acute pompholyx of the hands is secondary to a fungus infection on the feet. Scrapings should be taken from the skin of the feet and, if blisters are present, the roof of a blister can be cut away and sent for mycological examination. If fungus is found then the appropriate treatment is griseofulvin.

When the eruption has settled and if mycology is negative, patch tests are worth performing because occasionally a sensitivity to a contact allergen, for example a medicament, perfume or preservative in a handcream or rubber, may be uncovered. This may have precipitated the eczema or have exacerbated it. Alternatively, inappropriate treatment of a pompholyx on the feet with an antifungal agent may so irritate the skin as to initiate an autosensitization eczema on the hands.

There can be no doubt that many patients suffering from pompholyx of a non-reactive type have stressful lives and appropriate treatment may be helpful.

JUVENILE PLANTAR DERMATOSIS

Definition
A symmetrical eruption of the weight-bearing plantar surfaces of the feet in children, probably secondary to the occlusive nature of modern synthetic footwear.

Diagnostic features
- Children.
- Symmetrical, red, glazed and fissured.
- Plantar surfaces of the toes, forefoot and lateral sides of feet.
- Sparing of the toe webs and instep.
- Chronic.

Aetiology
The condition seems to be a relatively recent pheno-menon and is thought to be due to a change in composition of socks and shoes over the last fifteen years. Natural materials such as cotton, wool and leather are steadily being replaced by synthetic mater-ials such as nylon and plastics which are less porous. The loss of permeability is enhanced by various repellent coatings which are applied to shoes in order to improve their durability. A contact dermatitis to some part of the footwear has been suspected but patch testing has been unproductive.

The condition affects children and young adoles-cents, particularly those who continually wear the 'trainer' type of footwear. Some of the patients are atopic, but this is not by any means a consistent finding. They are often keen on football and other sports and it may be that the hot and humid environ-ment that these occlusive shoes produce, coupled with the friction to which the active child subjects the skin, sets up the disorder.

Clinical features
The condition is quite common and characteristic. The plantar surfaces of the weight-bearing areas of the foot are affected. The toe clefts and the instep are spared. The skin has a red, glazed and cracked appearance and the eruption is quite symmetrical (Fig. 3.32).

Differential diagnosis
Although the condition is frequently misdiagnosed as athlete's foot, the symmetry, the sparing of the toe webs and the negative mycology will differentiate the two.

Management
The management of this condition is difficult as many of the children refuse to change their footwear, and even if they do this does not necessarily produce a cure. However, they should be advised to adopt leather shoes and cotton socks, and change their shoes regularly throughout the day, returning to the old-fashioned principle of indoor and outdoor shoes. Periods of time free of footwear are advocated. Many of the children seem little troubled by the condition and it gradually disappears over a number of years as they enter adolescence.

(1) **Topical steroids.** These drugs do not seem to be of any great help, whatever potency is tried, although they may have some initial benefit but this soon wears off.

(2) **Emollients.** These are the treatment of choice.

LICHEN SIMPLEX (LOCALIZED NEURODERMATITIS)

Definition
An eczematous response to continual rubbing and scratching of a localized area of the skin.

Diagnostic features
- Very itchy.
- Localized and well defined.
- Unilateral.
- Lichenified.
- Elbows, ankles, neck and genitalia.
- Only responds to potent topical steroids.

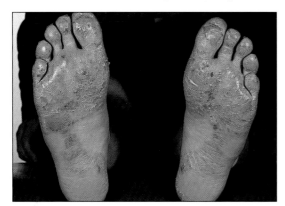

▲ **Fig. 3.32** *Juvenile plantar dermatosis. The childhood disorder affects the weight-bearing areas of the soles, is symmetrical, well-defined, red, glazed and fissured.*

Aetiology

This is a dermatological example of a 'habit tic' often initiated by some minor stressful life event. Continual rubbing and scratching results in thickening of the skin with exaggeration of the skin creases, a phenomenon known as lichenification. Lichen simplex can be induced in anyone, provided the stimulus to the skin is continued for long enough. Histologically, there is acanthosis and hyperkeratosis of the skin.

Clinical features

The condition may occur at any time during adult life. It is intensely itchy. There may be one or several well-defined patches of thickened skin, with marked accentuation of the skin creases (Fig. 3.33). These patches are unilateral, corresponding to the handedness of the patient, and are those that the patient can easily scratch and rub, such as the nape of the neck, just below the elbow, hand, inner aspect of the thigh, outer aspect of the lower leg, buttock, ankle and genitalia. Post-inflammatory hyper- or hypopigmentation are common in coloured races.

Management

(1) **Topical corticosteroids.** The condition responds to the most potent class IV topical corticosteroids. Class III steroids may also be effective, but usually they have to be applied under polythene occlusion. The only exception to the use of these strong steroids is when lichen simplex occurs on the face, when it responds to 2.5% hydrocortisone.

(2) **Systemic antihistamines.** Sedative antihistamines are often required to prevent the patient from scratching, particularly at night, whilst the steroid acts on the eczema. It is very important to point out to the patient that they should not scratch during treatment, because this only aggravates the disease.

(3) **Identification of precipitating factors.** The condition usually commences during a period of stress. Enquiries should be made regarding this, although the stress has often passed. The condition persists because the eczema once developed will only respond to anti-eczema therapy. In some patients, chronic neurosis is present and the condition having been treated then reappears elsewhere. In this case it is known as *lichen simplex chronicus*, for it is remarkably persistent over many years.

LICHEN STRIATUS

Definition

A self-limiting linear form of eczema occurring in children or young adults.

> **Diagnostic features**
> - Unilateral.
> - Limb or trunk.
> - Lichenoid papules.
> - Post-inflammatory hypopigmentation.

Aetiology

The pathology of the condition is that of eczema but the cause is quite obscure.

Clinical features

This is a distinctive relatively uncommon condition. The eruption is initially mildly pruritic and consists of lichenoid papules arranged in a linear or zosteriform distribution either along a limb (Fig. 3.34) or across part of the trunk. Post-inflammatory hypopigmentation subsequently develops.

Management

The condition resolves within a year. There is no specific treatment but class III topical steroids may alleviate the itch.

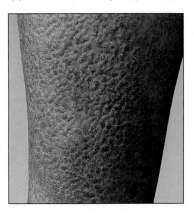

◀ **Fig. 3.33** *Lichen simplex. The patch is unilateral, well-defined and thickened with marked accentuation of the skin creases. Pigmentary abnormalities are common in coloured races.*

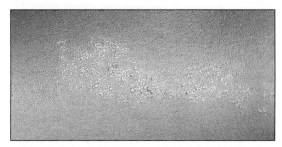

▲ **Fig. 3.34** *Lichen striatus. A linear eruption of lichenoid papules occur leaving behind temporary hypopigmentation.*

4 CONTACT DERMATITIS

INTRODUCTION

Contact dermatitis implies an eczematous reaction resulting from the interaction of an external substance with the skin. These reactions are categorized as irritant or allergic in origin (Fig. 4.1). The former can affect anyone, but the latter only occurs in the predisposed, is a delayed hypersensitivity allergic reaction and will recur everytime the allergen is encountered.

PRIMARY IRRITANT CONTACT DERMATITIS

Definition
Dermatitis which results from overexposure of the skin to an irritant substance.

Aetiology
An irritant dermatitis can occur in any individual, provided that the irritant agent is sufficiently concentrated and the exposure to it is prolonged enough. There is great variability in this response and certain individuals are more prone to it, particularly atopic subjects. It is not the result of an immunological reaction but of damage to the outer protective layer of the skin, the stratum corneum. Strong irritants such as caustics will clearly produce such a reaction, but this is not within the framework of this discussion.

DIFFERENCES BETWEEN PRIMARY IRRITANT AND ALLERGIC CONTACT DERMATITIS	
Primary irritant	Allergic
anyone	the predisposed
first exposure	subsequent exposures since it is an immunological reaction, which requires priming
atopic subjects vulnerable	no relationship to atopy
limited distribution	autosensitization and thus secondary spread may occur

▲**Fig. 4.1** *Differences between primary irritant and allergic contact dermatitis.*

The primary irritant dermatitis results from repeated insults to the skin which accumulate and eventually result in dermatitis. The reaction may occur anywhere on the skin. Dribbling in infants and lip licking and thumb sucking in children are examples of situations where primary irritant dermatitis may develop. However, the three main disorders which are commonly encountered and merit separate description are napkin dermatitis, housewife's hand dermatitis and a condition known as asteatotic eczema (eczema craquelé).

NAPKIN DERMATITIS

Definition
An eczematous response to prolonged exposure to body fluids, occurring in the napkin area.

Diagnostic features
- Redness, with or without scaling.
- Confined to the napkin area.
- Sparing of the genitocrural flexures.

Aetiology
It is not known why some babies are prone to this and others are not. It is not usually due to inexperience, for frequently the mother has brought up other babies without this problem. It is less common in breastfed babies and more common in those who have diarrhoea and are treated with antibiotics. The most vulnerable are those who attend crèches and daycare centres, where gastroenteritis is common. It is considered to be due to constant and prolonged immersion of the skin in urine and faeces, compounded by surrounding the sodden napkin with impervious plastic pants. Friction from the napkin and pants, and the maceration which results from the wet body fluids, abrade and disrupt the protective barrier of the skin. Urine that has been allowed to stand for several hours at body temperature will induce a dermatitis when applied to the skin, whereas fresh urine will not, so that prolonged periods without a napkin change may

be an important factor. Probably faecal lipases and proteases hydrolyse urinary urea which releases ammonia which in turn acts as an irritant. *Candida*

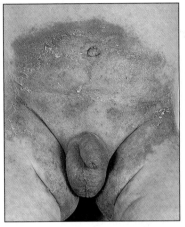

◄**Fig. 4.2** *Napkin dermatitis. The redness and scaling is largely confined to the area covered by the napkin. The genitocrural folds are spared.*

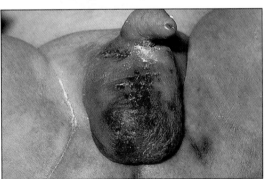

▲**Fig. 4.3** *Jacquet's napkin dermatitis. Erosions are present on the scrotum and penis resulting from failure to change the nappy.*

DIFFERENTIAL DIAGNOSIS OF NAPKIN ERUPTIONS

primary irritant dermatitis	eczema confined to napkin area with sparing of genitocrural folds
Jacquet's dermatitis	erosions and blisters in the napkin area
candidosis	uncommon — raw and macerated genitocrural folds with satellite pustules
psoriasis	rare — dry, red, well-defined patches with thick white scale; lesions elsewhere on torso
seborrhoeic eczema	genitocrural folds as well as napkin area; axillae, neck, face and scalp also involved
atopic eczema	face and flexures also involved

▲**Fig. 4.4** *Differential diagnosis of napkin eruptions.*

albicans is often isolated from napkin dermatitis but it is regarded as a secondary invader of macerated skin.

Clinical features

Napkin dermatitis begins during the first few months of life. There is a confluent erythema with some scaling on the convex surfaces covered by the napkin (Fig. 4.2). Thus, it involves the lower abdomen, pubic area, buttocks, genitalia and upper thighs, but spares the genitocrural flexures. The condition persists for a number of weeks and gradually fades as the infant becomes dry. Post-inflammatory hypopigmentation is common in coloured races and this takes several months to repigment. A more traumatic insult, often due to inexperience or neglect, results in blisters and erosions (Fig. 4.3; Jacquet's napkin dermatitis) from the soiled and sodden napkin being left in contact with the skin for many hours.

Differential diagnosis

The differential diagnosis of napkin eruptions is summarized in Figure 4.4.

Management

The condition is temporary so reassurance is important. Measures are directed at keeping the child as dry as possible. Babies void frequently, but as they grow older they do so less often, producing larger volumes of urine. Napkin changes should be frequent in the early stages and the child should be inspected every hour if possible. It does not seem to matter whether the napkin is disposable or washable; it is more important to have the child free of napkins and plastic pants as much as practicable. If the baby has been dry, then white soft paraffin or a combination of white soft paraffin and liquid paraffin should be applied as a water repellent and emollient, but if wet, the skin should be cleaned with water and a soap substitute, such as emulsifying ointment. Class I topical steroids are indicated: 1% hydrocortisone ointment should be applied sparingly to the area of the eczema, as percutaneous absorption is increased in infantile skin.

PRIMARY IRRITANT DERMATITIS OF THE HANDS (HOUSEWIFE'S DERMATITIS)

Definition

An eczematous eruption mainly on the backs of the fingers and hands occurring in those whose occupation requires frequent immersion of the hands in water and irritants.

Diagnostic features
- Eczema.
- Dorsa of the fingers and hands with sparing of the palms.
- Often past or family history of atopy.
- Often occupational, for example hairdresser, newly wed, or new-born child.

Aetiology
The disorder is common, primarily affecting young adult females. Although colloquially known as 'housewife's dermatitis', it occurs in any occupation in which there is frequent exposure to water and irritants such as detergents and shampoos. Hairdressers, nurses, chefs, cleaners and mechanics are amongst the vulnerable. It is estimated that fifty per cent of junior hairdressers develop some degree of primary irritant dermatitis of the hands during their apprenticeship, which largely consists of shampooing customers' hair. Many are nickel-sensitive subjects, the relevance of which is unexplained, but in an East German study it was found that if nickel-sensitive subjects were excluded from the profession, the incidence of hand eczema was greatly reduced. In addition, the condition is much more common in those that have a family or a personal history of atopy, especially atopic eczema.

Clinical features
The eczema usually begins under a ring and then spreads to the finger to which the ring has been changed. Gradually the backs of the fingers and hands are involved (Fig. 4.5) and there is a characteristic

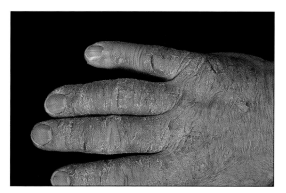

▲ **Fig. 4.5** *Primary irritant eczema. Ill-defined, dry, pink, fissured patches occur on the backs of the fingers and hands. Patch testing is necessary to rule out a contact allergen.*

sparing of the palms. The skin is itchy and ill-defined, pink, rough, fissured patches are found on examination. In severe cases with involvement of the skin around the posterior nail folds, nail growth may be disturbed, resulting in horizontal linear ridges across the nail plate (see Fig. 18.12)

Management
Reduction of exposure to water and irritants
The skin must be kept out of water as much as possible. For a housewife, this means a complete review of her daily routine. It is often useful to get her to write out a list of her previous day's activities and then discuss how much water exposure was really necessary. Washing machines should substitute for hand washing of clothes if possible. The preparation of meals which require cleaning of vegetables, for example, should be forbidden and other menus selected. Personal and social niceties, such as washing the hands prior to eating a meal or after urination should be temporarily discontinued.

Emollients
These should be used liberally.

Oral antihistamines
The eczema is pruritic and sedative antihistamines are sometimes required.

Topical glucocorticosteroids
Hydrocortisone is ineffective. Potent class III steroids are necessary. It is, however, important to instruct the patient to apply the ointment to the lesions only and not to spread it generally over the backs of the hands, thus reducing the possibility of side-effects.

Rest
Sometimes, a primary irritant dermatitis of the hands reflects an inability of a wife and mother to cope with her situation, such that she neglects herself and allows the skin to deteriorate. In a sense therefore it is a cry for help to her husband. She sees herself as servicing him, the house and the children and getting little attention in return. The condition rapidly responds to hospitalization, where the patient is given attention and everything is done for her. It is therefore helpful if the husband can be more involved in household duties and, probably more important, demonstrate that he cares for his wife. The condition tends to be a prolonged one in some patients and it is often because these factors are not put right that the condition continues.

Occupations

It may be necessary to change occupation. For example, a change from the operating theatre to outpatient duties may be all that is required for a nurse. For a hairdresser, the condition may improve when she becomes a senior and no longer has to wash the customers' hair. Sometimes, however, the profession has to be abandoned. As a matter of policy it is always sensible to advise atopics against entering a profession that requires this type of exposure.

Tar

Coal tar is not used as much as it should be to treat primary irritant eczema. Twenty per cent coal tar solution in emulsifying ointment is a very useful soap substitute.

ASTEATOTIC ECZEMA (ECZEMA CRAQUELÉ)

Definition

A dry, superficially fissured skin disorder, often on the shins of the elderly, precipitated by the drying effect of a cold winter or excess washing.

> **Diagnostic features**
> * Itching and soreness.
> * Dryness and cracking (crazy-paving appearance).
> * Especially found on the shins.
> * Responds primarily to emollients.

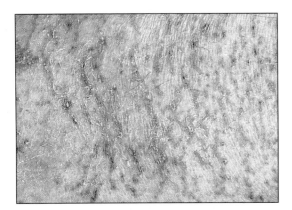

▲ **Fig. 4.6** *Asteatotic eczema. Sore dry red cracks occur characteristically on the shins of the elderly usually as a result of overzealous washing in winter.*

Aetiology

Asteatotic eczema is a disorder of the elderly. There is possibly a reduction in skin surface lipids and the condition is occasionally a presenting feature of myxoedema. The patients may have had a tendency to slight dryness of their skin all their lives, or the dryness has developed as they have aged, especially if they are sun-damaged. The histology is that of an eczema. It is a form of primary irritant dermatitis, which is usually precipitated by: (i) a cold winter with low relative humidity; (ii) admission to hospital and more frequent bathing of the skin than the patient is used to (usually daily baths by nurses); (iii) installation of central heating without adequate humidification, leading to a dry atmosphere; and (iv) diuretics.

Clinical features

The appearance is very characteristic, looking rather like mud that has dried in the sun and become cracked. Many superficial fissures are present (Fig. 4.6), criss-crossing over the skin surface. The skin is red, dry and scaly. The shins are the most characteristic site to be involved.

Management

The prognosis is usually good if the skin is properly cared for.

Emollients

These are crucial and time spent explaining lubrication is well rewarded. The doctor could actually apply an emollient to the skin at the consultation to emphasize the point.

Topical steroids

Class III steroids are of secondary importance and are often not required. If prescribed, they should be in an ointment not a cream form otherwise the dryness will be exacerbated.

Other measures

Bathing should be restricted to twice a week and emulsifying ointment used instead of soap. There should be no wool next to the skin.

ALLERGIC CONTACT DERMATITIS

Definition
This is a delayed hypersensitivity reaction which results in eczema. Once a predisposed individual has become sensitized, the potential to react persists indefinitely and the dermatitis will recur if the patient is re-exposed to the allergen.

Diagnostic features
- Usually acute with vesicles, blisters and weeping.
- Intermittent exacerbations forty-eight hours after exposure.
- Often no previous history of eczema.
- Face and eyelids often involved as a secondary phenomenon.
- Failure to respond adequately to topical steroids.

THE MOST COMMON NON-INDUSTRIAL ALLERGENS
rubber
perfumes
nail varnish
some plants
metal
dyes
cosmetics
medicaments
phosphorus sesquisulphide (matches)

◄**Fig. 4.7**
The most common non-industrial allergens.

Aetiology
This is a true allergic phenomenon, corresponding to type IV hypersensitivity (Gel and Coombes classification). The reaction does not happen with the first exposure, for the immune system requires priming. The allergen is usually a low molecular weight chemical which links with a protein. It is processed by Langerhans' cells and macrophages and then transported via the lymphatics to the paracortical area of the lymph nodes. Here the thymus-derived lymphocytes are primed and then returned to the skin via lymphatics or blood vessels ready to react with the antigen. This priming takes approximately 7–10 days. On subsequent exposure to the antigen this cell-mediated reaction results in a dermatitis within 48–72 hours.

The most common antigens outside of industry are given in Fig. 4.7. The most common industrial agents are chromates in cement, resins in the plastic industry, dyes, rubber and glues. The diagnostic clue to an industrial dermatitis is an eczema on exposed areas of the skin which tends to remit at the weekend or during a holiday, when the patient is not at work. Other workers may be similarly affected. Since this diagnosis may lead to litigation and unemployment, expert advice is required, often from a dermatologist specializing in industrial medicine.

There are many contact allergens and referral to a dermatologist is almost always necessary because patch tests are required. If the allergen is not identified promptly and the patient continues to be exposed, a chronic dermatitis may result despite removal of the antigen at a later date.

Clinical features
The patient usually gives a history suggesting an acute eczema, describing intense irritation, blisters and weeping of the skin. Often the face is involved, particularly as part of an autosensitization process (Fig. 4.8), which is a reaction of the skin to a contact dermatitis elsewhere on the body. The clue to the diagnosis of allergic contact dermatitis is the distribution of the eczematous eruption, the lack of any past history of eczema as a child and the failure to control the eruption adequately with topical steroids until the allergen is removed. The clinical features of certain common examples of contact dermatitis are described here.

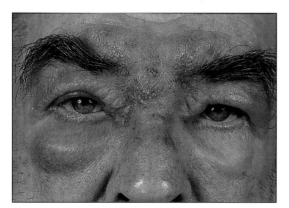

▲**Fig. 4.8** *Contact dermatitis. The inflammatory reaction in contact dermatitis is often acute or subacute. The face is often involved secondary to autosensitization.*

Contact dermatitis due to metal

Metal dermatitis is the commonest cause of contact dermatitis and predominantly affects females. Nickel and cobalt are constituents of jewellery which is not solid gold or silver, and of a host of other items (Figs. 4.9–4.11). The diagnosis is suspected by the sites involved (Fig. 4.12).

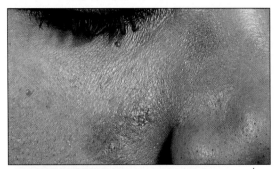

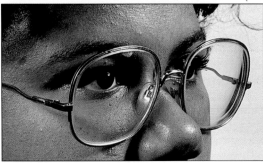

▲ **Figs. 4.9 & 4.10** *Contact dermatitis to metal spectacle frames. This patient presented with a patch of eczema with post-inflammatory pigmentation on her cheek (Fig. 4.9) which was due to her metal spectacles (Fig. 4.10).*

COMMON SITES AND SOURCES OF METAL DERMATITIS	
Site	Source
earlobes	earrings
cheeks	metal spectacle frames
neck	necklace and/or catch
wrists	bracelet, watch strap
waist and umbilicus	jean studs
elbow	chain on bag
lower leg	zip in boots
around eyes	autosensitization

▲ **Fig. 4.12** *Common sites and sources of metal dermatitis.*

COMMON SITES AND SOURCES OF RUBBER DERMATITIS	
Site	Source
hands	gloves, tyre-mechanics
feet	shoes, especially soles
waist	elastic in underwear
chest	elastic in brassière
face	bathing cap, snorkel mask or autosensitization

▲ **Fig. 4.13** *Common sites and sources of rubber dermatitis.*

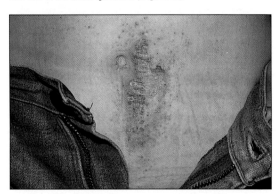

▲ **Fig. 4.11** *Nickel contact dermatitis. This patch of eczema was secondary to metal in the zip and studs of her jeans.*

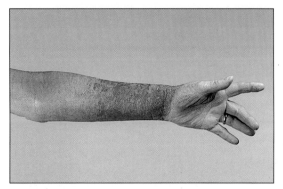

▲ **Fig. 4.14** *Rubber glove contact dermatitis. The dermatitis occurs around the wrists and on the backs of the hands. The palms are usually spared.*

Contact dermatitis due to rubber

This dermatitis is common in industry, but is frequent even in domestic surroundings. The allergen is usually a rubber accelerator or antioxidant, rather than the rubber itself. The common sites of rubber dermatitis are given in Fig. 4.13. Rubber gloves are the most frequent source. The eczema occurs on the backs of the fingers and hands and around the wrists, where the eruption may be sharply delineated. The palms are often spared (Fig. 4.14), presumably because the allergen has more difficulty penetrating the very thick stratum corneum. Sensitization may be a complicating factor in patients who already have a primary irritant or constitutional eczema and who have been using rubber gloves to protect their hands. Shoe dermatitis from rubber occurs on the parts of the soles which are weight-bearing, so that the instep is usually spared, and on the dorsa of the feet and toes, with sparing of the toe-web spaces. Rubber in clothing is usually easy to suspect because the distribution of the eruption corresponds so well to the article of clothing worn.

Contact dermatitis due to perfumes and cosmetics

Common allergens are given in Figure 4.15. Cosmetics rarely cause allergic contact dermatitis considering how extensively they are used. Many act as irritants rather than true allergens, particularly in atopic subjects, and patch tests are negative. Once the dermatitis has been treated and has settled down, the cosmetics can be used again without further problems. Perfumes are the most common allergens and the dermatitis occurs at the site of application, usually the neck and wrists, and on the face from the perfume sprayed into the atmosphere. However, many substances are perfumed, so that the dermatitis may occur on the hands

COMMON COSMETIC ALLERGENS
perfume and perfumed articles
lanolin
preservatives in creams
(e.g. parabens, Dowicil 200)
deodorants (formaldehyde)
nail varnish
hair dyes

◀**Fig. 4.15**
Common cosmetic allergens.

from perfumed soap or in the axillae from perfumed deodorants. The latter also contain formaldehyde and because the axillae are occluded areas, permitting enhanced penetration, sensitization is frequent.

Preservatives are added to creams to prevent bacterial contamination. Parabens was a common preservative to which allergic contact dermatitis occurred, but it is now being replaced by formaldehyde-releasing preservatives such as Dowicil 200 and the incidence of hypersensitivity to these agents is increasing. Lanolin is gradually being removed from many face creams as it is a well-recognized sensitizer. Hair dyes (paraphenylenediamine) occasionally sensitize, and in the past dyes in clothing similarly produced problems that are uncommon nowadays. New sensitizers are always appearing and a recent one was musk ambrette, an ingredient of aftershaves, which produced a photosensitivity reaction.

Contact dermatitis due to nail varnish

Nail varnish dermatitis is worth considering separately, because although cosmetic dermatitis is readily suspected, nail varnish dermatitis is rarely so, either by the patient or the practitioner. The reason is that the eruption occurs at the sites of the contact with nail varnish, such as the face, neck, jaw and upper chest, rather than on the fingers as might be assumed. This is because women apply the nail varnish so carefully to the nails, which do not sensitize, without touching the surrounding skin. The eruption, like other forms of contact dermatitis, may be acute or subacute, sometimes causing closure of the eyes and swelling of the face. Often oval patches corresponding to the finger nails can be quite clearly seen on the cheeks or jaw. The allergen is santolite (aryl-sulphonamide formaldehyde).

Contact dermatitis due to medicaments (dermatitis medicamentosa)

Iatrogenic contact dermatitis is common (see Fig. 4.16) and could be avoided if certain classes of compounds were not used on the skin. Local anaesthetics and topical antihistamines are common sensitizers. Dermatologists rarely use either for that reason. Local anaesthetics are often prescribed for pruritus ani by well-meaning surgeons, but sensitization ultimately occurs in a significant number of subjects. Topical antihistamines are available over the counter and are used for all manner of eruptions, including insect bites. They are of no proven value and are best avoided.

Topical antibiotics, such as neomycin and its cross-reactants, soframycin and framycetin, rarely cause problems except when prescribed for varicose eczema and varicose ulcers (Fig. 4.17). These conditions are particularly vulnerable to dermatitis medicamentosa for reasons that have not been adequately explained. Otitis externa, which is a form of seborrhoeic dermatitis affecting the ear, may also react to topical antibiotics. Topical antibiotics are extensively prescribed in various acne preparations but rarely give problems in this site. They are also prescribed in combination with topical steroids, but again contact sensitization is unusual, except in the case of varicose eczema (Fig. 4.17). The diagnosis should be suspected if an eczematous eruption, which ordinarily would respond to such a preparation, deteriorates. Chloramphenicol used in eyedrops does give rise to sensitization, but uncommonly considering its widespread use and it therefore should not be discredited.

Phosphorus sesquisulphide (match) dermatitis

Phosphorus sesquisulphide is a constituent of 'strike anywhere' non-safety matches, for example Swan Vesta (in the UK), and is present in the striking head of the match and the strike side of the box. This is a disorder of males essentially and is rarely suspected by the patient. The face is involved (Fig. 4.18) as the fumes spread up to it after the match is struck. The outer thigh or breast is affected, corresponding to a trouser or shirt pocket in which the matches are kept (see Fig. 4.19). The palm of the hand may be involved from holding the box. The condition will flare up in any public place where smokers use such matches.

COMMON SITES AND SOURCES OF DERMATITIS MEDICAMENTOSA	
Site	Condition and medicaments
legs	varicose eczema and ulcers (antibiotics and lanolin)
eyes	ophthalmological conditions (chloramphenicol eye drops) and autosensitization
ears	otitis externa (antibiotics)
anus	pruritus ani (local anaesthetics and ethylenediamine)

▲ **Fig. 4.16** *Common sites and sources of dermatitis medicamentosa.*

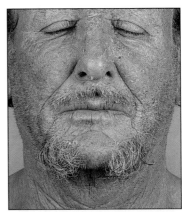

◀ **Fig. 4.18** *Phosphorus sesquisulphide (match) dermatitis. The dermatitis occurs on the face from the fumes and at sites where the matchbox is close to the skin.*

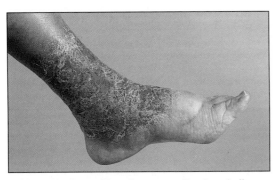

▲ **Fig. 4.17** *Dermatitis medicamentosa. Certain topically applied drugs are common sensitizers, particularly when applied to varicose eczema.*

COMMON SITES AND SOURCES OF MATCH DERMATITIS	
Site	Source
face	fumes
breast	box in shirt pocket
thigh	box in trouser pocket
palm	holding box
ears	cleaning with matchstick

▲ **Fig. 4.19** *Common sites and sources of match dermatitis.*

Management of contact dermatitis

The diagnosis of a suspected contact dermatitis should always be confirmed by patch testing. There are approximately thirty allergens which are encountered commonly enough to constitute a battery of tests which are applied to the skin. Other relevant potential allergens are added to this battery, for example parts of the shoe, if a foot eruption is being investigated, and the patient's cosmetics and nail varnish, if a facial dermatitis is under review. The chemicals are put into aluminium wells fitted into an adhesive tape, and then stuck onto the patient's back. They are removed after 48–72 hours, and the skin is inspected for a patch of dermatitis corresponding to the application of the allergen (Fig. 4.20). Some reactions are delayed and it is wise to inspect the skin a further 48 hours later. This testing procedure requires experience and is normally done by the dermatologist. Care is required in interpretation of the results, because irritant reactions may occur. This always happens if shampoos are patch tested. An irritant reaction will have disappeared by the second reading, whereas an allergic reaction will still be present. Some suggest that all patients with eczema should be patch tested, because clinical acumen is not always correct, but this is not always practical and there is a danger of sensitizing a patient to an allergen during the procedure. The advantage of patch testing is that it demonstrates to patient and doctor the cause of the dermatitis.

Clearly the patient will recover if the antigen is permanently removed. Sometimes a substitute may be used, for example certain firms specializing in hypoallergic products make santolite-free nail varnish and fragrance-free cosmetics. However, certain points are worth making. In nickel dermatitis, for example, some patients have a liking for clothes with metal adornments and find these hard to give up. It is important to tell them that clothing in between the metal and the skin does not prevent the reaction, as sweat leaches out the metal. Painting the metal with nail varnish is also unsatisfactory as it quickly wears off.

Patients with rubber sensitivity should be advised to change to polyvinyl chloride (PVC) gloves, preferably lined with cotton, and all-leather or PVC shoes. The elastic in underwear should be removed and lycra brassières are recommended. Patients should be reminded of other sources of rubber, for example squash balls, tyres and rubber undersheets and pillows.

Public places may be a source of exposure so the patient with match dermatitis should be aware that someone may be using phosphorus sesquisulphide matches in a bar or restaurant, and patients with perfume sensitivity should take care in the perfume departments of large stores and duty-free shops at airports.

Iatrogenic dermatitis medicamentosa could be avoided if doctors refrained from treating varicose eczema and ulcers with topical antibiotics and avoided using ethylenediamine-containing ointments and topical anaesthetics and antihistamines.

PLANT CONTACT DERMATITIS

Definition

A delayed hypersensitivity allergic contact reaction to a plant.

> **Diagnostic features**
> *Primula and* **Rhus** *dermatitis*
> - Acute, weeping, vesiculo-bullous.
> - Finger tips and hands.
> - Forearms.
> - Other areas touched by fingers, such as face (especially eyelids) and genitalia.
>
> *Bulb dermatitis*
> - Chronic eczema with dryness, hyperkeratosis and fissuring.
> - Finger tips.
> - Under finger nails.
>
> *Chrysanthemum and airborne dermatitis*
> - Chronic lichenified eczema.
> - Face, neck, hands, forearms (exposed skin).
> - Occupational.

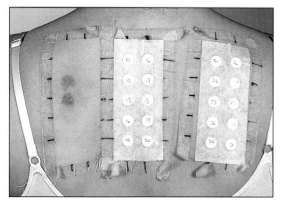

▲ **Fig. 4.20** *Patch tests. A battery of suspected and common allergens are applied to the back for 48 hours. Two positives are present.*

Aetiology

The plants responsible for the allergy vary depending upon the local flora. The most common in North America are members of the genus *Rhus*, especially poison oak and ivy. In the UK, primula is the commonest due to a quinone (primin) in the hairs on the leaves, stems and flowers. Chrysanthemums and other Compositae contain sesquiterpene lactones in their stems and leaves which sensitize florists and gardeners more often than those who receive them occasionally as gifts. Tulips, garlic and onion bulbs contain a natural fungicide, alpha-methyl gamma-butyrolactone, and produce dermatitis on the finger tips. Airborne contact dermatitis may result from some species, for example the American ragweed *Ambrosia*, and in India there is an epidemic from the weed *Parthenium hysterophorus* imported unwittingly from Texas.

Clinical features

The clinical features vary depending on the source. Primula and *Rhus* dermatitis is acute, either papulo-vesicular or vesiculo-bullous in morphology and streaky and patchy in configuration. Bulb dermatitis is a chronic dry hyperkeratotic eczema of the tips of the fingers and under the nails, whereas chrysanthemum dermatitis is a chronic lichenified eczema of the exposed parts simulating an airborne contact dermatitis.

Management

Patch testing is necessary to establish the diagnosis and strict avoidance of the allergen is required to avoid recurrences. Potent topical steroids are necessary to treat the eruption, and systemic steroids may be necessary for a severe attack of *Rhus* dermatitis.

PHOTOCONTACT DERMATITIS

Introduction

Photocontact dermatitis is an interaction between a photosensitizing chemical and ultraviolet light which produces either a toxic or an allergic response. Photo-toxic reactions are non-immunological and anyone can develop the reaction given the right circumstance of sufficient exposure to the chemical and ultraviolet light. The reaction may be either local or systemic. The latter is considered under drug eruptions (see Chapter 15). The common local reactions are phyto-photodermatitis and Berloque dermatitis.

Phytophotodermatitis

Definition

This is a reaction between a plant chemical and ultraviolet light, resulting in acute blistering and pigmentation.

Diagnostic features
- Acute, vesiculo-bullous eruption.
- Linear streaks.
- Post-inflammatory hyperpigmentation.
- Summer months.

Aetiology

The chemical is a furocoumarin containing 5-methoxy-psoralen, which is crushed onto the skin, commonly either by lying in a meadow or by cutting back weeds on a summer's day. There is a direct interaction between long-wave ultraviolet light and the psoralen, and an inflammatory reaction takes place.

The main plants responsible are parsnips, giant hogweed, cow parsley, dill, angelica, fennel, celery, *Amni majus*, lime, bergamot and orange. *Amni majus*, which grows along the Nile valley, is of some interest. It has been known in Egypt as a phototoxic agent for centuries and is used to treat vitiligo. It contains a psoralen which is now used to treat psoriasis as part of photochemotherapy (PUVA).

Clinical features

The degree of inflammatory response varies but it is usually vesiculo-bullous (Fig. 4.21) and is always followed by hyperpigmentation which consists of a bizarre network of streaks so characteristic as to constitute a spot diagnosis.

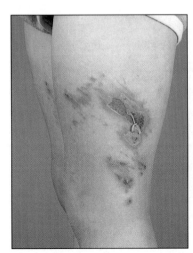

◄**Fig. 4.21** *Phytophoto-dermatitis. A bizarre streaky vesiculo-bullous eruption occurs on sites which have been in contact with weeds containing furocoumarins which have interacted with sunlight.*

Management

A potent topical steroid may be indicated in the acute stages but explanation is usually all that is required.

Berloque dermatitis

Definition

An interaction between 5-methoxypsoralen in colognes and perfumes and long-wave ultraviolet light results in post-inflammatory pigmentation.

Diagnostic features
- Bizarre streaky hyperpigmentation.
- Usually on the side of the neck.

Aetiology

Berloque dermatitis has a similar mechanism to phyto-photodermatitis but is due to an interaction between oil of bergamot, which contains 5-methoxypsoralen, and long-wave ultraviolet light. Oil of bergamot is present in many colognes and perfumes.

Clinical features

The acute inflammatory stage of Berloque dermatitis often does not occur at all and the patient presents with a bizarre streaky hyperpigmentation, which is presumably post-inflammatory in origin. The pigmentation may occur anywhere on the body where the perfume has come into contact with the skin, but the side of the neck is most typical (Fig. 4.22). The pigmentation slowly fades after a number of months.

Management

Explanation is usually sufficient.

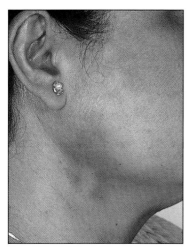

◄ **Fig. 4.22** *Berloque dermatitis. This dermatitis is due to an interaction between sunlight and oil of bergamot, which is present in many perfumes. The side of the neck is the commonest site.*

Photoallergic contact dermatitis

Definition

A delayed hypersensitivity cell-mediated immunological response between an allergen and ultraviolet light, which only occurs in predisposed individuals.

Diagnostic features
- Eczema.
- Light-exposed areas.

Aetiology

The skin requires to be primed and subsequently re-exposed to the allergen. The sensitivity is life-long and the dermatitis will recur every time the patient is exposed to the chemical and sunlight. The best known example of this problem occurred thirty years ago. Certain bacteriostatic substances, namely tetrachloro- (or bromo-) salicylanide, were added to toiletries and soaps, and in particular Lifebuoy soap. The eczematous eruption occurred on exposed areas of the skin on bright sunny days when there were still traces of the chemical from the soap on the skin. This was a true photoallergic contact dermatitis. The condition is no longer encountered in the UK, but occasionally small epidemics of cases occur when the chemical is added to soaps by manufacturers who are unfamiliar with its chemistry. Bithionol and hexa-chlorophane occasionally cause a similar problem. A scent containing musk ambrette was added to after-shave preparations and colognes a few years ago and a photocontact dermatitis occurred on exposed areas, particularly the face. The eruption is becoming less common as the concentration of the musk ambrette is reduced or it is removed.

Topical medicaments containing sulphonamides and promethazine when applied the skin may act as photocontact allergens but there is no need to prescribe them, so the problem should not really occur.

Systemic agents occasionally cause photocontact dermatitis, particularly in workers manufacturing drugs such as phenothiazines, and in patients taking, for example, promethazine hydrochloride or sulpho-namides to which they have been sensitized by a topical route.

Clinical features

The eruption is mainly eczematous and occurs on exposed parts of the skin such as the face, 'V' of the neck, backs of the hands and, in women, the lower legs. Areas which are protected from sunlight, for example behind the ears, and under the eyebrows, the nose, the chin and the hair, are spared.

Management

It is important to establish the antigen by photopatch testing. The allergens are applied to the back in the usual way for 48 hours and then irradiated after removal of the patches and the results read 48 hours later.

The allergen must be avoided for life because otherwise these patients may become persistent light reactors and develop a condition called actinic reticuloid, even though they subsequently avoid the photoallergen.

5 PSORIASIS

INTRODUCTION

Although there may be a unifying explanation for psoriasis, it is not a homogenous disease clinically. There are various states of the disorder, for example chronic and stable or acute and unstable. The latter may result in generalized erythroderma or pustulation. Bacterial infection may precipitate a short-lived entity known as guttate psoriasis. These clinical variants are described separately here for the sake of clarity. Also since psoriasis can affect any site on the body and can sometimes be quite difficult to diagnose if it appears on, say, the hands or genitalia alone, I have further subdivided the clinical features by site as well. This subdivision is relevant therapeutically because different sites require different modes of therapy. Finally, psoriasis may affect the nails (Chapter 18) and joints.

Definition

Psoriasis is a common chronic benign hyperproliferative condition of the skin, which is often inherited and sometimes associated with disorders of the joints and nails. It is usually characterized by symmetrical, well-defined red plaques, with a thick silvery scale, but there are a number of morphological subtypes.

Aetiology

Psoriasis appears to affect 1–2% of the British and North American populations and both sexes equally. No race is exempt, but whereas it is common in the Indian subcontinent, it is rare in the West Indian, American black, the Japanese and the pure American Indian. One-third of patients recall a family history. It is most probably inherited as an autosomal dominant with incomplete penetrance. A strong association with the human leucocyte antigens (HLA) B13 and B17 has been reported in psoriasis, and with HLA B27 in pustular psoriasis. Offspring of a psoriatic have a three-fold increased chance of developing the disease. It may commence at any age from infancy (napkin or diaper psoriasis; Fig. 5.1) to old age, but adolescence, early adult life and late middle-age are the most frequent times.

Psoriasis is one of several disorders which may develop in sites of injury (the Koebner phenomenon). Thus napkin psoriasis is probably a manifestation of a primary irritant dermatitis in an infant with a psoriatic diathesis. Scratching of the skin, injury, a surgical incision (Fig. 5.2) or tight-fitting clothing may all induce the appearance of psoriasis.

Amongst various contributory factors, streptococcal infections are well recognized as precipitating guttate psoriasis. The effect of other infections is less well established. Alcohol, antimalarials and lithium may exacerbate the disease. Practolol, a beta-blocker now withdrawn, produced an eruption which had several psoriasiform features.

Although many patients benefit from ultraviolet

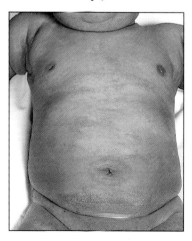

◀ **Fig. 5.1** *Psoriasis. It may commence in infancy, particularly around the napkin area with spread elsewhere.*

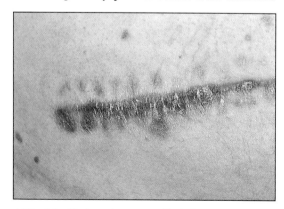

▲ **Fig. 5.2** *Koebner phenomenon. Psoriasis may appear on skin damaged by trauma, in this case around surgical incision.*

irradiation, which may explain the seasonal improvement in summer, not all do. Excess ultraviolet irradiation resulting in sunburn may produce a Koebner phenomenon.

The histopathology in the chronic stable variety is characteristic (see Fig. 5.3). The earliest changes are seen in the papillary dermis. The capillaries are dilated and have proliferated. They are surrounded by polymorphonuclear leucocytes and some mononuclear cells. The polymorphs enter the epidermis and form small microabscesses, and if these are present in large numbers the clinical picture is pustular psoriasis. In the epidermis there is acanthosis (thickening of the epithelium) and hyperkeratosis, both due to excess keratin production. It was van Scott's pioneering work that established that the epithelium was mitotically hyperactive. The basal cell layer is increased in volume and mitotic figures are present. The granular cell layer is absent and there is parakeratosis (retention of the nuclear remnants in the stratum corneum). The whole epithelium is thrown into folds and the epidermal ridges (rete ridges) are elongated, clubbed and fused at their borders. The pathology is now known to represent an epithelial hyperproliferation, and studies of cell transit through the epidermis indicate that cell replacement occurs roughly seven times faster than normal. Thus, the psoriatic basal cell is shed in about four days, whereas a normal one is shed in 28 days. The 'normal' skin in the psoriatic patient is also mitotically active, but not to the same degree. The scales which are shed so freely and constitute such an embarrassment in psoriasis are a direct result of the overactivity of the epithelium. The erythema of the skin is due to the dilatation and proliferation of the capillaries in the papillary dermis.

The problem is to glean the cause of this pathology. The inflammatory cells in the dermis are probably of prime importance, but it is not established whether it is the polymorphs or monocytes (and this includes Langerhans' cells) which are responsible. Numerous biochemical abnormalities have been found in psoriasis, but there is difficulty in establishing whether they are responsible primarily for the disease or are simply epiphenomena. In the 1970s disorders of cyclic AMP were thought to be responsible, and in the 1980s prostaglandin metabolism and especially leucotriene activity are under intense review.

Clinical features

Although usually chronic, psoriasis is a dynamic disease. It waxes and wanes in intensity throughout life. It may be exceedingly troublesome at some stage, early adulthood for example, and then lessen, or even go into complete remission. It may be extremely limited or widespread, such that psoriasis may mean different things to different people. It may affect a single area such as the scalp, hands, genitalia, joints or nails without disturbance elsewhere. It may be quite stable, and then suddenly become red, angry and sore. It may be symptomless or intensely itchy and uncomfortable. It is therefore not enough just to make a diagnosis of psoriasis. It needs to be classified, for example by type and site, for this will determine the treatment and outcome.

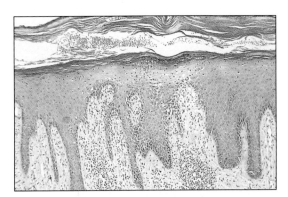 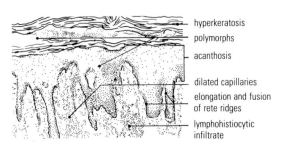

hyperkeratosis
polymorphs
acanthosis

dilated capillaries
elongation and fusion of rete ridges
lymphohistiocytic infiltrate

▲ **Fig. 5.3** *Pathology. The epidermis is thickened and hyperkeratotic. The rete ridges are elongated and fused. There is a dermal and epidermal infiltrate and dilated capillaries.*

PSORIASIS VULGARIS

Diagnostic features
- Well-defined red plaques.
- White or silver scales.
- Symmetrical.
- Extensor surfaces.

This is the most common and stable form of psoriasis. The lesions are symmetrical, very well defined and slightly raised (Fig. 5.4). They are deep red in colour and have a thick white or silvery scale (see Fig. 1.7) which when scraped away (grattinage) leaves tiny bleeding points from the dilated superficial capillaries. The size and shape of the plaques vary enormously. Small plaques may coalesce into large ones. Healing takes place centrally (see Fig. 1.28), so that annular configurations result. The sites commonly affected are the scalp and extensor surfaces of the elbows, knees, sacrum and the limbs, but of course it may occur anywhere on the skin.

The diagnosis is probably one of the easiest in dermatology. It is also one of the most responsive forms of psoriasis to therapy, particularly to dithranol.

SUBACUTE OR ACUTE PSORIASIS

Diagnostic features
- Bright red, well-defined plaques.
- Little or no scale.
- Sore.

Psoriasis may become sore and inflamed. It is bright red, has little surface scale and is tender to touch (Fig. 5.5). The cause may be obscure but it often results from injudicious treatment such as inappropriate use of dithranol or sudden withdrawal of very potent class IV topical steroid therapy, or a severe physical or emotional illness. It is an unstable and dangerous stage because it may herald an impending erythroderma or even an episode of generalized pustular psoriasis. It is not easy to treat. Bland preparations and bed rest are called for and, more often than not, systemic therapy.

ERYTHRODERMIC PSORIASIS

Diagnostic features
- Universal redness and scaling.
- Often nail and hair growth disturbance.

This may be an end-result of subacute or acute psoriasis, but it occasionally arises out of the blue. The term *erythroderma* implies that virtually the whole cutaneous surface is involved. (Psoriasis is one of the most common causes, but eczema, mycosis fungoides and drug eruptions may also result in erythroderma.) The skin is a deep red colour (erythroderma), and may be scaly (exfoliative psoriasis). The redness results from capillary proliferation. Usually there are areas of both erythroderma and exfoliation present (see Fig. 5.7). The scale is thick and white, which serves to distinguish it from other forms of erythroderma. The condition may lead to temporary

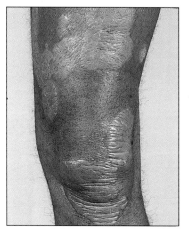

◀**Fig. 5.4** *Psoriasis vulgaris. The lesions are very well defined and a deep red colour, even in pigmented races. The lesions heal centrally.*

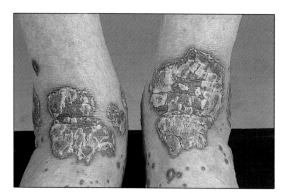

▲**Fig. 5.5** *Acute psoriasis. The skin is tender and bright and fiery red. Pustulation may follow. Systemic therapy is usually necessary.*

loss of hair and to disturbances in nail growth, producing horizontal ridging and occasionally loss of nails.

The patient is often unwell with a fever and leucocytosis. He feels cold and shivery and covers himself with blankets to keep warm. Generalized vasodilatation leads to excessive loss of body heat and central hypothermia. The increased cutaneous blood flow also produces a high cardiac output, and may lead to heart failure, particularly in those with a compromised myocardium. There is increased percutaneous loss of water, because the epidermal barrier to water loss is impaired. Increased loss of protein and iron through the exfoliating scales may lead to hypoproteinaemia and iron deficiency anaemia. Derangement of the epidermal barrier also causes increased epidermal permeability so that great care has to be taken with topical applications, particularly topical steroids, because systemic absorption is likely to be high. Patients often use large quantities of topical steroids in this condition and must be weaned off them carefully, otherwise adrenal failure may occur.

There was an appreciable mortality associated with this disease, but modern systemic therapy is life-saving.

PUSTULAR PSORIASIS

There are two forms of the disease, one localized to the palms and/or soles, and the other generalized. The former is relatively common and is an important differential diagnosis of skin eruptions involving the hands and feet. Generalized pustular psoriasis is not a common event, but may occur during the course of a common disease and may proceed extremely rapidly. It must be recognized early because of its serious nature.

Pustular psoriasis localized to the palms and soles

Diagnostic features
- Yellow pustules which turn brown.
- Occur on a red background.
- Often symmetrical.
- Palms and soles.
- There may be typical psoriasis elsewhere.

This is characterized by yellow pustules which turn brown, occurring on a well defined background of erythema (Fig. 5.6). Sometimes there are obvious psoriatic scales present within the plaque, but on other occasions these are absent. There may or may not be typical psoriasis elsewhere. The plaques on the palms and soles are remarkably symmetrical. The disorder is very difficult to treat with the usual local

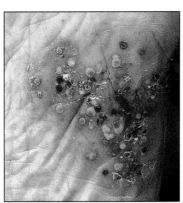

◀**Fig. 5.6** *Localized pustular psoriasis. Sterile yellow pustules, which become brown, occur on a well-defined background of erythema on the palms or soles.*

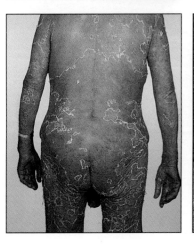
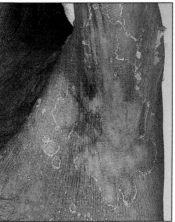

◀**Figs. 5.7 & 5.8** *Generalized pustular psoriasis. This patient is erythrodermic. In addition there is extensive peeling of the skin following small sterile pustules visible in the axilla (Fig. 5.8).*

measures. If it fails to go into remission after a number of months or so, and is particularly distressing to the patient, it may be necessary to commence treatment with systemic agents.

Generalized pustular psoriasis (of von Zumbusch)

Diagnostic features
- High fever, leucocytosis.
- Extensive crops of small sterile pustules.
- Skin is generally bright red and sore.

This disorder is rare but it does have an appreciable mortality. The cause of the pustulation may not be obvious, but is usually due to mismanagement. Systemic steroids or large quantities of very potent topical steroids may precipitate the disease if they are reduced or withdrawn quickly. Systemic steroids should never be used to treat psoriasis, but they are sometimes given for a co-existing condition: if they are reduced quickly by a physician unaware of this danger, generalized pustulation may result. Similar cases have been seen in recent times in patients who have been using large quantities of very potent class IV steroids and who have been unwisely advised to stop them immediately. Occasionally, localized palmar/plantar pustular psoriasis may become generalized.

Extensive sheets of small, sterile, yellow pustules cover the skin, which is fiery red and sore (Figs 5.7 & 5.8). The patient feels ill, has a fever and a leucocytosis. The pustulation may cease spontaneously in mild cases, but in others continues. The dangers of the disease include secondary bacterial infection of the skin, urinary tract and lungs, leading to septicaemia, dehydration, electrolyte imbalance, hypocalcaemia and hypoalbuminaemia. The patient requires hospitalization and usually systemic therapy. Methotrexate is effective but should be administered in much smaller amounts than for other forms of psoriasis because bone-marrow toxicity is much more likely than in other forms. Retinoids are also effective and etretinate is probably now the drug of choice.

GUTTATE PSORIASIS

Diagnostic features
- Follows a streptococcal throat infection.
- Rapid evolution.
- Very small red papules, with thick white scales.
- Mainly on trunk and limbs.
- Resolution within four months.

This is a common disorder of adolescents or young adults. The prognosis is usually excellent. It commences two to three weeks after a severe streptococcal throat infection despite adequate antibiotic therapy. The onset is acute with an eruption of very small, drop-like ('guttate') papules all over the trunk and limbs (Fig. 5.9). The lesions are a deep red colour, and often have the characteristic silver scale on their surface. The condition resolves completely in most cases within four months. In some patients the psoriasis never recurs. In others, it is followed by the insidious onset of psoriasis vulgaris. Because of the widespread nature of the lesions, treatment with ointments is often impractical, and the condition is ideally managed with tar baths, followed by exposure to ultraviolet light.

PSORIATIC ARTHROPATHY

Joint involvement occurs in a minority of patients who have psoriasis of the skin or nails. Occasionally, however, joint involvement identical to that which may accompany psoriasis occurs without any cutaneous evidence of the disease. The patients are usually seronegative and there may be a family history of psoriasis, which helps to distinguish the condition from rheumatoid arthritis. It is beyond the scope of this text to detail the changes in the joints.

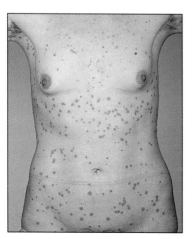

◄**Fig. 5.9**
Guttate psoriasis. Small drop-like (guttate) red scaly papules occur on the trunk and limbs after a severe throat infection.

SITES OF PSORIASIS

Psoriasis can occur anywhere on the skin, but classically on the elbows, knees, trunk and limbs, when it is
generally very easy to recognize. However, certain
sites regularly cause diagnostic confusion and may be
difficult to treat.

SCALP
The scalp is very commonly involved, and the difficulty diagnostically is that the hair obscures the
lesions. The plaques are discrete and red and have a
considerable silver scale. They are remarkably symmetrical. Often they extend beyond the hair-bearing
areas, onto the glabrous skin. The condition rarely
results in hair loss, but scalp psoriasis is particularly
difficult to treat.

FACE
Fortunately the face is usually spared, perhaps due
to its continual exposure to ultraviolet irradiation.
However, if it is affected, even a mild degree can
cause considerable embarrassment. The lesions are
well-defined, deep red, and have a thick scale. The
disease rarely occurs in isolation on the face, so the
diagnosis should not be too difficult. It may be
confused with seborrhoeic eczema but is distinguished
by its lack of response to hydrocortisone.

FLEXURES
Psoriasis may occur in the major flexures as part
of general cutaneous involvement, but it may predominantly affect the flexures, and this is particularly
so in the obese where occlusion and friction produces
a Koebner phenomenon. Middle-aged and elderly
patients, especially women, are particularly susceptible. The plaques are well defined and a deep red
colour, but they lack the characteristic silver scale.
Occasionally patients may have a coincidental fungal
infection in the flexures, and it is always wise to take
samples to rule out tinea or candida, for clearly
antipsoriatic treatment would not be appropriate and
steroids in particular would be detrimental.

Flexural psoriasis is difficult to treat. Dithranol
aggravates the condition, and topical steroids are only
partially successful. In widespread intractable cases,
systemic therapy should be considered.

HANDS AND FEET
The visibility of psoriasis on the hands and the
abnormal texture felt on shaking the hands of the
patient with psoriasis are serious social disabilities.
Involvement of the palms and fingertips may interfere
with manual dexterity and involvement of the feet can
make walking painful and difficult. The diagnosis of
psoriasis on the dorsa of the hands and feet is quite
straightforward. When it is present on the palms and
soles alone it may be more difficult, particularly if
there is no evidence of the disease elsewhere, because
the thickened stratum corneum transforms the typical
appearance. The lesions are extremely well defined
and symmetrical and usually of a deep red colour. The
scale is thick and white on the hands, but may be
yellowish on the feet. There are none of the vesicles or
exudates found in eczema, but fissuring is common. It
is extremely resistant to local topical therapy and
systemic therapy may be appropriate. The condition
is sore rather than itchy. The nails may be involved,
which may help in the diagnosis.

GENITALIA
If genital psoriasis occurs in the presence of psoriasis
on the body, the diagnosis is not difficult. However, it
sometimes occurs in isolation or in association with
minor involvement of the scalp. The lesion is well
defined, red and symmetrical, but silver scales may
well be absent.

MANAGEMENT OF PSORIASIS

Psoriasis, like any chronic disease with a limited
number of therapeutic options, calls for considerable
skill in management. It is important to ascertain a
number of facts about the patient's disease.

(1) **The extent.** Patients vary greatly in their tolerance
of the disease: some are remarkably phlegmatic,
others never adjust to it, while most lie somewhere
in between. It is important to establish how bad they
consider their condition and how much they expect
from treatment.

(2) **Function.** Psoriasis of the palmar surfaces may
impair the ability to work. Psoriasis of the fingertips
may interfere with manual dexterity and that on the
plantar surfaces may make it difficult to walk.

(3) **Visibility.** Fortunately psoriasis is usually not
present on exposed parts of the skin but if it is then
the treatment may need to be more aggressive. There
is untold suffering, even for those in whom it is not
visible, when it comes to making adult physical
relationships. Psoriasis on the hands may preclude a
patient from working in a restaurant or with food,

even though there is no danger of infection. Psoriasis therefore may interfere with livelihood.

(4) Symptoms. For most patients the disease does not itch, but it may become itchy or sore and will need to be treated accordingly.

(5) Type of psoriasis. Guttate psoriasis has a good prognosis, but patients with erythrodermic, pustular or subacute psoriasis, or those who have had multiple admissions to hospital, often require systemic therapy.

(6) Age and physical health. It is often easier to treat elderly patients with extensive psoriasis because the dermatologist can justify prescribing systemic therapy more readily than in a young person with many decades to live.

(7) Past treatments. Most patients who have had their psoriasis for some time will have tried all the available topical remedies. If they have found any particular therapy helpful, it may well be worth trying again.

(8) Use of steroids. Any patient who is using more than 30g of a potent topical steroid a week, or who is continually requesting 100g tubes of ointment, needs reassessment.

(9) Factors which influence the disease. It is always worth enquiring what factors the patient considers to be relevant. Those that regularly influence psoriasis include: (i) *Sunlight.* Many find sunlight beneficial and, if so, ultraviolet light can be used as treatment. (ii) *Stress and unhappiness.* Although it is difficult to prove that undue stress exacerbates psoriasis (although all clinicians will have seen this happen), personal distress may make the psoriasis less easy to bear. In this case, simple psychotherapy may be of enormous benefit. (iii) *Alcohol.* Patients with extensive psoriasis often drink heavily. It is difficult to assess which comes first, but there can be little doubt that excessive alcohol consumption worsens psoriasis. They should be advised to abstain or reduce consumption.

Treatments can be divided into those which are topical and safe, and those which are systemic and potentially dangerous. Since the disease is a chronic one, treatment must never in the long term do more harm than good. This is a fundamental consideration in the choice of therapy. Also, psoriasis is a dynamic disease, and thus the treatment which is effective on one occasion may not be appropriate on another. Similarly, a drug which agrees with one patient may not agree with another.

Topical therapy
The local remedies for psoriasis are summarized in Figure 5.10

Useful points
- Tar is not used enough.
- Frequent repeat prescriptions of potent steroids are hazardous.
- Hydrocortisone is ineffective even on the face.
- Dithranol is often used incorrectly.

Treatments
TAR
Tar is a complex mixture of substances produced from coal. It is effective in psoriasis but its mode of action is unknown: whereas other remedies can be demonstrated to be antimitotic, this has not consistently been shown to be the case with tar. It has been used for at least a century; it smells and is messy, but is extremely useful and safe. There are many excellent proprietary preparations, usually based on coal tar extract in an appropriate cream, lotion, solution, gel, emulsion or shampoo. A useful extempore preparation is coal tar solution (5%, 10% or 20%) in emulsifying ointment used as a soap. Tar is particularly useful when used in combination with ultraviolet light, salicylic acid or topical steroids.

(1) With ultraviolet light. Tar is a photosensitizer. Goeckerman popularized a treatment with tar baths followed by exposure to ultraviolet B, which is particularly indicated for guttate psoriasis and psoriasis vulgaris.

(2) With salicylic acid. Salicylic acid is a keratolytic and therefore aids removal of psoriatic scales and improves the penetration of medicaments combined with it. Coal tar and salicylic acid ointment is suitable for chronic plaque psoriasis; for the scalp, ung. cocois co. is discussed later.

(3) With steroids. Although tar is remarkably safe, it occasionally irritates the skin and causes a folliculitis, and it should be avoided in the flexures, on the

LOCAL REMEDIES FOR PSORIASIS	
tar	alone with ultraviolet B with salicylic acid with topical steroids
topical glucocorticosteroids	alone
dithranol	alone with topical steroids
ultraviolet B	alone

▲ **Fig. 5.10** *Local remedies for psoriasis.*

genitalia and in complicated, unstable or erythro-dermic psoriasis. Combination with a topical steroid can prevent this and improve therapy.

Tar is not a carcinogen when used to treat psoriasis, although it is a carcinogen in experimental animals and also in workers who are continually exposed to it.

GLUCOCORTICOSTEROIDS

Potent and very potent steroids do have an effect in psoriasis, although it is often short-lived. Either only the scale is removed or the disease relapses quickly when the steroids are withdrawn. Many therefore would say that topical steroids should be avoided in psoriasis as they are only temporarily effective and abuse and side-effects are common. However, this is a counsel of perfection because steroids are cosmetically acceptable and easy to use, whereas tar and dithranol require time and patience. They are indicated for the patient with (i) limited areas of psoriasis, or (ii) psoriasis of the scalp, face and flexures. Hydrocorti-sone is ineffective in psoriasis and so, except for the face, are the moderately potent class II steroids.

Topical steroids are often prescribed in combi-nation with tar or dithranol.

(1) With tar. Proprietary preparations are available but they contain virtually homeopathic amounts of hydrocortisone (0.25% or 0.5%). Extempore combi-nations mixed by an experienced pharmacist are preferable, for example 3% coal tar solution mixed with a potent steroid such as betamethasone 17 valerate for the body or a class II steroid such as clobetasone butyrate for the face.

(2) With dithranol. There are no proprietary versions of this, but there is good evidence that an extempore formulation of 0.1% dithranol in quarter-strength clobetasol propionate with subsequent increments of dithranol (0.25% and 0.5%) may be effective.

DITHRANOL (ANTHRALIN, CIGNOLIN)

Dithranol is a derivative of chrysarobin (yellow ara-roba) which was derived from the bark of the araroba tree, which is indigenous to South America and Southern Asia. Chrysarobin was known as Goa powder because it was exported from Brazil to the Portuguese colony. It was originally used in the treatment of ringworm but was found to be effective in psoriasis when the latter was mistaken for ringworm and treated with chrysarobin. It has been used since the beginning of the century to treat psoriasis and is an antimitotic agent. It is effective for chronic stable psoriasis and is the standard inpatient therapy. Dith-ranol is made up in Lassar's paste (2% salicylic acid,

25% starch, 25% zinc oxide in soft paraffin) and applied daily, starting at 0.1% and gradually increasing through 0.25% to 0.5%; occasionally higher concen-trations are prescribed. It has to be used with care because:
- it may cause erythema and burning of the normal skin (Fig. 5.11), so should only be applied to the lesions;
- it stains clothing and sheets, as well as bath enamel;
- it stains the patient's skin temporarily (Fig. 5.12), but this clears within ten days of stopping therapy.

Dithranol should not be used:
- in the flexures, because burning is inevitable;
- on inflamed psoriasis, for it will aggravate it and may even induce pustulation;
- anywhere near the eyes (it has to be used with extreme caution on the face and this is best left to the specialist).

In hospital, dithranol in Lassar's paste is applied by the nurse. The areas are then covered with talc in an attempt to reduce spreading onto normal skin, and then covered with tube-gauze dressings. The dith-

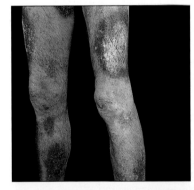

◀**Fig. 5.11** *Dithranol burn. Burning has occurred around the plaques of psoriasis because dithranol has been used in too high a concentration and has been allowed to spread onto normal skin.*

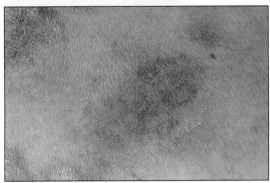

▲**Fig. 5.12** *Dithranol-treated psoriasis. The dithranol has cleared the psoriasis but temporarily stained the skin brown.*

ranol is left on until washed off the next day with arachis oil in the bath. The patient also uses a tar soap (for example, 20% coal tar in emulsifying ointment), and a couple of hours later has ultraviolet-B phototherapy. This is known as the Ingram regime and is suitable for chronic stable psoriasis; most patients are free of the disease after three weeks in hospital. However, the disease often returns over the ensuing months, and 50% have reverted to their initial state by the end of a year.

Unfortunately many patients abandon the drug as outpatients, unless they have had previous experience of it as inpatients. It is very important to explain its use and particularly to indicate that it must be restricted to the lesions alone and not used in the flexures or on the face. Certain precautions are emphasized below. Several proprietary preparations are now available and are somewhat easier to use than Lassar's paste. A helpful modification is for the patient to apply the dithranol carefully, leave it on for 30 minutes and then wash it off. This 'short contact therapy' is ideal for day-care centres which exist in some provincial towns in the UK (for example, Leeds and Newcastle-upon-Tyne) as a result of the late Dr John Ingram's pioneering work. The United States and continental Europe have also developed such centres in the last decade. They allow the patient to continue working, while attending a centre where a trained nurse applies the drug which is washed off half an hour later. This avoids the expensive and time-wasting practice of a three-week stay in hospital.

Useful points for dithranol therapy

- Start with a low dose (0.1%).
- Careful application to avoid erythema (burning).
- Do not use in flexures or on face.
- Use only in psoriasis vulgaris.
- Warn about staining.

ULTRAVIOLET LIGHT

Many patients observe that their psoriasis improves or even clears completely in the sun. It is thus logical to use artificial methods of ultraviolet irradiation, if natural sunlight is not available.

Ultraviolet B (290–320nm), is commonly employed. Many standard lamps used in hospital physiotherapy departments (for example, the widely used Theraktin UV lamp) also deliver ultraviolet C (<290nm) which causes burning before ultraviolet B does and therefore limits the potential time of the exposure to ultraviolet B. Better lamps are now available, which do not deliver ultraviolet C. The skin should be tested before starting treatment to determine the exposure time required to produce the minimum amount of reddening (erythema) 6–24 hours later. This is known as the minimum erythema dose and is the starting dose, which should be gradually increased with each visit. A tar bath one hour before the ultraviolet B will enhance its effect and is an excellent treatment for psoriasis vulgaris and guttate psoriasis. Repeated courses are permissible. Ultraviolet A (320–400nm) has no effect on its own in psoriasis; sun beds are therefore of no benefit.

Topical treatment of various sites
SCALP

(1) Potent topical steroids. These are used initially either in a gel or liquid form. Class III steroids are often ineffective, so that it may be necessary to increase to a class IV steroid and even these are sometimes unsatisfactory. The patient must be warned against allowing the drug to spread onto the forehead, where it may cause a steroid-induced acne.

(2) Tar. Tar-containing shampoos should be used as a routine. Several proprietary shampoos are available.

(3) Ung. cocois co. In resistant cases ung. cocois co. is a particularly helpful formulation. It consists of 60% coconut oil, 13% emulsifying wax, 12% coal tar solution, 9% yellow soft paraffin, 4% precipitated sulphur, 2% salicylic acid. It should be applied at night to the scalp which is then covered with a scarf or bath hat, and washed out the next day with a tar-containing shampoo. Although it is unpleasant, patients will use it for a limited period when they see that it works. It is easier to persuade them to do this if the treatment with the cosmetically acceptable topical steroids has failed. Dithranol can be added to the ung. cocois co., starting at 0.1% concentration (but not in white-haired individuals, because it stains).

It has to be admitted that even these measures fail. Psoriasis of the scalp is not easy to defeat. Patients can get disheartened if treatment is not effective immediately especially if it is unpleasant, so they give up without a proper trial. Applications by a skilled practice nurse can then make all the difference.

FACE

(1) Steroids. Hydrocortisone is ineffective and psoriasis is the exception to the rule that powerful steroids should not be used on the face. However, if potent steroids are going to be used, it is important that it is impressed upon the patient that they must apply these drugs sparingly and accurately to the areas affected for it is all too easy to induce acne.

(2) Tar. Tar applied to the skin of the face sometimes irritates but it is always worth trying. Combination with a mild steroid may reduce this and proprietary preparations are available. Combination with a class II steroid may be even more effective, for example an extempore formulation of 3% coal tar in clobetasone butyrate.

(3) Dithranol. Dithranol burns and therefore it is unwise to use it on the face except under daily supervision, which usually means when the patient is hospitalized. It is usual to start at very low doses such as 0.05%.

(4) Ultraviolet light. This is a good therapy for psoriasis of the face, and patients can use their own UVB lamps. It is extremely important however to explain to them the difference between UVA and UVB. Burning does not occur with UVA; it may occur with even small exposures to UVB. The length of exposure depends on the skin type and the manufacturer's instructions. It is important for the patient to understand that exposure begins initially in doses of seconds rather than minutes, and that the eyes must be protected with the appropriate glasses.

FLEXURES AND GENITALIA
(1) Dithranol and tar are contraindicated. Dithranol inevitably burns, and tar tends to irritate.
(2) Steroids. Potent steroids are usually required, but it is important to remember that flexures are perfect habitats for fungi and it may be that the latter are present rather than psoriasis.

BODY AND LIMBS
These are usually the easiest areas to treat with dithranol if the psoriasis is stable.

HANDS AND FEET
Psoriasis of the hands and feet is one of the most difficult disorders to treat in the whole of dermatology. The thickened stratum corneum of these areas limits the penetration of any drug considerably.
(1) Steroids. Class IV steroids are indicated and usually polythene occlusion is required in addition, but even this is unsatisfactory.
(2) Tar. Tar in the form of a soap may be of some benefit, particularly with the painful fissuring and cracking that occurs.
(3) Dithranol. Increasing doses of dithranol in Lassar's paste are certainly worth trying. Combination with a potent steroid (dithranol in a quarter-strength clobetasol propionate) is an alternative.

Systemic therapy is often required in this disorder.

NAILS
Essentially there is no effective treatment for psoriasis of the nails, but spontaneous resolution may occur. There was a vogue for treating the nail-fold of patients with severe nail dystrophies with intralesional steroids, but the disease tended to relapse. It is always worth remembering that a patient with psoriasis can get a coincidental tinea or candida infection in the nails which may be treatable.

Systemic therapy
The decision to employ systemic therapy is always a difficult one, for on the whole it is a long-term commitment as the disease usually returns to its previous state on cessation of therapy. The decision is best made by the specialist, guided by the family practitioner's knowledge of the patient's personal circumstances. Indications for systemic therapy are listed in Figure 5.13.

Although there are a number of possible systemic agents, those most commonly used by specialists are discussed below. It will be appreciated that although they are all effective, they have potentially ominous side-effects, and patients require constant supervision.

METHOTREXATE
This has been available since the early 1950s when it was noted that psoriatics who were being treated for leukaemia with aminopterin (a related drug) were cleared of their skin disease. Methotrexate is given *once a week* in a dose of 0.2–0.4mg/kg, which on average totals about 25mg; it is sometimes given in divided doses over a 36-hour period once a week, based on the knowledge of the kinetics of the epi-

INDICATIONS FOR SYSTEMIC THERAPY	
definite	erythrodermic psoriasis
	generalized pustular psoriasis
relative	subacute psoriasis
	extensive flexural psoriasis
	extensive psoriasis vulgaris
	(i) in the elderly or incapacitated
	(ii) where multiple admissions have failed
	(iii) interference with function, personal
	happiness or livelihood

▲ **Fig. 5.13** *Indications for systemic therapy.*

dermal cell cycle in psoriasis. Much lower doses are used in generalized pustular psoriasis.

There are minor immediate side-effects associated with the drug. Many patients feel slightly nauseous or unwell for a number of hours after taking their weekly dose, and to reduce these symptoms it is best to take the drug in the evening. The drug also occasionally causes headaches and gastrointestinal haemorrhage. It is a cytotoxic drug and bone marrow toxicity is a potential hazard, but it rarely gives rise to haematological side-effects in the dose prescribed for psoriasis. Occasionally, however, mistakes are made and in error the patients are given the drug daily with very serious consequences. The real hazard of the drug, if used for a number of years, is hepatotoxicity. Liver function must be monitored by blood tests, scans and liver biopsy, and it is unwise to prescribe the drug for a patient who abuses alcohol.

Oligospermia is a side-effect; but although fertility is decreased, a child of the man taking methotrexate should be quite normal. The drug is teratogenic in early pregnancy, and so all female patients should take contraceptive precautions if they are sexually active. Conception is probably safe three months after cessation of systemic therapy, but patients should be advised to wait longer.

ETRETINATE (TIGASON)

The retinoids are the major therapeutic advance in dermatology in the 1980s. It has long been recognized that vitamin A deficiency results in dry skin, follicular hyperkeratosis and epithelial squamous metaplasia, which is reversible with vitamin A supplements. Vitamin A was known to be beneficial in acne but generally disappointing in psoriasis, particularly because of toxicity (hypervitaminosis A), so a screening programme of synthetic analogues of vitamin A was instituted for drugs with an improved risk versus benefit ratio. This resulted in etretinate.

The drug is given in a dose of 1 mg/kg and is effective in all forms of psoriasis, particularly in erythrodermic and generalized pustular psoriasis and in extensive psoriasis in the elderly. All patients suffer from dryness of the skin and lips during therapy, but this is rarely a significant problem. The drug is metabolized by the liver, and increases the serum triglycerides and cholesterol. Liver disease and hyper-

lipidaemia are therefore relative contraindications for the drug. A diffuse interosseous calcification has occasionally been observed. The drug is a teratogen and pregnancy is strictly contraindicated during therapy, and afterwards for at least one year. The long-term side-effects are yet to be assessed. In the UK it is only prescribable by specialists.

PHOTOCHEMOTHERAPY (PUVA)

On its own, long-wave ultraviolet light (UVA) is ineffective in psoriasis, but in combination with 8-methoxypsoralen (P) it is highly effective in certain individuals. The psoralens are photosensitizers. The drug is given orally in a dose of 0.6 mg/kg, and two hours later the skin is irradiated with UVA. The technique is known as PUVA or photochemotherapy. The dose of UVA (Joules/cm^2) depends on the skin type of the patient. Unfortunately, as might be predicted, the treatment is a cutaneous carcinogen and it is likely that this side-effect will only begin to be obvious 10 or 20 years from now. At present PUVA is best reserved for older individuals, although it does require regular attendance at the hospital.

PUVA is usually given three times a week for the first 5 weeks to obtain complete clearance of the psoriasis, and then once every 7–10 days for maintenance, which is tedious for the less mobile. It is popular with younger patients because of its cosmetic acceptability plus the accompanying tan. However, it is wise to exclude those with type 1 and type 2 skins, that is those who sunburn easily, for they are most at risk of skin cancer later. It is also sensible to exclude those who have had a prior history of radiotherapy or cutaneous malignancy, or those who have been exposed to arsenic to treat their psoriasis. Photochemotherapy is effective in dark skins, although the resultant general increase in pigmentation is often unacceptable to the patient.

It is most important that the patients wear protective glasses from the moment that they take their 8-methoxypsoralen tablets until 24 hours later, as cataracts and other ocular abnormalities are likely to be hazards otherwise. The therapy is no help for inaccessible sites of the body, such as the flexures and the scalp. The most common side-effects are burning of the skin and itching. The latter can be eased by the regular use of emulsifying ointment in the bath.

6 PITYRIASIS ROSEA AND LICHEN PLANUS

INTRODUCTION

Two unrelated disorders, both of unknown aetiology, are described together in this chapter. They are commonplace and merit comprehensive description.

PITYRIASIS ROSEA

Definition

A short-lived condition affecting young adults which evolves rapidly on the trunk after the initial patch that heralds the attack.

> **Diagnostic features**
> - Herald patch.
> - Symmetrical, oval, pink patches.
> - Characteristic peripheral scale.
> - Restricted to trunk and proximal limbs.

Aetiology

The disease is common. It affects both sexes equally and occurs in adolescence and early adult life. It is seen more frequently in the autumn and winter. The histology is that of an eczema, but its aetiology is obscure. Most favour a viral cause, because second attacks are unusual, suggesting the acquisition of immunity. On the other hand, outbreaks among associates of the patient are exceptional, so it is not infectious, and sophisticated microbiological investigatory techniques have been unrewarding.

Clinical features

The initial lesion is a pink (rosea) oval patch approximately 3–6cm in diameter. It has a scale (pityriasis) which occurs like a collarette towards the periphery (Fig. 6.1) but not at the margin of the lesion. It is followed after a few days, sometimes later, by an eruption of similar but much smaller lesions and hence is known as the herald patch. It occurs anywhere on the skin within the area usually affected by the condition (Figs 6.2 & 6.3). The herald patch is one of the enigmas of dermatology, as it occurs in no other skin disease. The earliest lesions of the subsequent eruption are pink papules, which occasionally can be mistaken for insect bites, but the papule rapidly spreads outwards to produce oval macules varying from 1 to 3cm in size. This stretching outwards produces a characteristic collarette of scale.

The distribution of the rash is essentially that of a T-shirt and shorts; indeed Lassar (1889) thought that clothing might be its cause, but this has not been substantiated by patch tests. Thus, the neck, trunk, upper arms and thighs are affected. The lesions occur in a symmetrical distribution. The patient is otherwise completely well and there are no preceding symptoms. The condition lasts approximately 6 weeks and then fades, rarely recurring. In pigmented skins, post-inflammatory hyperpigmentation (Fig. 6.4) may occur and this takes many months to disappear.

For the specialist, the diagnosis is generally very straightforward, because he usually sees the patient after the rash has spread, and it is suspected from the history: enquiry usually elicits the answer that one patch appeared first. However, for the general practitioner the diagnosis can be more difficult, because the herald patch may remain solitary for several days or even weeks before the subsequent lesions appear; not surprisingly, *in view of its oval or ring shape it may be misdiagnosed as ringworm*.

Occasionally confusion may arise when the eruption is not quite true to form.

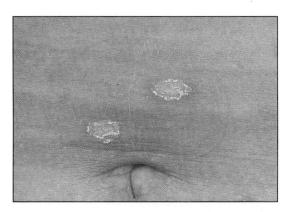

▲ **Fig. 6.1** *Pityriasis rosea. The individual lesions are oval and pink (rosea) and have a peripheral collarette of scale.*

- The herald patch is sometimes absent.
- The eruption may be very florid indeed, with coalescence of many of the pink patches. However, the collarette of scale on the lesion should provide the diagnosis.
- In sun-tanned individuals it may be restricted to sun-spared areas, such as the breasts, axillae, pubis and buttocks.
- In coloured skins, particularly Negroes, the eruption may be more widespread, occurring on the forearms and lower legs in addition to the usual distribution. The morphology of the lesions, however, remains the same, although the pinkness may be difficult or impossible to discern. This variant is more persistent and lasts several months. It is known as an *eczematide*. Post-inflammatory hyperpigmentation is the rule.

Differential diagnosis
Tinea and the herald patch
The herald patch on its own is a difficult diagnosis.

The differential is that of any annular or discoid patch especially ringworm. However, in ringworm, particularly animal ringworm, the margin of the annular patch is more inflammatory and raised and there is a tendency for central healing. Scrapings of the skin mounted in potash should reveal hyphae. However, if the peripheral collarette of scale is detected and pityriasis rosea is suspected, the diagnosis may be confirmed when the rest of the eruption develops a few days later.

Truncal eruptions
There are a number of eruptions involving the trunk which sometimes cause diagnostic confusion. These include secondary syphilis, pityriasis versicolor, guttate psoriasis, seborrhoeic eczema and drug eruptions.

Management
It is not sufficient to tell the patient that the eruption will disappear within a few weeks. Most patients are concerned about infectivity and also whether the rash will appear on the face. It is not infectious, and although it characteristically occurs on the neck, it very rarely affects the face.

Many patients are asymptomatic but a few suffer severely from itch. It is wise therefore to prescribe a class III glucocorticosteroid for this. Topical steroids do not modify the eruption, but they do alleviate the itch.

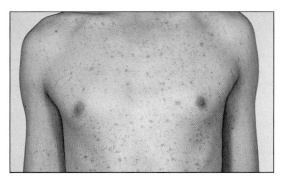

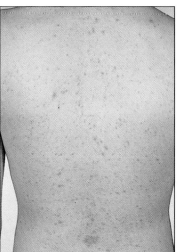

▲ Figs 6.2 & ◀ **6.3** *Pityriasis rosea. The eruption predominantly affects the trunk. It begins with a single ('herald') patch which is larger than the subsequent red oval patches and is visible in this patient on the lower back (Fig. 6.3).*

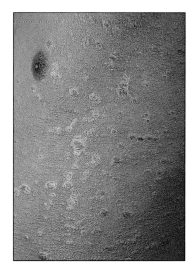

◀ **Fig. 6.4** *Pityriasis rosea. In coloured skins the pink colour is often absent but there are oval patches with peripheral scaling and post-inflammatory hyperpigmentation as they heal.*

LICHEN PLANUS

Definition
A relatively common pruritic mucocutaneous disorder, displaying a highly characteristic purple colour and distinctive papular morphology, which lasts a number of months and occasionally years, and clears leaving temporary post-inflammatory hyperpigmentation.

Diagnostic features
- Very itchy.
- Purple, flat-topped, shiny, polygonal papules.
- May occur anywhere, but particularly on the wrists, ankles, forearms, lower legs, genitalia, umbilicus and sacrum.
- Lace-like patterning on the buccal mucosa.
- Koebner phenomenon.
- Leaves hyperpigmentation as it heals.

Aetiology
The disease is relatively common. The specialist will see one case every ten days and a family practitioner one or two a year. Men and women are equally affected. All races are susceptible but in particular, for some unaccountable reason, Nigerians. It can present at any time but usually between the ages of 30 and 60 years.

The cause is unknown, but there are a number of intriguing features regarding its nature. Its pathology is striking, and a skin biopsy may provide the diagnosis when the dermatologist has missed it.

There is an intense band-like infiltration of the upper dermis by thymus-derived lymphocytes (Fig. 6.5), that push the epidermis upwards, thus forming the characteristic papule of lichen planus. The lymphocytes destroy the basement membrane and basal cell layer of the epidermis, shifting melanin into the dermis, which accounts for the post-inflammatory hyperpigmentation. The rete ridges are flattened out and have a saw-tooth appearance. Degenerating cells which contain immunoglobulins stain pink with eosin and are known as 'colloid bodies'.

Lymphocytes thus dominate the histology and are responsible for considerable destruction, but their purpose here is a mystery. Interestingly, lesions identical to lichen planus clinically, histopathologically and immunologically occur in the early stages of the graft versus host reaction between immunocompetent donor cells and recipient tissues in patients undergoing bone marrow or other transplantation.

The disease is seen in association with various autoimmune disorders such as primary biliary cirrhosis, chronic active hepatitis and diabetes mellitus.

Certain drugs, in particular penicillamine (especially when prescribed for primary biliary cirrhosis), arsenic, gold, methyldopa and para-aminosalicylic acid, produce eruptions which simulate lichen planus. Antimalarials, especially mepacrine hydrochloride, were responsible for outbreaks of lichen planus in troops taking them during the Second World War; this eruption had a tendency to be quite chronic and produce scarring. A lichenoid eruption also occasionally occurs as a form of allergic contact dermatitis on the hands in those who come in contact with colour developer in photography.

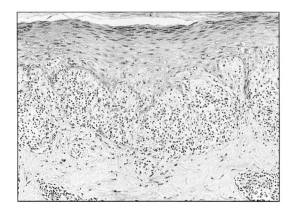

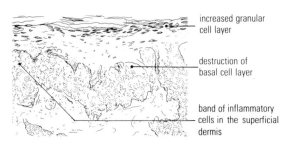

increased granular cell layer

destruction of basal cell layer

band of inflammatory cells in the superficial dermis

▲ **Fig. 6.5** *Histopathology of lichen planus. There is a band of inflammatory cells, predominantly lymphocytes and* histiocytes, in the superficial dermis, which destroys the basement membrane and basal cell layer of the epidermis.

Clinical features

The eruption begins abruptly. It is usually very itchy and the patient, who is in every other respect perfectly well, presents early. The individual lesions are so distinctive and the colour so arresting, that the diagnosis may be suspected immediately and almost established by examining a single papule.

The lesion is a mixture of blue and red, and is thus purple (Fig. 6.6) or 'violaceous'. The lesions are papular, between 1 and 3mm in diameter, polygonal in shape and flat-topped and shiny (Fig. 6.7) when viewed in a good light. Fine, white tracery may be visible on the surface, so-called Wickham's striae (Fig. 6.8). The application of mineral oil will highlight these striae. The papules are usually quite discrete, but they may become confluent, producing plaques and annular lesions. Linear and other arrangements may result from trauma to the skin, a phenomenon described by Koebner (Fig. 6.9). As the lesions heal, post-inflammatory hyperpigmentation

(Fig. 6.10) results. This may last a few weeks in a Caucasian, many months in an Asian, and years in a Negro, constituting a very considerable cosmetic problem.

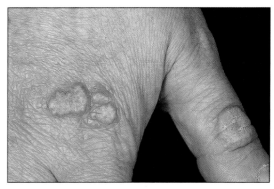

▲**Fig. 6.8** *Lichen planus. Polygonal flat-topped purple papules may merge into each other, producing plaques. Wickham's striae (fine, white lines) are visible on the surface.*

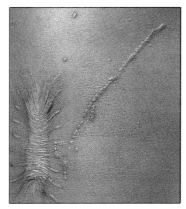

◀**Fig. 6.9** *Lichen planus. Lichen planus may occur in a linear manner in areas of trauma (Koebner phenomenon).*

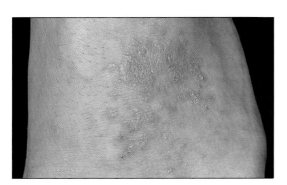

▲**Fig. 6.6** *Lichen planus. The lesions have a very characteristic purple or 'violaceous' colour.*

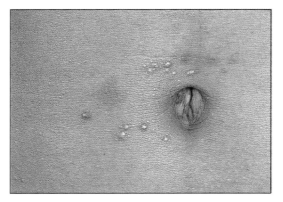

▲**Fig. 6.7** *Lichen planus. The papules are flat-topped and shine in a good light. The area in and around the umbilicus is a common site. Post-inflammatory pigmentation occurs.*

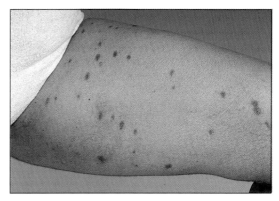

▲**Fig. 6.10** *Lichen planus. Post-inflammatory hyperpigmentaon is usual and may be very persistent in coloured skins.*

The distribution of the eruption will help to confirm the diagnosis. It is symmetrical and although it can occur anywhere on the skin, it has a predilection for the wrists, hands, forearms, ankles, shins, umbilicus, lumbosacral region and genitalia (Fig. 6.11). In many cases the mouth is involved as well, but curiously this is uncommon in Negroes. The mouth lesions consist of a delicate lace-like white patterning, producing streaks or dots (Fig. 6.12) on the inner surface of the cheeks, lips, tongue or gum margins. They are usually asymptomatic.

There is a tendency for fresh lesions to appear over the course of 9–18 months, but ultimately the condition goes into complete remission and it is unusual for second attacks to occur.

Clinical variants

There are a number of variants of the disease, some of which are extremely rare, such as involvement of the nails and the scalp, both of which may result in scarring and permanent damage. The more common types include:

(1) **Annular.** Although ring-shaped lesions may be a feature of ordinary lichen planus, occasionally there may be just a few scattered asymmetrical circular lesions on the body which are often mistaken for ringworm. Careful examination reveals that there is no scaling, and that the margins of the lesion are made up of the characteristic, flat-topped shiny papules with their red/blue hue (Fig. 6.13).

(2) **Hypertrophic.** Lesions may occur on the fronts of the shins (Fig. 6.14) during an attack of lichen planus, but they then persist indefinitely despite the disappearance of the rest of the rash. The variant is more

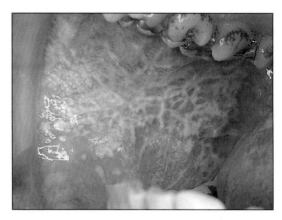

▲ **Fig. 6.12** *Lichen planus. In the mouth a lace-like patterning of white lines and dots occur, especially on the buccal mucosae.*

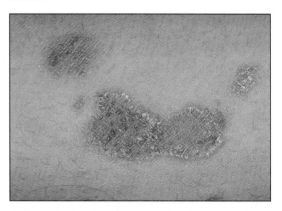

▲ **Fig. 6.13** *Annular lichen planus. Annular configurations occur. The purple papules at the margin are the clue to diagnosis. Post-inflammatory pigmentation has occurred centrally.*

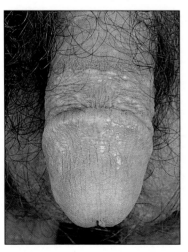

◀ **Fig. 6.11** *Lichen planus. Purple shiny papules are present on the glans and shaft of the penis. Occasionally the genitalia and mouth are the only sites involved.*

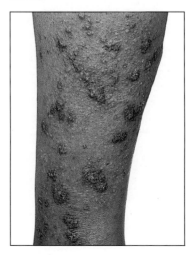

◀ **Fig. 6.14** *Hypertrophic lichen planus. Persistent thickened pigmented plaques (which may not be purple in Negroes) occur especially on the shins.*

common in black skins. The lesions are well-defined, thickened (hypertrophic) plaques. Their purple colour suggests their identity, but a biopsy may be necessary to substantiate it. The lesions are difficult to treat even with intralesional steroids.

(3) Oral lesions are common but occasionally they occur alone or in association with genital lesions. Very rarely erosive or ulcerative lesions are present on the gums, buccal mucosae and tongue. Usually tell-tale white streaks are present around the ulcers, which helps in the diagnosis, but a biopsy and careful follow-up are frequently necessary, because very occasionally malignant transformation occurs.

(4) Palmar or plantar lichen planus is rare in isolation, but is difficult diagnostically because the thickness of the stratum corneum may obscure the purple colour and instead the lesions appear yellow and warty (Fig. 6.15). It is always worth studying the palms and soles of patients who have lichen planus elsewhere, to fix in the mind this clinical appearance.

Differential diagnosis

The diagnosis is mostly based on clinical observation and annular lesions may be easily diagnosed, but biopsy is unequivocal if there is doubt, because the histology is so specific. The diseases which cause confusion are guttate psoriasis, lichenoid forms of eczema and, because of its itchy nature, scabies.

Management

The patient needs to know that the condition is neither serious nor infectious and that it is not a life-long affliction. The average patient is free of it within a few months — 50% are clear within nine months and 85% within 18 months. The remainder usually have variants such as complicated oral lesions or hypertrophic plaques. Ordinary lichen planus very rarely recurs. Lichen planus may be treated by:

(1) Topical steroids. Therapy has been revolutionized by class IV steroids. The itch is quickly alleviated and the active purple papules are flattened and become pigmented. It is important to point out that the steroid will not help the post-inflammatory hyper-pigmentation, so there is no point in treating a specific lesion once the itching has subsided. *Hydrocortisone is quite ineffective and even class III steroids are relatively useless*, unless used under polythene.

(2) Systemic steroids. These are sometimes necessary for particularly widespread and troublesome cases, or those involving important functional areas such as the hands and feet. Although there are no hard and fast rules, 30–35 mg prednisolone is a reasonable starting dose, with reductions of 5 mg per week, until 15 mg is reached, and then reductions by 2.5 mg weekly. Occasionally second courses are required.

(3) Antihistamines. Sedative antihistamines are occasionally required for itch.

Treatment of specific variants

(1) Hypertrophic lichen planus. This is a difficult disorder to manage but treatment centres around steroids, either very potent topical steroids enhanced by polythene occlusion, or intralesional triamcinolone.

(2) Oral lesions. Topical steroids are applied in special formulations which facilitate their adherence to the oral mucosae. Triamcinolone acetonide in ora-base is the one usually used, but if this fails then a class IV steroid ointment can be applied direct to the lesions. Occasionally, systemic steroids are required for ulcerative lichen planus but their long-term effects are disappointing and side-effects are common.

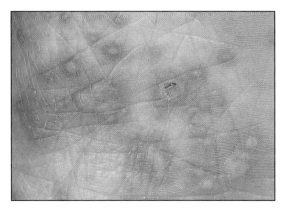

▲ **Fig. 6.15** *Lichen planus. On the palms and soles the purple colouration may be difficult to discern and the lesions appear yellow and thickened.*

7 NAEVI

INTRODUCTION

Naevi are benign proliferations of cells which are normally present in the skin. Thus a melanocytic naevus (commonly referred to as a mole) is a benign proliferation of melanocytes which are normal constituents of the basal cell layer of the epidermis. Similarly, an epidermal naevus is a benign proliferation of keratinocytes, and a sebaceous naevus of sebaceous glands. Clearly any structure in the skin may be the origin of a naevus. Only common ones are discussed here. The exact aetiology of these 'mistakes' is unknown. Some naevi are present at birth but others develop within the first decades of life, for example Becker's epidermal naevus.

Naevi are extremely common and all individuals have such blemishes on the skin, sometimes in profusion. Patients consult doctors about them for cosmetic reasons or because they are anxious as to their nature. Many of the lesions can be diagnosed by simple inspection and the physician can predict whether the lesion is benign or potentially malignant, and whether it will resolve spontaneously, is best left alone, can be simply removed, or requires the skills of a plastic surgeon.

EPIDERMAL NAEVUS

Diagnostic features
- Well-defined plaque or plaques.
- One or more centimetres long.
- Often linear arrangements.
- Rough warty fissured surface.

Clinical features
This lesion is usually present at birth or arises within the first decade, and may increase in size at puberty. It is quite benign. A well-defined raised plaque with a rough warty surface, with prominent fissuring, it sometimes forms a linear arrangement (Fig. 7.1). It is a brown or yellowish colour.

Management
The naevus is often indistinguishable clinically from a basal cell papilloma (seborrhoeic wart) other than by the history of its existence since childhood. This is important, because whereas the seborrhoeic wart can be removed simply by curettage and cautery or by cryotherapy, an epidermal naevus can only be excised.

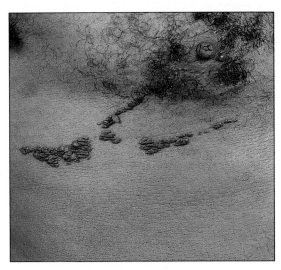

▲ **Fig. 7.1** *Epidermal naevus. The lesions are well-defined plaques with a warty surface often distributed in a linear manner.*

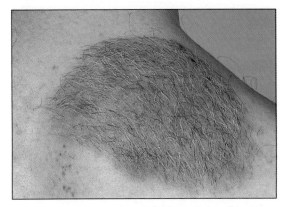

▲ **Fig. 7.2** *Becker's naevus. The shoulder is a common site for this pigmented hairy naevus which appears in adolescence.*

BECKER'S NAEVUS

Diagnostic features
- Pigmented and hairy patch.
- Shoulder, scapula or front of chest.
- Onset in adolescence.

Clinical features
The lesion appears during adolescence. It is flat initially but may thicken. It is pigmented and subsequently has thick coarse hairs in it (Fig. 7.2).

Management
There is no treatment.

SEBACEOUS NAEVUS

Diagnostic features
- Yellow plaque with small, rounded elevations.
- One or more centimetres in diameter.
- Often present on the scalp.
- Increases in size at puberty.
- Occasionally premalignant.

Clinical features
This is a common naevus of the head and neck region, which is usually present at birth. It is an androgen-sensitive tumour and increases in size in infancy as the sebaceous glands do, but subsequently regresses until puberty when it again grows to reach its maximum size. The lesion is a raised, hairless, yellow or orange plaque which is surmounted by many small, rounded elevations (Fig. 7.3).

Management
There is an increased risk of change to a basal cell carcinoma in later life. Prophylactic excision is therefore advisable in the second or third decade by a plastic surgeon.

MELANOCYTIC NAEVI

Introduction
Melanocytic naevi are commonly referred to as 'moles'. They are exceedingly common and probably occur in all Caucasians. They consist of a benign proliferation of melanocytes having arisen from the neural crest early in fetal life. Some melanocytic naevi are present at birth (*congenital naevi*) and are permanent. Most, however, develop gradually during childhood, more rapidly during adolescence, fairly slowly during the first half of adult life and then disappear in the forties, so that it is rare to find acquired pigmented naevi in the elderly.

In childhood, most melanocytic naevi proliferate at the junction of the epidermis and the dermis, forming nests of cells and are known as *junctional naevi*. Subsequently, these melanocytes migrate into the dermis. If there are nests of melanocytes both in the dermis and at the junction with the epidermis, they are known as *compound naevi* (Fig. 7.4), but if the nests are exclusively in the dermis, they are known as *intradermal or cellular naevi*.

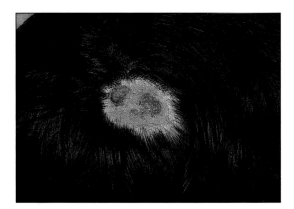

▲ **Fig. 7.3** *Sebaceous naevus. A yellow plaque is present in the scalp with hair loss. Two basal cell carcinomas have developed within it.*

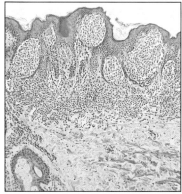
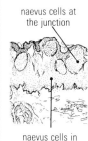

naevus cells at the junction

naevus cells in the dermis

▲ **Fig. 7.4** *Compound melanocytic naevus. Numerous collections of melanocytic naevus cells are present in the dermis and at the junction of the epidermis with the dermis.*

Congenital melanocytic naevi tend to be similar histologically to compound naevi with extension of the nests into the reticular dermis and subcutaneous fat.

The melanocytes in a *blue naevus* are situated deep in the reticular dermis. Incident light on the heavily pigmented cells at this level is reflected back to the naked eye as a blue rather than brown colour (a property of light, known as Tindel's effect). The naevus is regarded as a failure of melanocytes to arrive at the dermo-epidermal junction from the neural crest.

The *halo naevus* is a benign pigmented naevus, surrounded by a patch of vitiligo which leads often to elimination of the naevus and eventual repigmentation of the skin. The condition is probably an autoimmune phenomenon because there is a dense inflammatory cell infiltration of the naevus and antibodies against the cytoplasm of malignant melanoma cells are present in the serum.

Innumerable myths surround moles, largely because of their association with malignant melanoma. The following are the correct versions of such myths:

- Moles of the palms, soles and genitalia are not potentially dangerous and do not need to be removed. Ten per cent of young men have moles on the palms, soles or genitalia and yet malignant melanoma is uncommon in these sites.
- Electrolysis of hair from compound naevi is not dangerous.
- Excision of a benign mole does not provoke malignant change.

The myth that excision is dangerous presumably must have arisen after a malignant melanoma, misdiagnosed as a benign mole, was removed and subsequently metastasized. Eighty per cent of malignant melanomata arise from previously normal skin and not from moles at all. The rest arise either from congenital naevi, dysplastic naevi (chapter 9) or occasionally from ordinary acquired moles.

Congenital melanocytic (pigmented) naevus

Diagnostic features
- Present at birth.
- Larger than one centimetre.
- Round or oval.
- Even distribution of pigment.
- Various surface changes.

Clinical features

This naevus is present at birth, occurring in about 1% of all newborn infants, and persists throughout life. It varies greatly in size (Fig. 7.5), reaching many centimetres in some cases and very occasionally covering most of the integument (*giant hairy pigmented naevus*). However, the majority are small, although always greater than 1cm in size, and this distinguishes them from acquired junctional naevi, to which they are otherwise similar. The lesion is usually raised, sometimes with small, raised pebbly (mamillary) projections. It may be smooth, warty, lobular or cerebriform. The lesion is round or oval with accentuated surface skin markings. It varies in shade from a light tan to medium or dark brown, often with two colours, the darker shade being distributed centrally (Fig. 7.6). The arrangement of the colours is generally uniform. Sometimes the lesions are hairy.

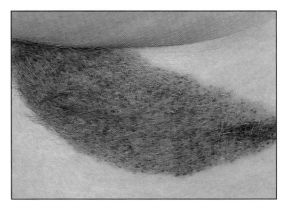

▲ **Fig. 7.5** *Congenital melanocytic naevus. One per cent of Caucasians are born with one. Lesions vary in size. Prophylactic excision is impracticable here.*

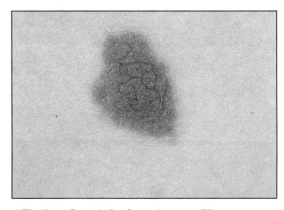

▲ **Fig. 7.6** *Congenital melanocytic naevus. There are two shades of pigment which are uniformly distributed. It is mostly raised with, in this case, mamillary projections on the surface.*

Management

The major concern regarding the congenital melanocytic naevus is its premalignant potential. This is an area of controversy. Certainly there is a greatly increased risk of malignant melanoma in those rare cases of congenital giant hairy pigmented naevi (*bathing trunk naevi*). However, the risk in ordinary congenital naevi is very low considering that melanoma is uncommon and yet 1% of the population have these naevi.

The best advice is that these naevi should be excised if this is technically possible without mutilation and cosmetic ill-effect, which in practice encompasses only the smaller ones (Fig. 7.7). Since the leg is a common site for malignant melanoma in women and the trunk in men, one should always consider removing congenital naevi in these areas.

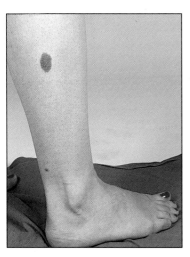

◀ **Fig. 7.7** *Congenital melanocytic naevus. The lesion has an even colour, is larger than 1cm and was present at birth. The risk of malignancy is slight but the leg is a common site for melanoma, so prophylactic excision is reasonable.*

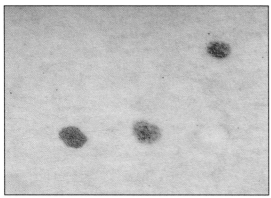

▲ **Fig. 7.8** *Junctional melanocytic naevi. These benign acquired naevi are relatively uniform in distribution of colour and regular in outline.*

Junctional melanocytic naevus

Diagnostic features
- Flat.
- Less than 0.5cm in diameter.
- Round or oval.
- Uniform distribution of pigment(s).

Clinical features

Junctional melanocytic naevi are the most common of the acquired moles, which develop in the first three decades of life. They are quite asymptomatic, never itch and are usually no bigger than 0.5cm in size. They are either flat or slightly raised, and have a single colour or are two-toned. The important distinction from malignant melanoma is that the arrangement of pigment within the lesion is uniform. The shape is generally but not entirely even, being either oval or round (Fig. 7.8). Although close inspection is very important, it is often helpful to examine such a mole from a distance initially, since this gives a better idea of whether the arrangement of colour and shape is uniform and regular in contrast to the disordered appearance of a malignant melanoma. The surface is usually smooth and the skin creases are generally preserved.

Any naevus with junctional activity has the potential for malignant change, but this is rare in comparison with their prevalence, for it is estimated that the average Caucasian has at least 25 moles. Some authorities believe that individuals with a large number of junctional naevi have an increased risk of developing malignant change, but personal observations show that most patients with malignant melanoma have if anything fewer moles than average.

Management

Junctional naevi may be excised for cosmetic reasons or if there is doubt about their nature, otherwise they should be left alone to save the patient from unnecessary and unsightly scars.

Compound naevus

Diagnostic features
- Raised.
- Less than 0.5cm in diameter.
- Round or oval.
- Even distribution of pigment(s).

Clinical features

These moles are pigmented and raised (Figs 7.9 & 7.10). They are composed (compounded) of naevus cells at both the dermo-epidermal junction and in the dermis.

Management

These may be excised for similar reasons as junctional naevi.

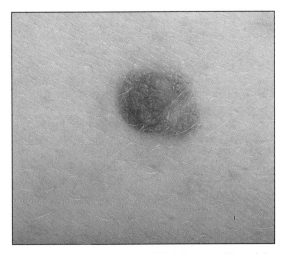

▲ **Fig. 7.9** *Compound naevus. The lesion is roughly oval, has two colours and is raised centrally and evenly pigmented. The naevus cells are present both in the dermis and at the dermo-epidermal junction.*

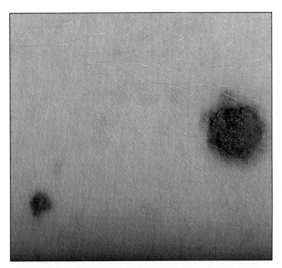

▲ **Fig. 7.10** *Compound naevus. The lesion is mainly dark brown with a lighter rim. It is raised centrally. The lower lesion is flat and is a junctional naevus.*

Intradermal (naevo-cellular) naevus

Diagnostic features
- Flesh-coloured.
- Soft, raised and round.
- Sometimes hairy.
- Commonly on the face.

Clinical features

These lesions are mainly flesh-coloured (Fig. 7.11) since all the naevus cells are present in the dermis. They are particularly common on the face and sometimes constitute a cosmetic problem. They are small, soft and dome-shaped, and sometimes display surface telangiectasia.

Management

They have no malignant potential. Smaller ones can be satisfactorily removed by shaving them off flush to the skin and gently cauterizing their base.

Blue naevus

Diagnostic features
- Blue or blue-black colour.
- Round, raised, smooth surface.
- Soft papule or nodule.
- Found on the face, hands and feet.

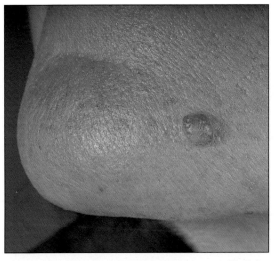

▲ **Fig. 7.11** *Intradermal (naevo-cellular) naevus. The lesion is common on the face and is often multiple. It is a flesh-coloured papule.*

Clinical features

The lesion is usually less than 0.5cm in diameter. It is a round blue papule or nodule (Fig. 7.12) with a smooth surface. It may occur anywhere on the skin but in particular on the hands, feet, head and face. It is quite benign with no malignant potential.

Management

The lesion may be excised for cosmetic reasons.

Mongolian blue spot

Diagnostic features
- Flat, blue, extensive.
- Buttocks, sacrum.
- Infancy.

Clinical features

The lesion is extensive, flat and blue in colour (Fig. 7.13). The site is characteristic.

Management

Reassurance that the lesion disappears in due course is all that is required.

Halo naevus (Sutton's naevus)

Diagnostic features
- White halo.
- Surrounding a pigmented naevus.
- Youth.

Clinical features

The condition is common in the first two decades, and sometimes gives rise to alarm although the lesion is quite harmless. There is a completely white area of depigmentation which surrounds a pigmented melanocytic naevus, in a very uniform manner (Fig. 7.14). The naevus eventually disappears and the depigmentation repigments.

Management

As the lesion is harmless, explanation is all that is required. It certainly does not need to be excised.

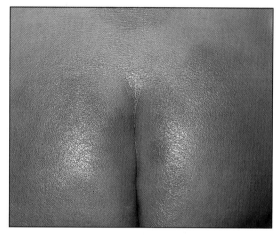

▲**Fig. 7.13** *Mongolian blue spot. A flat blue extensive discolouration occurs in the lumbar sacral area. It is common in mongoloid or negroid babies and is transitory.*

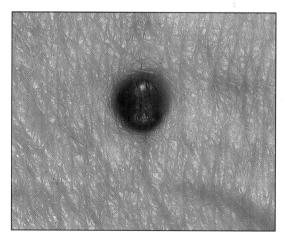

▲**Fig. 7.12** *Blue naevus. The papule is an even blue or blue-black colour. The back of the hand is a common site. It is benign with no malignant potential.*

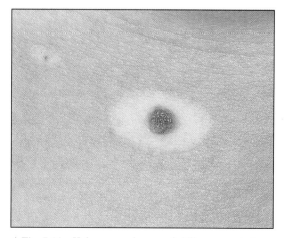

▲**Fig. 7.14** *Halo naevus. An area of vitiligo surrounds the melanocytic naevi. The moles will disappear and the skin will eventually repigment.*

JUVENILE MELANOMA (SPITZ NAEVUS)

Definition
An uncommon, but important, benign pigmented naevus of childhood.

> **Diagnostic features**
> - Red-brown papule.
> - Childhood or adolescence.
> - Commonly on the face.
> - Sometimes erroneously reported as malignant by pathologists.

Clinical features
The lesion is a solitary, well-defined dome-shaped, red-brown papule (Fig. 7.15) or nodule, with a smooth surface, often occurring on the face. The condition is uncommon but requires mention because pathologists, particularly if not given any clinical details, may report it as a malignant melanoma. The features which should alert the general practitioner that it is not a melanoma, are that it occurs in childhood and adolescence (when malignant melanoma is very rare) and when such a diagnosis was totally unexpected from the clinical features.

Management
Simple excision is usually required for cosmetic reasons.

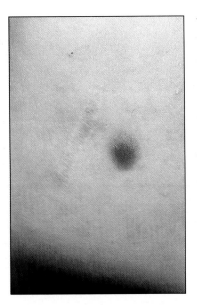

◀ **Fig. 7.15**
Juvenile melanoma. A red-brown papule is present on the cheek of a young boy. The scar is from excision of a previous one. The histology may be misinterpreted as malignant but is completely benign.

VASCULAR NAEVI

Strawberry naevus
Definition
A rapidly growing, benign vascular tumour or angioma, appearing shortly after birth, attaining quite sizeable proportions, and gradually resolving over the ensuing few years.

> **Diagnostic features**
> - Rapid growth after birth.
> - Red or purple round nodule.
> - Eventual spontaneous resolution.

Clinical features
The lesion may be present at birth or arise shortly afterwards, and reaches its maximum size (which varies greatly) within the first 6 months of life. It is a sharply circumscribed, bright red or purple, rounded, domed tumour (Fig. 7.16). The surface may be smooth, lobulated and sometimes become partially ulcerated. It may be solitary or multiple. The head and neck are the most common sites but it may occur anywhere on the body. It is slightly more common in the premature. It is presumably a failure of embryonic angioblastic tissue to establish contact with the normally developing vascular network.

The lesion varies in its composition. It may be superficial consisting predominantly of capillary proliferation, or it may be a mixture of capillaries and a cavernous element. In the latter case the lesion has a deeper subcutaneous element. Rarely, the lesion may be virtually all subcutaneous. This is important for prognosis, for the superficial lesions practically all resolve spontaneously and completely by the seventh birthday. Even the deep lesions resolve completely in

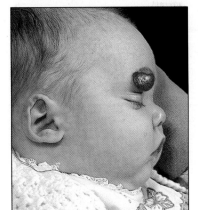

◀ **Fig. 7.16**
Strawberry naevus. A purple dome-shaped nodule appearing shortly after birth, which resolved spontaneously.

most cases, but a few, although resolving considerably, may leave some residual disfigurement.

Management

Masterly inactivity is what is required for the strawberry naevus. Well-meaning friends and relatives may press the parents into demanding that something should be done, which is perfectly understandable, especially when the lesion is on the face. However, it is important to note that the infant is blissfully oblivious of the problem until much older, when the lesion is normally fading well. The desire to operate or X-irradiate must be firmly resisted. Serial photographs to illustrate the ultimate resolution of the problem in other children are very useful.

Occasionally the lesion bleeds but this usually responds to simple pressure.

The surface of the angioma may erode but on the whole this is of no significance. If the lesion does not resolve completely, any baggy redundant folds of skin may be excised by a plastic surgeon when the child enters the second decade. Occasionally, large lesions obstruct the airway or interfere with feeding or vision. Intralesional or systemic steroids may then be indicated.

Very rarely a haemorrhagic diathesis occurs (Kasabach–Merritt syndrome) with thrombocytopenia due to platelet sequestration and consumption of clotting factors within the angioma. There is bleeding into the angioma and an urgent referral to hospital is indicated.

Port-wine stain (naevus flammeus)
Definition

A permanent vascular naevus present at birth, which is a serious cosmetic disability if present on the face and is very occasionally associated with intracranial angiomas, congenital glaucoma, and limb hypertrophy.

Diagnostic features
- Purple.
- Flat patch.
- Unilateral.
- Especially on the face and neck.
- Permanent.

Clinical features

The lesion is present at birth and is completely flat, but may become raised later. The lesion is discoloured, usually purple, and varies in size from a few millimetres to several centimetres. It is usually unilateral. It can occur anywhere on the body, but the nape of the neck and the face are particularly common sites. On the face it frequently covers the distribution approximating to the sensory branches of the trigeminal nerve (Fig. 7.17) and occasionally may be associated with ipsilateral intracranial leptomeningeal angiomatosis, resulting in epilepsy, contralateral hemiparesis and/or mental retardation (Sturge–Weber syndrome). If it is complicated by limb hypertrophy, it is known as the Klippel–Trenaunay–Weber syndrome. Computerized axial tomography has greatly improved the diagnosis of intracranial angiomas.

Management

Management is unsatisfactory. Surgery, cryotherapy, thorium X, grenz rays and tattooing are among the treatment failures. The argon laser offers promise for the future. Darker, well-established lesions, have shown favourable responses, but it is a slow, tedious, expensive and not widely available technique. Cosmetic camouflage remains the simplest practical proposition (Fig. 7.18). Most centres have access to an expert in cosmetic camouflage who will determine

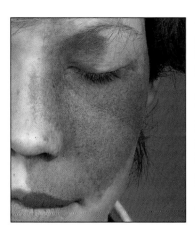 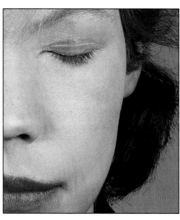

◀ **Figs 7.17 & 7.18** *Port-wine stain. The lesion is present at birth and permanent. Instruction in cosmetic camouflage may be very helpful (Fig. 7.18).*

the correct skin colouring for the individual patient, and teach the patient how to make up and disguise the lesion.

Salmon patches
Definition
A temporary vascular blemish present at birth and disappearing within one year.

> **Diagnostic features**
> - Pink patch.
> - Forehead, eyelid or lip.
> - Present at birth.
> - Fades.

Clinical features
Salmon patches are extremely common. The lesion is a much paler pink than the port wine stain. It occurs most commonly on the forehead, glabella, upper eyelids and lips. It usually fades within the first year of life.

Spider naevus
Definition
A localized arterial dilatation of the skin.

> **Diagnostic features**
> - Central minute red papule.
> - Tiny linear channels radiating outwards.
> - Common on the face.

Clinical features
The lesion has a central, dilated vessel, from which radiate tiny linear channels (Fig. 7.19). It arises spontaneously, usually in childhood or early adult life. It may occur singly, or be multiple. It occurs anywhere on the skin in the distribution of the superior vena cava. Many appear during pregnancy, and then subsequently disappear afterwards, or are precipitated by oral contraceptives.

Management
The lesion is usually of no significance in children or young adults but multiple lesions are sometimes associated with liver disease. The lesion is very simple to treat. The central arteriole is obliterated with a cold cautery needle, and then cauterized. There is barely any discomfort. A small scab forms which disappears within a few days. The spider naevus quite often recurs, but treatment can be repeated.

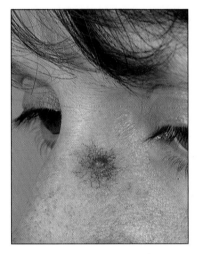

◀**Fig. 7.19**
Spider naevus. There is a central arteriole with tiny radiating linear channels.

8 BENIGN SKIN LESIONS

INTRODUCTION

Benign lesions of the skin and its appendages, rather like naevi, are very common indeed and patients consult about them for similar reasons. The lesions that have been included in this chapter are those which are commonly referred to pigmented lesion clinics as possible melanomas and certain minor blemishes which can be easily treated by the family practitioner.

Common lesions such as cysts, lipomata and neurofibromata, which are rarely misdiagnosed or cause alarm, have been excluded.

SEBORRHOEIC WART (SEBORRHOEIC KERATOSIS, BASAL CELL PAPILLOMA)

Definition
An exceedingly common benign abnormality of basal cell maturation consisting of a well-defined, raised, rough-surfaced papule or plaque.

Diagnostic features
- Well-defined.
- Raised.
- Uniform colour.
- Various shades of brown.
- Rough, fissured or stippled surface.
- Often itchy.

Aetiology
Although very common in the elderly, seborrhoeic warts are becoming quite common in young and middle-aged Caucasians who have at some stage in their lives enjoyed solar exposure. They result from a failure of keratinocyte maturation, leading to an accumulation of immature yet benign cells within the epidermis. Neighbouring melanocytes may transfer melanin to the abnormal keratinocytes so that the lesions are usually pigmented, varying in colour from a light tan to dark brown or black.

Clinical features
The lesion has a variety of clinical appearances and it is this that causes the confusion. Lesions may be big or small and may occur singly or in large numbers (Figs 8.1 & 8.2): a study of lesions in any one individual will confirm their variety.

The essential features are that the lesion is fairly well-defined with a rough surface, which is fissured (see Fig. 1.31) or stippled in appearance. It almost appears to have been stuck onto the skin. The colour varies enormously and depends on the amount of

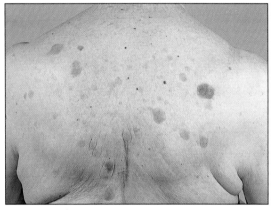

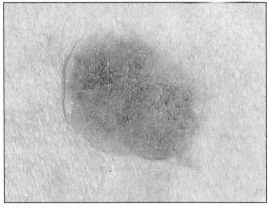

▲ **Figs 8.1 & 8.2** *Seborrhoeic warts. They often occur in large numbers. A close-up (Fig. 8.2) shows a very well-defined, essentially tan-coloured lesion with a rough, fissured surface.*

melanin taken up by the immature keratinocytes: yellow, tan, brown or black in colour (Fig. 8.3) or various shades in between. The lesion is usually raised, but it may be hardly raised at all. Indeed, histologically, it may be difficult to distinguish the flat

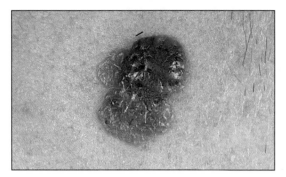

▲ **Fig. 8.3** *Seborrhoeic wart. The lesion is well-defined and although quite dark has a rough stippled surface, which distinguishes it from a melanoma.*

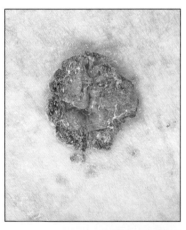

◀**Fig. 8.4** *Irritated seborrhoeic wart. The lesion is inflamed and has bled. The lesion is well-defined with a fissured surface.*

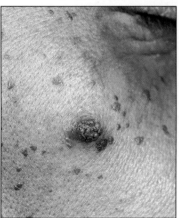

◀**Fig. 8.5** *Dermatosis papulosa nigra. These pigmented papules occur on the face in Negroes and are inherited. Histologically they are seborrhoeic warts.*

solar lentigo (see Fig. 1.2) from a seborrhoeic wart, such that they may well be just different parts of the same pathological process. Sometimes, the lesions may be pedunculated, especially around the eyes or in the flexures. They may be asymptomatic but they often itch and sometimes become red and inflamed (Fig. 8.4).

The lesions usually occur only on areas that have at some stage been exposed to the sun. They are thus rare on the buttocks, inner aspects of the arms, or inner aspects of the thighs.

They also occur in early adult life as an inherited condition on the face in Negroes (Fig. 8.5) and consist of pigmented papules which may be pedunculated. They are known as *dermatosis papulosa nigra*.

Management
The lesion is the most common differential diagnosis of a malignant melanoma, so reassurance is often all that is required. It may be removed surgically or with cryotherapy.

(1) Surgery. The seborrhoeic wart is very simply removed under local anaesthesia by curettage and cautery. This technique leaves behind tiny pinpoint bleeding on the underlying skin, which is highly characteristic. Cautery to stop the bleeding should be gentle, because the seborrhoeic wart is an epidermal abnormality without dermal involvement and thus no scarring should occur. Pedunculated lesions may be removed with scissors.

(2) Cryotherapy. Liquid nitrogen is a simple non-invasive technique which is particularly effective for small lesions. Its advantage is that many seborrhoeic warts can be frozen rapidly, but the disadvantage is that there is no specimen for histopathological examination.

HYPERTROPHIC SCARS AND KELOIDS

Definition
Hypertrophic scars and keloids are a hyperproliferative response of connective tissue to trauma.

Diagnostic features
- Smooth surface.
- Firm.
- Papule, nodule or plaque.
- Sites of inflammation or injury.

Aetiology

These lesions are usually an abnormal response of the skin to inflammation, infection or trauma, especially burns. They occur:

- In certain families.
- Especially in Negroes.
- After surgery in certain sites of the body. These include the chin, neck, shoulders, upper trunk, back and sternum (Fig. 8.6). It is often not appreciated that even excellent surgery will often result in hypertrophic scars or widened scars in these areas. The ear lobes are particularly vulnerable to keloid formation (Fig. 8.7), particularly in the Negro, after ear-piercing.
- In certain skin disorders: (i) *Acne*, which may be

quite minor, particularly on the sternum. (ii) *Ingrowing hairs*, particularly under the neck in the Negro. (iii) *Folliculitis* on the back of the scalp (Fig. 8.8), again particularly in the Negro.

Clinical features

Hypertrophic scars and keloids are raised and firm and have a smooth shiny surface. The histology of the two is similar, and the terms are sometimes used synonymously, but a hypertrophic scar is confined to the area of trauma, whereas a keloid spreads beyond this and has a worse prognosis. They can be extremely unsightly.

Management

The lesions are very difficult and disappointing to treat. Corrective surgery is frequently followed by recurrence, and resulting scarring may be of a greater size than previously. Some advocate prior radiotherapy or local compression, but results are still usually poor.

Certainly intralesional triamcinolone is worth trying, particularly for hypertrophic scars. It is best to use a 1cm^3 syringe, i.e. a small-bore syringe with a wide-bore needle so that maximum pressure can be exerted. Tapes impregnated with steroids (for example Haelan tape, UK — flurandrenolone) are useful. They may be applied to the hypertrophic scar and left in position for the whole day, during which time the steroid is slowly released into the scar.

The family practitioner can help his patient best by discouraging the removal of lesions for 'cosmetic' reasons in areas known to give poor scarring such as the chest and back.

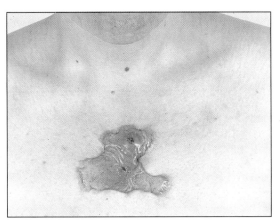

▲ **Fig. 8.6** *Keloid. The sternum is a common site for keloid formation either after surgery or acne. Keloids spread beyond the area of trauma; hypertrophic scars are limited within it.*

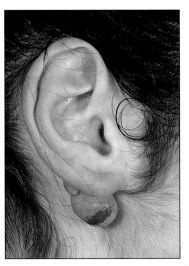

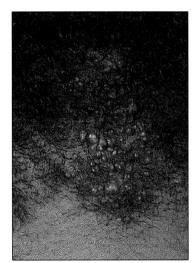

◀**Fig. 8.7** *Keloid. Keloids secondary to ear lobe piercing are common, especially in Negroes. They recur larger if excised.*

◀**Fig. 8.8** *Nuchal keloids. Firm papules occur at the back of the scalp secondary to folliculitis in Negroes. They may become confluent and result in hair loss.*

DERMATOFIBROMA (HISTIOCYTOMA, SCLEROSING HAEMANGIOMA)

Definition
A very common skin tumour occurring frequently on the lower legs and thought to be reactive in origin, possibly to a long-forgotten insect bite.

Diagnostic features
- Firm.
- Papular, occasionally nodular.
- Smooth surface.
- Often pigmented.
- Attached to overlying skin but relatively mobile within it.
- Present especially on legs.

Aetiology
It is quite possible that the lesion represents a reaction to a long-forgotten insect bite, the reactive process involving fibroblasts, endothelial cells and histiocytes. It does occur most commonly on the lower legs, and the patients often remark that they have been prone to insect bites.

Clinical features
The lesion is common and sometimes quite deeply pigmented, so it assumes importance in the differential diagnosis of malignant melanoma. The lesion is a raised papule or nodule between 0.5 and 3.0cm in diameter, with a smooth surface (Fig. 8.9). It is quite firm and can be gripped between the finger and thumb and moved within the skin, but it is adherent to the overlying skin. It varies somewhat in colour, being red brown, brown or sometimes very dark brown indeed. It may be single or multiple and may occur anywhere on the body, especially the lower limbs (Fig. 8.9).

Management
The lesions may be excised for diagnostic or cosmetic reasons, although those on the lower limbs are often followed by a less than perfect scar.

PYOGENIC GRANULOMA (GRANULOMA TELANGIECTATICUM)

Definition
An extremely common benign vascular papule occurring in the young, possibly as a response to injury.

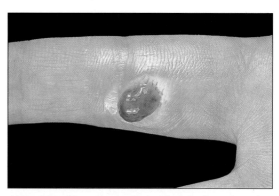

▲**Fig. 8.10** *Pyogenic granuloma. The lesion is a red papule or nodule which is friable and bleeds easily. The finger is a common site.*

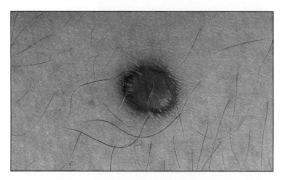

▲**Fig. 8.9** *Dermatofibroma. The lesion is a firm pigmented papule which is attached to the overlying skin but relatively mobile within the skin. Multiple lesions may be present especially on the legs.*

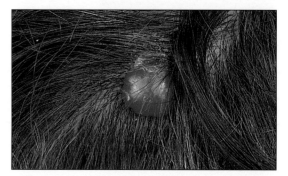

▲**Fig. 8.11** *Pyogenic granuloma. The scalp is a common site. The lesion can be removed by curettage and cautery under local anaesthesia.*

Diagnostic features
- Sudden onset.
- Red papule or nodule.
- Bleeds.
- On finger, face or scalp.

Aetiology

The lesion affects both sexes and occurs mostly in children and young adults but it can occur at any time. It is possibly a result of trauma, but many patients have no recollection of any injury. The pathology suggests that the condition is a reactive one. It consists of widely dilated blood-filled channels surrounded by proliferating capillary buds. It should be noted that, despite its name, the condition is neither granulomatous in pathology nor pyogenic in origin.

Clinical features

The patient presents early since the lesion is sudden in onset and tends to bleed. It is a friable red or purple papule (Fig. 8.10) or nodule. It may occur anywhere on the skin, including the mucosal surfaces, but it is most common on the fingers, around the nail, on the face and in the scalp (Fig. 8.11).

Management

The lesion can be quite simply removed by curettage and cautery under local anaesthesia; it often bleeds profusely, despite cautery, but firm pressure on the

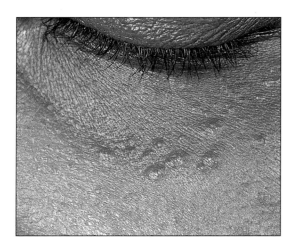

▲ **Fig. 8.12** *Syringomata. They are flesh-coloured papules around the eyes and are composed of sweat ducts.*

lesion by a co-operative patient is all that is usually required to stem the flow.

SYRINGOMA

Definition

A benign tumour of sweat ducts, which is usually multiple on the face.

Diagnostic features
- Small flesh-coloured papules.
- Around eyes, neck and front of chest.
- Commence in second decade.

Aetiology

The cause is unknown. They consist of a double line of cells similar to those which line sweat ducts.

Clinical features

They are usually multiple around the eyes (Fig. 8.12). They are small smooth-surfaced flesh-coloured papules.

Management

They are harmless but can be diathermied.

COMMON MINOR LESIONS OF THE SKIN

Grouped together here are a number of conditions which rarely appear in undergraduate texts, for they are quite clearly not serious, and yet they are very common. They often present for cosmetic reasons, and are easily dealt with by a family practitioner. Sometimes patients are over-preoccupied with them, which may be a manifestation of an affective disorder.

Milia (whiteheads)
Definition

A small, white or cream-coloured papule occurring most commonly on the face.

Aetiology

The lesion is a minute epidermal cyst. It occurs:
- Commonly in the young as part of the acne process.
- After any blistering process which involves the dermo-epidermal junction, for example bullous pemphigoid or mild sunburn.
- Commonly as a result of chronic solar damage.

Clinical features

The lesion is simple to diagnose. It is a 'whitehead' or minute white or cream-coloured papule (Fig. 8.13), which is firm in consistency.

Management

Milia often disappear spontaneously in the young after a number of months, but they can be easily removed by breaking the skin surface with a sterile needle and scraping out the tiny cyst.

Skin tags (fibro-epithelial polyps)
Definition

A very common small soft pigmented papule, which is often pedunculated, occurring around the neck and in the flexures.

Aetiology

The cause of skin tags is quite unknown. They occur in both sexes and increase in incidence with advancing years. Some patients seem particularly prone to them, especially during pregnancy. The histology is rather uninspiring, a tag being a polyp and consisting of mature keratinizing squamous epithelium, overlying a fibrovascular core. Sometimes clinically identical lesions turn out histologically to be seborrhoeic warts or melanocytic naevi.

Clinical features

The lesion may be solitary, particularly in the groin or axillae. It is flesh-coloured or pigmented, usually pedunculated and always soft. Alternatively, there may be a profusion of lesions, particularly around the neck (Fig. 8.14): in this site, they may be very minor protrusions but nevertheless be cosmetically unacceptable to the patient.

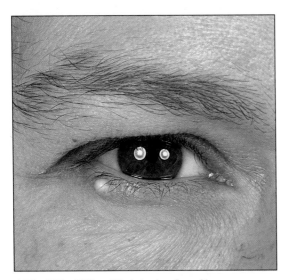

▲ **Fig. 8.13** *Milium. The lesion is a firm white or cream coloured papule occurring most commonly on the face. It is a minute epidermal cyst. They are frequently multiple.*

Management

Small lesions can be cauterized without anaesthesia. The discomfort is momentary and no worse than the prick of a local anaesthetic. Liquid nitrogen is also effective. More pedunculated lesions can be removed with scissors or a cutting cautery under local anaesthesia.

Campbell de Morgan spots (cherry angiomata)
Definition

Red or purple macules or papules, occurring on the trunk, that are simple haemangiomata.

Aetiology

The cause of these lesions is unknown. Although more common in the elderly, they also occur quite frequently from the fourth decade onwards, contrary to their synonym of 'senile haemangiomata'.

Clinical features

The lesions are usually multiple. There may be tiny pin-point red macules, or more obvious, discrete, red smooth-surfaced papules (Fig. 8.15).

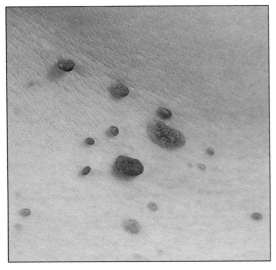

▲ **Fig. 8.14** *Skin tags. The lesions are either tiny raised dots or pedunculated pigmented soft papules, often in profusion around the neck.*

Management

The lesions are of no medical significance but over-concern about them suggests anxiety or depression. They can be cauterized.

Angiokeratoma

Definition

A small, benign red papule on the scrotum, composed of dilated blood vessels, with a hyperkeratotic surface.

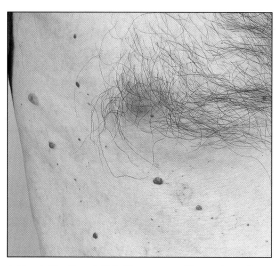

▲ **Fig. 8.15** *Campbell de Morgan spots. These red macules or papules occurring on the trunk are simple angiomata. Preoccupation with them often indicates an affective disorder.*

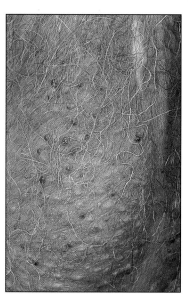

◀ **Fig. 8.16** *Angiokeratoma. This is a small red papule with a rough surface. They are often multiple on the scrotum and are quite harmless.*

Clinical features

Solitary lesions occur on the limbs in the young. Multiple lesions occur commonly on the scrotum (Fig. 8.16).

An extensive diffuse variety occurs in *Fabry's disease*, a rare inborn error of glycosphingolipid metabolism. It is accompanied by acroparaesthesia and severe episodic cutaneous and abdominal pain.

Management

The simple types are quite harmless. Solitary lesions may be excised.

Fordyce spots

Definition

Multiple, small yellow papules, occurring in and around the mouth. They represent normal but visible sebaceous glands.

Clinical features

Fordyce spots are very common and may be regarded as a normal variant. They occur inside the mouth, especially on the buccal mucosae and on the lips. They are discrete, very slightly raised, yellow lesions (Fig. 8.17), and many patients are quite unaware of their presence.

Management

Simple reassurance should be enough, but some patients are overconcerned about them and this is usually a manifestation of an affective disorder.

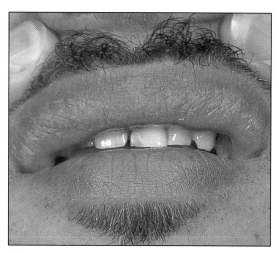

▲ **Fig. 8.17** *Fordyce spots. Multiple small yellow papules occur as a normal variant on the lips and buccal mucosae. They are sebaceous glands. Morbid overconcern with them does occur.*

Senile sebaceous hyperplasia
Definition
A small yellow papule with a central depression occurring on the face, consisting of numerous mature hyperplastic sebaceous glands.

Clinical features
Despite its name, the condition may occur from the thirties onwards. There may be several lesions. They occur on the face and are quite benign, but they are often mistaken for basal cell carcinomata; however their yellow colour (Fig. 8.18) helps to distinguish the two.

Management
Reassurance is usually enough, but the lesions can be cauterized under local anaesthesia.

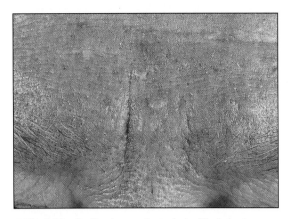

▲**Fig. 8.18** *Senile sebaceous hyperplasia. The lesion is a small yellow papule with a central depression occurring on the face, especially the forehead. They may be multiple.*

9 SOLAR DAMAGE AND SKIN CANCER

INTRODUCTION

The incidence of skin cancer is increasing in the West, yet there is considerable ignorance regarding it and its primary cause, sunlight, amongst the British public, rather akin to that regarding lung cancer and cigarette smoking 30 years ago. There is a general belief that there is so little sunshine in the UK that it does not constitute a problem, but there are a dozen sunny days in each summer and each one of these can burn and damage an Anglo-Saxon skin. Skin cancer is a British and North European disease: it may be more common in Americans and Australians, but it is their British or Northern European cutaneous phenotypes which makes them prone to it.

The problem is compounded by the dictates of fashion, the ease of access to the sun and the increasing longevity of the population. Even if solar protection soon becomes the norm, there is nothing that can be done to reverse damage already done, so the problem is likely to be with us well into the 21st century.

The propensity for solar damage depends upon:
- The patient's skin type.
- The cumulative exposure to ultraviolet light.
- The intensity of exposure.
- The age of exposure.

The skin types are numbered in Figure 9.1. Types 1 and 2 are most susceptible. Ultraviolet induced skin cancer does not occur in the Negro (type 5). The red-headed, blue-eyed, fair-skinned individual who burns and freckles easily is most at risk, but appearances are deceptive. Thus, although dark-haired, brown-eyed and olive-skinned peoples are usually exempt, it is their response to sunlight that matters. If they burn, their skin type may be 1 or 2 and therefore they will be in a high risk group.

The amount of exposure is important. The link between sunlight and skin cancer was first established in those whose occupations took them into the sun, viz. sailors. Thus solar keratoses and squamous cell carcinomata occur as a result of chronic exposure and these are commonest in those who spend a lot of time outdoors and become chronically weather beaten. The intensity of exposure is also relevant. Thus certain forms of malignant melanoma are most common in workers who are ensconced in their offices or factories most of the year and who expose their white, non-tanned skin intensely on vacation, often burning in the process. The timing of exposure may be important. Much of the damage may be done in childhood. Thus indigenous Australians are more prone to malignant melanoma than Anglo-Saxons who emigrate to Australia in their teens. Indeed it is an important part of the management of the problem to advise patients who have skin cancer of the potential danger to their children and grandchildren through having inherited a similar skin type.

Useful points to consider in the diagnosis and management of skin cancers are given in Figure 9.2.

SKIN TYPES	
Type 1	Always burns, never tans
Type 2	Always burns, sometimes tans
Type 3	Sometimes burns, always tans
Type 4	Never burns, always tans
Type 5	Negro skin

▲ **Fig. 9.1** *Skin types.*

SKIN CANCERS: USEFUL POINTS
Always refer direct to a dermatologist rather than specifically to a surgeon or radiotherapist. A multi-disciplinary approach to skin cancer, coordinated by a dermatologist, is best
Always examine the rest of the skin for other cutaneous malignancies
Review such patients annually. A patient with one skin cancer may well develop another later
Be alert for the incidental diagnosis. Skin cancers are often visible, especially on the face

▲ **Fig. 9.2** *Useful points to consider in the diagnosis and management of skin cancers.*

Physical signs of solar damage

All the changes to be described can be seen in an accelerated form in the rare disorder, *xeroderma pigmentosum*, a condition of extreme photosensitivity due to an enzymatic failure to repair ultraviolet light-damaged epidermal DNA, which results in multiple types of skin cancer beginning in childhood.

Sunburn

This is entirely preventable with modern sun screens, but it is still the major culprit in initiating solar damage. It is caused by ultraviolet B (UVB; 290–320 nm) and results in painful erythema (Fig. 9.3) and sometimes oedema and blistering. It is followed by desquamation (peeling).

Freckles (ephelides)
Definition

A freckle is an increase in melanin production without melanocytic proliferation.

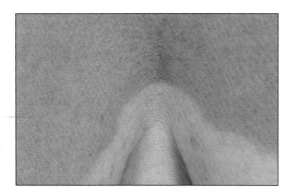

▲ **Fig. 9.3** *Sunburn. The painful erythema of sunburn which damages epidermal DNA is preventable with sunscreens.*

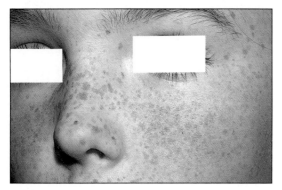

▲ **Fig. 9.4** *Freckles (ephelides). Freckles are transitory pigmented macules, occurring in the sun, on the face in childhood.*

Clinical features

Freckles occur in children with type 1 and type 2 skins, predominantly on the face and especially on the cheeks and over the nose (Fig. 9.4). They increase in number in the summer but diminish during the winter. Although often regarded as a healthy sign, freckling is actually one of the first indications of solar damage. It may be considered to be a result of over-stimulation of pigment cells by ultraviolet light.

Lentigines
Definition

A lentigo is a benign proliferation of melanocytes along the basement membrane.

Clinical features

A lentigo is a later complication of solar damage and is a permanent pigmented lesion. Lentigines occur on the sun exposed areas, particularly the face, backs of the hands (see Fig. 1.2), arms, front of the chest (Fig. 9.5), upper back and shoulders. A lentigo is an even-coloured macule or patch varying from light tan to dark brown in colour. It may be quite flat or just slightly raised with a matt appearance, such that distinguishing it from a seborrhoeic wart may be impossible. On the backs of the hands lentigines are known as 'liver' or 'age' spots by patients, but in reality they have nothing to do with either. They do not occur on solar-protected sites, such as the inner aspect of the upper arms, and it is worth pointing this out to patients who disbelieve the rôle of the sun.

Solar elastosis

Gradually damage occurs to the elastic fibres in the dermis, producing microscopically a rather dramatic

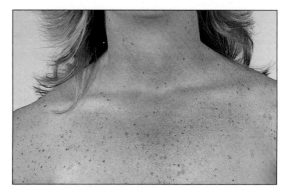

▲ **Fig. 9.5** *Lentigines. These are permanent even-coloured macules or patches indicating sun damage.*

picture of disarray, known as solar elastosis. Clinically a number of appearances may result.

(1) Cutis rhomboidalis nuchae. This bizarre term is perhaps better though unkindly known as 'peasant's neck'. The skin is thrown into exaggerated coarse folds, particularly around the neck, but with impressive sparing of the sun-shielded area under the chin (Fig. 9.6).

(2) Atrophy of the skin. The skin loses its elasticity, particularly on the dorsal aspects of the hands, forearms and shins. It is dry, wrinkled and thin. The blood vessels are vulnerable and purpura results from the least trauma (Fig. 9.7).

(3) Comedones, milia and yellow plaques. Blackheads, whiteheads and yellow plaques are common features of chronically sun-damaged skin.

SOLAR KERATOSIS (ACTINIC KERATOSIS)

Definition

A premalignant disorder of the epidermis occurring on solar-damaged skin.

Diagnostic features
- Red.
- Well-defined, slightly raised, rough papule or plaque.
- Adherent scale.
- Solitary or multiple.

Clinical features

The lesion starts as a minute area of telangiectasia which is rarely observed by the patient but proceeds to a well-defined, red papule or plaque, with a rough (often remarked upon by the patient), very adherent, yellow/brown scale (see Fig. 1.5), which can only be removed with difficulty, leaving a raw bleeding surface. Lesions are often multiple and are found in the chronically solar exposed areas of the skin, viz. the face, ears, backs of the hands, forearms and shins. Because hair is protective, the scalp of a man who has been bald from a young age is particularly vulnerable. *Solar keratoses on the bald scalp are often misdiagnosed as eczema.*

Solar keratoses are potentially malignant after a number of years. The lesion may gradually become thickened and squamous cell carcinoma results. However the prognosis is usually good, because the lesions rarely metastasize.

Management

(1) Liquid nitrogen or its equivalent is very effective. Only a minor degree of inflammation without blistering is required. An application in the order of 15 seconds is usually sufficient.

(2) Surgery. Curettage and cautery are effective, but scarring may result, which is unlikely with cryotherapy. This method, however, does have the advantage of permitting histological examination of the material removed. All indurated lesions are likely to have progressed to very early squamous cell carcinomata and should be excised and submitted for histology.

(3) Topical therapy. It was first noticed in South Africa, during the treatment of lung cancer with systemic 5-fluorouracil, that solar keratoses in these patients became red and inflamed and subsequently became detached. The drug was then used topically and found to be effective. It is an antimetabolite

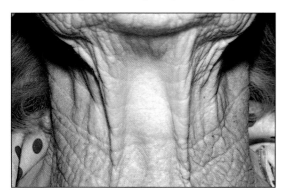

▲ **Fig. 9.6** *Solar elastosis. Yellowing and furrowing of the skin results from chronic solar response. The protected area under the neck is undamaged.*

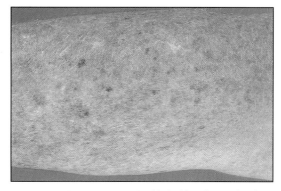

▲ **Fig. 9.7** *Solar purpura. The skin is thin, pigmented and dry. Purpura and scars result from the least trauma.*

which blocks the incorporation of thymidine into DNA. It is particularly suitable for multiple lesions, especially on the face. However it is less effective on the hands and forearms, possibly because penetration into the skin is not so good. Combination with topical retinoic acid, however, improves this penetration. The application of 5-fluorouracil twice daily results in an intense inflammatory reaction (Fig. 9.8), which can be disquieting to the patient. Experience in its use is therefore required, as is very careful explanation of its effects to the patient. The inflammation does not occur immediately, but usually after about 10 days. It is sometimes useful to employ a stop/start policy of one week's active treatment followed by one week's rest, for a total of 4 weeks of active treatment. The drug has no effect on normal skin, and a major advantage in severely sun-damaged skin is that it destroys the earliest microscopically abnormal cells before they have given rise to macroscopically obvious skin changes. It produces excellent cosmetic results (Figs 9.9 & 9.10).

CUTANEOUS HORN

Definition
A clinical description of a horny outgrowth of skin, with no pathological meaning.

Clinical features
This is a purely descriptive term indicating marked keratin cohesion which gives rise to a horny outgrowth (Fig. 9.11) which does not in any way identify its aetiology. It may be caused by a viral wart, seborrhoeic wart, solar keratosis, keratoacanthoma or squamous cell carcinoma. Examination of the base of the lesion may be helpful in determining its origin. A flat or very slightly raised red base suggests a keratosis, a well-defined warty base suggests a seborrhoeic wart, and a red indurated base, a squamous cell carcinoma.

Management
Surgical removal and submission for histological examination is the treatment of choice.

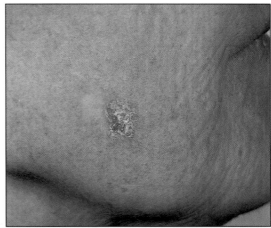

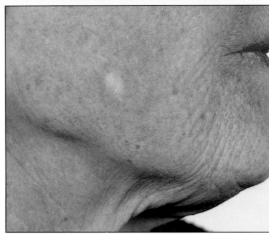

▲ **Figs 9.9 & 9.10** *Solar keratosis. This solar keratosis, previously treated with curettage and cautery leaving a white scar (upper), recurred but was treated successfully with 5-fluorouracil without leaving any mark (lower).*

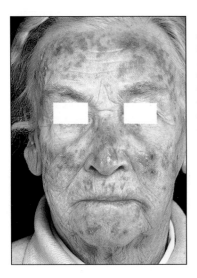

◀ **Fig. 9.8** *5-Fluorouracil reaction. A temporary disconcerting erythema occurs around the solar keratoses during treatment.*

BOWEN'S DISEASE (INTRAEPIDERMAL CARCINOMA) OF THE SKIN

Definition

An intraepidermal carcinoma of the skin which occasionally proceeds to squamous cell carcinoma.

Diagnostic features
- Well defined plaque.
- Red with an adherent scale.
- Solitary.

Aetiology

The disorder is relatively common. A solitary plaque on an exposed site is likely to be due to excess ultraviolet irradiation, but arsenic ingestion should be suspected in patients with multiple lesions on covered sites. Only five per cent of patients with Bowen's disease recall arsenic ingestion, but statistically significant quantities of arsenic may be found in their skins. Arsenic has been used therapeutically as Fowler's solution for psoriasis and syphilis, in combination with bromide for epilepsy and chorea, and in Gay's solution as a treatment for asthma in the US. It is used industrially as a weed killer, pesticide, sheep dip and fungicide. It was incorporated in many children's tonics including Parrish's food, and also in many homeopathic preparations. Arsenic may also predispose to internal malignancy.

Clinical features

The lesion is a well-defined, very slightly raised, red plaque, with a rough adherent scale (Fig. 9.12). It grows very slowly and if it is due to ultraviolet light it is usually solitary, and the most common sites are the face, backs of the hands, lower legs and the backs of the fingers. *On the fingers it is frequently misdiagnosed as an eczema or a psoriasis*, but it is always unwise to make such a diagnosis in a solitary persistent lesion and biopsy is advisable. In cases where arsenic is implicated, the lesions may be multiple and occur asymmetrically on the trunk.

Although the lesion is potentially capable of developing into a squamous cell carcinoma, this is unusual. However, malignant change is suggested if the lesion becomes thicker and more indurated and the surface becomes eroded or ulcerated.

Management

(1) **Cryotherapy.** Liquid nitrogen should be applied for 30 seconds. Recurrences are not uncommon and retreatment may be necessary.

(2) **Surgery.** (a) Curettage and cautery are satisfactory. (b) Excision is the best treatment if primary closure is practicable.

(3) **Radiotherapy.** The lesion is radiosensitive but scarring and sometimes radionecrosis result, especially in lesions on the dorsum of the hand.

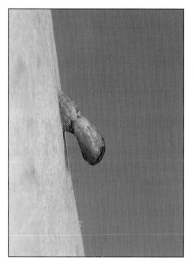

◀Fig. 9.11
Cutaneous horn. This is a descriptive term indicating marked keratin adhesion, in this case due to a small keratoacanthoma.

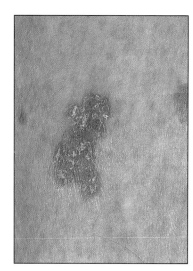

◀Fig. 9.12
Bowen's disease (intraepidermal carcinoma of the skin). The lesion is a very well-defined, slightly raised, red plaque with a rough adherent scale.

(4) Topical therapy. 5-Fluorouracil cream twice daily for 5 weeks is effective (Figs 9.13 & 9.14), but recurrences do occur so follow-up is wise. Excellent cosmetic results may be obtained.

KERATOACANTHOMA

Definition

A rapidly growing benign tumour of Caucasian skin occurring mainly on exposed areas, which involutes spontaneously within 4 months.

Diagnostic features
- Rapid growth.
- Well-defined, dome-shaped papule or nodule.
- Central, keratin-filled crater.
- Involutes spontaneously to leave a pitted scar.
- Sun-exposed skin.

Aetiology

Keratoacanthoma is quite a common tumour. It affects older age groups, and has a 3:1 incidence of males to females. Chronic solar overexposure is the common cause, but transplant recipients taking immunosuppressive drugs long-term are prone, as well as individuals exposed to pitch and tar. Histologically the condition has many features in common with a squamous cell carcinoma but its behaviour is different in that it involutes spontaneously.

Clinical features

The history is most important. The lesion starts 'as a spot' which continues to grow alarmingly and rapidly in size. The papule becomes a very well-defined uniform nodule, either red- or flesh-coloured. It stands proud and elevated away from the surrounding normal skin and has a central keratin-filled crater (Fig. 9.15). It is usually 1.5–2.0cm in size but may be larger. It gradually accumulates more keratin and begins to involute and heal, leaving behind a pitted scar (Figs 9.15 & 9.16). The whole process takes about 4 months.

The commonest sites are light-exposed areas — the face, particularly the nose and cheeks, and the dorsum of the hands and forearms. It is seen in Caucasians with type 1 or type 2 skins.

Management

The lesion should be removed either by curettage and cautery or by primary excision and closure. The problem is that site constraints are such that if the lesion has been allowed to grow too large it is difficult to remove surgically without major plastic repair, particularly on the face, *so the patient should be referred quickly.* However if surgery is technically difficult (since the diagnosis can usually be made with confidence and confirmed by a skin biopsy), the keratoacanthoma can be left and allowed to heal spontaneously. Any unsightly scar can be rectified later. Nevertheless any clinician is happier if the lesion can be completely removed since the diagnosis is easier to confirm histologically if the entire lesion is examined, rather than a biopsy specimen, especially as the condition can occasionally masquerade as squamous cell carcinoma.

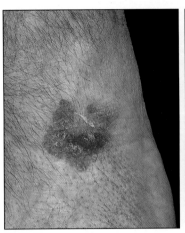 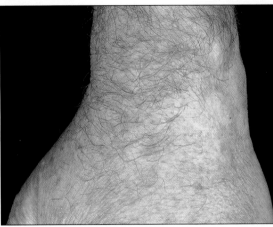

◀**Figs 9.13 & 9.14** *Bowen's disease. This lesion (left) would have required a skin graft if excised surgically. It was successfully treated with 5-fluorouracil with no recurrence 6 years later (right).*

SQUAMOUS CELL CARCINOMA

Definition
A malignant tumour arising from squamous epithelium which may eventually metastasize.

Diagnostic features
- Solitary.
- Indurated plaque or nodule.
- Surface may become crusted or ulcerated.
- Usually solar exposed sites.

Aetiology
This is a relatively uncommon tumour in the UK, but which is increasing in frequency. It is potentially dangerous, because after infiltrating locally, it may metastasize to lymph nodes resulting in carcinomatosis. It is twice as common in males and tends to occur in older age groups. The incidence and aetiology varies in different parts of the world. The causes are as follows:

(1) **Ultraviolet irradiation.** This is by far the most common cause in Caucasians. The highest incidences in the world are in Texas and Queensland. The lesion may start *de novo* in chronically sun-damaged skin and ultimately metastasize, or arise from a preceeding solar keratosis or Bowen's disease when metastasis is unusual.

(2) **X-irradiation.** In the days before the danger of X-rays was appreciated, radiologists were at risk of developing this tumour, particularly on the hands, and even nowadays it is occasionally seen in dentists who perform their own radiography without taking adequate precautions. Previous X-ray treatment of diseases such as psoriasis, ringworm, acne and ankylosing spondylitis may be followed by the development of squamous cell carcinoma.

(3) **Polycyclic hydrocarbons.** Tar, mineral oils, pitch and soot are carcinogens to which individuals may be exposed industrially. Soot was the first carcinogen to be identified: Percival Pott established it as the cause of squamous carcinoma of the scrotum in adults who as children had ascended chimney stacks to sweep them.

(4) **Scars.** Squamous cell carcinoma may be a late sequela of scarring either from burns, for example, thermal injury due to sitting too close to a fire (erythema ab igne) or from warming devices placed on the skin or from skin diseases which result in scarring, for example epidermolysis bullosa, lupus vulgaris or very occasionally chronic varicose ulcers.

(5) **Certain genetic skin diseases.** (i) *Albinism*: there is an enzymatic failure to produce the photoprotective pigment, melanin, and squamous cell carcinoma ultimately may result, especially in albinos who live in sunny climates. Interestingly, squamous cell carcinoma is not a problem with vitiligo, a disease in which melanocytes which produce the melanin are absent. (ii) *Xeroderma pigmentosum*: this is an enzyme deficiency which results in failure to repair DNA following solar injury. It results in the early evolution of skin cancer.

(6) **Skin disease affecting the mucosae.** Lichen planus, affecting the oral cavity, and lichen sclerosus et atrophicus, affecting the genitalia, are very rarely premalignant.

(7) **Human papilloma virus.** The wart virus has been implicated in the development of squamous cell carcinoma of the vulva.

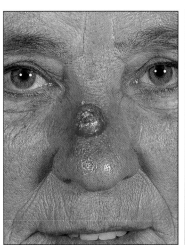 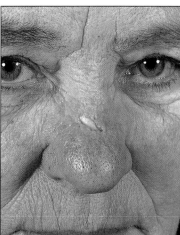

◀**Figs 9.15 & 9.16**
Keratoacanthoma. There is a well-defined nodule (left), which is elevated from the surrounding normal skin, with a central keratin crater on the nose. The nodule has resolved spontaneously to leave a pitted scar (right).

Clinical features

The lesion starts as a thickening of the skin and becomes an indurated plaque. It grows laterally and vertically, gradually becoming fixed and nodular (Fig. 9.17). Eventually the surface becomes crusted or ulcerated (Fig. 9.18). Ulcers often have a purulent base, which is revealed if the crust is removed. The margin is firm and more raised than that of a basal cell carcinoma and is often everted and irregular in shape. It grows more rapidly than a basal cell carcinoma but not as fast as a keratoacanthoma.

Most lesions occur on sun-exposed areas, thus the face, ears (Fig. 9.19), lower lip and the extensor surfaces of the hands, forearms and lower legs are the commonest sites. Apart from the face, these are all unusual sites for a basal cell carcinoma. The surrounding skin usually has signs of actinic damage.

The importance of squamous cell carcinoma is that it may metastasize to lymph nodes and end fatally. The factors governing prognosis are:

(1) **The preceding lesion.** Squamous cell carcinomata arising in a solar keratosis or in cutaneous Bowen's disease rarely metastasize. Those arising *de novo* or from other causes, for example chronic scarring disorders and X-irradiation, are more likely to do so.

(2) **Site.** Lesions on the ear and the vermillion of the lip often metastasize. Those on the external genitalia and anus, including those that develop from mucosal Bowen's disease, also may metastasize.

(3) **Degree of differentiation.** Clearly, a well-differentiated squamous cell carcinoma has a better prognosis than a poorly differentiated one.

(4) **The depth of invasion** of the tumour at the time of diagnosis.

Management

Squamous cell carcinoma should be managed jointly by a plastic surgeon and a radiotherapist. Surgical excision is the treatment of choice, but radiotherapy is also effective in many cases. Treatment will depend on the nature, size and site of the tumour, the presence or absence of metastasis, and the health of the patient.

BASAL CELL CARCINOMA

Definition

A common locally destructive malignant tumour of the skin derived from basal cells from the lower epidermis.

Aetiology

Basal cell carcinoma is the commonest malignant tumour of the skin. Although undoubtedly its prevalence increases with solar exposure, and although it is more common in skin types 1 and 2, ultraviolet light is not the sole cause. Firstly, although it is very common on the head and neck, it is unusual on other light-exposed areas such as the backs of the hands and forearms, unlike solar keratoses and squamous cell carcinomata. Secondly, the inner canthus and eyelids, sites which are more shielded from sunlight than others on the face, are frequently involved. Thirdly, it does appear on solar-protected areas, such as the vulva. The situation is not fully explained, but it may be that the basal cell layer of the pilosebaceous

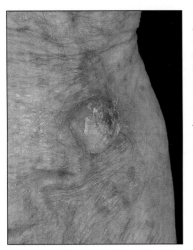

◀**Fig. 9.17**
Squamous cell carcinoma. An indurated nodule is present. The back of the hand is a solar-exposed and common site for keratoses and squamous cell carcinoma.

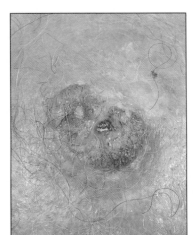

◀**Fig. 9.18**
Squamous cell carcinoma. The lesion is ulcerated and has a purulent base. The margin is indurated and more raised than that of a basal cell carcinoma.

follicles on the face is more susceptible to the effects of ultraviolet light. Pathologically the tumour is composed of islands of basal cells, originating from the basal cell layer of the epidermis and from adnexal structures.

Basal cell carcinomata are still being seen in patients who had ringworm of the scalp accidentally overtreated with X-irradiation many years previously. Patients treated for ankylosing spondylitis with X-irradiation may also develop basal cell carcinoma after a latent period of a number of decades. It is also probable that patients with lymphoma and particularly with Hodgkin's disease (since it is now curable), who have been treated with X-rays, will develop basal cell carcinomata in the irradiated areas.

Clinical features

The basal cell carcinoma occurs most commonly on the face and is most frequent in the elderly, but with the changes in the recreational activities discussed earlier, it is now occurring in young and middle-aged adults.

It grows slowly, is painless and consequently is frequently ignored by the patient who sometimes allows it to grow to proportions which require complex therapy. This is particularly so in the elderly and is becoming a considerable problem with an increasingly geriatric population. The basal cell carcinoma rarely metastasizes but it is locally invasive and destructive. This is of particular importance when the lesion is situated near to the eye, nose or ear. If neglected, the tumour may infiltrate deeply through tissue planes into the cranial cavity, with serious consequences. Because of its location on the face, it

should be possible to diagnose the lesion incidentally, when the patient attends the family practitioner for some unrelated problem. There are five clinical subtypes of basal cell carcinoma, each discussed separately below.

Subtypes of basal cell carcinoma

The rodent ulcer

Diagnostic features
- Well-defined papule or nodule.
- Rolled, pearly, telangiectatic margin.
- Eroded or ulcerated centre.
- Painless.
- The face.

Clinical features

Patients often remark that the lesion tends to bleed and subsequently scabs, but never quite seems to heal. They note that it is painless and therefore consider it to be harmless. The lesion commences as a small papule which subsequently becomes nodular and ulcerates centrally. The margin of the ulcer is well defined, slightly raised and rolled, with a colour similar to that of a pearl. Tiny blood vessels (telangiectasia) may be seen coursing over this margin (see Fig. 1.32) and this sometimes makes the lesion appear red. However, compression blanches the tumour and reveals the characteristic pearly colouration.

The term 'rodent ulcer' is expressive, in that the tumour grows inexorably, eroding and gnawing away at the skin (Fig. 9.20), which is rather fancifully reminiscent of the behaviour of a rat.

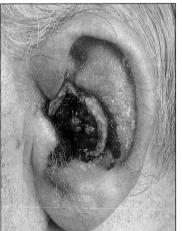

◀**Fig. 9.19**
Squamous cell carcinoma. The ear is a common site. The ulcer has a haemorrhagic crust and an everted margin.

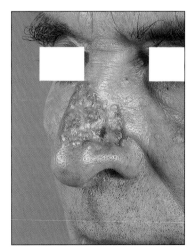

◀**Fig. 9.20**
Rodent ulcer. The lesion is locally malignant. It is frequently neglected, despite its visibility, because it is painless.

Pigmented basal cell carcinoma

This lesion has similar features to a rodent ulcer but the margins of the tumour are heavily pigmented (see Fig. 1.32) and thus occasionally it is mistaken for a malignant melanoma (Fig. 9.21).

Cystic basal cell carcinoma

Diagnostic features
- Nodular.
- Pearly colour.
- Smooth, telangiectatic surface.
- Lobulated.
- The face.

Clinical features
In this variant, the central part of the tumour does not break down and ulcerate until late in its evolution. It often achieves a great size, often being mistaken for a benign cyst. It is a well-defined papule which gradually becomes a lobulated nodule, which is pearly in colour with a smooth telangiectatic surface (see Fig. 1.6).

Morphoeic basal cell carcinoma

Diagnostic features
- Plaque.
- Pearly.
- Telangiectatic surface.
- Scar-like.
- The face.

Clinical features
This type is the most dangerous basal cell carcinoma and is the one *most likely to be misdiagnosed as a scar*, for it does not appear as a tumour at all, but as a slightly elevated, smooth, firm plaque (Fig. 9.22). Indeed, the term 'morphoea' means sclerodermatous or hardened skin. Telangiectasia and the pearly colour are important features. The lesion spreads insidiously and is invariably diagnosed late. Nests of tumour cells infiltrate well beyond the apparent clinical margins of the plaque, as well as infiltrating deeply into the dermis and subcutaneous tissues. It can therefore be difficult to discern the limits of the tumour, so that incomplete excision is not unusual.

Superficial basal cell carcinoma

Diagnostic features
- Well defined.
- Red, scaly plaque.
- Fine, rolled, telangiectatic, pearly border.
- Often multiple.
- Especially on the trunk.

Aetiology
Many patients with multiple plaques have received arsenic, often unwittingly as children, just like those with Bowen's disease. UV explains most solitary lesions. It is called 'superficial' because of its pathological appearance. Basal cells are seen as buds, often still attached to the epidermis, but dipping into the superficial dermis.

Clinical features
This lesion is frequently misdiagnosed because it is a plaque and not the anticipated nodule, and because it often occurs on the trunk or limbs. It is a slightly raised, red plaque with an adherent scale. It is very well defined, and careful inspection of its margin in a good light should reveal a very thin, rolled, telangiectatic pearly border (Fig. 9.23). After a number of years, the lesions may thicken and become nodular and ulcerated. *The superficial basal cell carcinoma is often mistaken for a patch of psoriasis*, just as Bowen's disease is mistaken for eczema. However solitary lesions, or multiple, asymmetrical lesions, sparing the classic sites for psoriasis (elbows, knees and scalp), should alert the physician to the correct diagnosis. Biopsy will resolve the difficulty. An occasional problem is a patient who has psoriasis which has previously been treated with arsenic, and has both conditions.

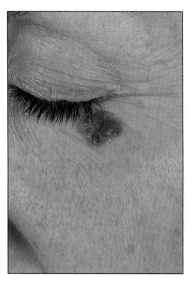

◀ **Fig. 9.21**
Pigmented basal cell carcinoma. Although heavily pigmented, the lobulated and rolled margin suggests carcinoma and not melanoma.

Diagnosis and management of basal cell carcinoma

Diagnosis

(1) **Histology.** The diagnosis can either be established by a skin biopsy or following definitive surgery.

(2) **Cytology.** This is a simple and efficient technique. The lesion is scraped with a sharp scalpel blade and the cells which are so removed are smeared onto a slide and fixed in a similar way to those of a cervical smear. Clumps of malignant basal cells can easily be identified after appropriate staining.

Management

The basal cell carcinoma is best managed by a dermatologist. Direct referral to a surgeon or radiotherapist by a family practitioner is an implied decision to treat accordingly. The average general surgeon does not have enough experience of the diagnosis and surgery of the disease and, worse, may delegate the lesion to be excised by a junior doctor. Radiotherapy is not always the appropriate treatment. Many dermatologists work closely with plastic surgeons and radiotherapists, and difficult cases may be managed in a combined clinic.

There are a number of effective remedies for this tumour and for many patients each one is as good as the other. The choice of treatment depends on the size, site and nature of the lesion and the physical condition of the patient. The latter is a very important assessment for the family practitioner to make and to comment on when referring the patient.

Curettage and cautery

This is the most common technique used by the dermatologist. It is suitable for small papular lesions less than 1 cm in diameter, and can also be used for superficial basal cell carcinomata of the skin. It is particularly suitable for the elderly and the infirm. The tumour mass is soft and friable and comes away easily when scraped with the curette. The surrounding fibrous stroma is more resistant and should be cauterized, and then scraped away again. Healing occurs within three weeks, with surprisingly little scarring, so this is an effective therapy in experienced hands. It is a very simple therapy from the patient's point of view and can be done quickly at the time of the consultation under local anaesthesia.

It is contraindicated for:

- Lesions greater than 1 cm in diameter.
- Lesions around the eyes, nostrils and ears.
- Deeply ulcerated lesions.
- Morphoeic basal cell carcinomas.

Otherwise recurrences may occur.

Plastic surgery

This is the treatment of choice in healthy individuals with:

- Lesions around the eye, nose and ear.
- Morphoeic basal cell carcinomas.
- Recurrence after radiotherapy.
- Younger individuals.

The plastic surgeon has the skills to excise adequately and to repair, either primarily or with a graft or rotation flap. The cosmetic result is usually excellent.

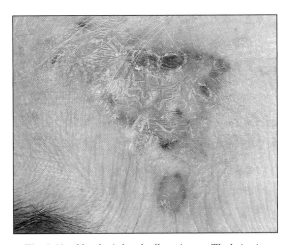

▲ **Fig. 9.22** *Morphoeic basal cell carcinoma. The lesion is a scar-like plaque with a slightly raised and rolled, and in this case partly pigmented, margin.*

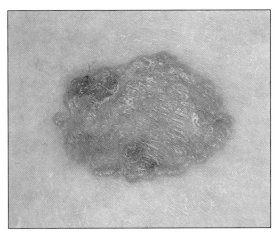

▲ **Fig. 9.23** *Superficial basal cell carcinoma. The lesion is a plaque with a well-defined rolled pearly margin.*

The success of the operation, that is, adequate clearance, can be confirmed by the pathologist.

Radiotherapy

Modern techniques of fractionating the dose have greatly improved the cosmetic results. Previously, single doses of irradiation resulted in scarring and sometimes radionecrosis. Radiotherapy is particularly suitable for:
- The elderly, and 'the timorous'.
- Large lesions.
- Surgical failures.

It should, however, be noted that radiotherapy cannot be repeated and should be avoided in:

(1) **Certain sites.** Irradiation of the ear, lower leg and back of the hand may result in radionecrosis. If possible, basal cell carcinomata of the lower eyelid should not be irradiated because this leads to loss of eyelashes, stenosis of the lachrymal duct and epiphora. These may be avoidable with plastic surgery.

(2) **Certain types.** (a) Morphoeic basal cell carcinoma is relatively radio-resistant and of course there is no histological proof that it has been eradicated after radiotherapy. (b) Superficial basal cell carcinoma may be effectively treated with radiotherapy, but it leaves a poor cosmetic result with prominent radiodermatitis.

Mohs' chemosurgery

This is barely available in the UK and in the US is limited to highly specialized centres. It is probably the best treatment for extensive invading destructive lesions and surgical failures. The principle of the technique is microscopic control at the time of the removal of the tumour, so special laboratory facilities are required. The undersurface of each layer of excised tissue is examined by frozen section until the margins and base are deemed free of tumour. It is painstaking, and is cost/time ineffective, for the majority of patients.

Topical cytotoxic agents

5-Fluorouracil is contraindicated, except for the treatment of superficial basal cell carcinomata. It is effective but recurrences are much more common than with Bowen's disease or solar keratoses.

Cryosurgery

Ordinary liquid nitrogen applied with a cotton wool bud is not effective, but liquid nitrogen cryoprobes and cryojets are used by some dermatologists. However, it is a fairly unpleasant therapy and probably has no great advantages over the others. It should only be used for uncomplicated tumours.

MALIGNANT MELANOMA

Definition

The commonest potentially fatal skin cancer, which paradoxically if diagnosed early is curable. It arises from melanocytes probably as a result of over-stimulation by ultraviolet light and may metastasize via lymphatics and the circulation.

Diagnostic features
Suspicious symptoms (CHANGE)
- Increased growth.
- Darkening or change in colour.
- Changes in shape.
- Sometimes itching or bleeding.

Suspicious signs (IRREGULARITY)
- Greater than 0.5 cm in size.
- Uneven distribution of shades and colours.
- Irregular outline or notching.
- Nodule formation (usually black).

Aetiology

Although malignant melanoma is still not very common in the UK, consultations regarding the possibility that a lesion might be one are very common indeed. The lesion is becoming much more common world-wide. The incidence has doubled in a decade in Scandinavia and Australia. It has quadrupled in the Caucasians, without rising at all in the Hispanics, living in Arizona. Similar increases are being seen in the UK

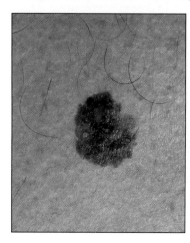

◄**Fig. 9.24** *Superficial spreading malignant melanoma. The back is the commonest site in men.*

where the incidence is approximately five new cases per 100,000, but this may be an underestimation. Queensland, Australia has the highest incidence in the world, 40 cases per 100,000. In the UK approximately a thousand patients die of the disease every year, which is a similar number to those who die of carcinoma of the cervix.

Ultraviolet light is the most important cause, and the incidence of malignant melanoma in those with the susceptible skin increases with proximity to the equator. The red-haired, blue-eyed, freckled individual with poor tanning and high burning capability has the greatest predisposition. The type of exposure is thought to be important. Whereas solar keratoses, and basal and squamous cell carcinomata occur in those who spend a lot of time out of doors and are chronically exposed, the superficial spreading and nodular malignant melanoma are much more evident in indoor than in outdoor workers. It is therefore suggested that intense but infrequent exposure once or twice a year, on vacation, may be more important than chronic continuous exposure. The exception is the lentigo maligna melanoma, which is a disorder of the elderly and seems to be related to chronic solar exposure.

Malignant melanoma is rare in childhood and adolescence, most common in the thirties and forties, but is seen frequently enough in the twenties. The lower leg is the commonest site in women and the back in men. The lower leg may be more vulnerable in females because they go stockingless in the summer and because modern stockings make for poor physical protection from ultraviolet light. The truncal distribution in males may be explained by the tendencies of men to take their shirts off when mowing the lawn (Figs 9.24 & 9.25) or working outside.

The acral lentiginous melanoma is rare in Caucasians but is the most common in Orientals and Negroes, and trauma may be a factor.

Nodular malignant melanoma is twice as common in males and usually presents after 40. It is the tumour most likely to have metastasized to a regional lymph node by the time of presentation.

Malignant melanoma metastasizes via the lymphatics to lymph nodes and via the bloodstream to the brain, lung, liver, bones and skin, and is ultimately fatal.

Previously, the prognosis was thought to be very poor indeed, but many believe that no one should die from malignant melanoma, provided the diagnosis is made early enough. Regrettably, too many patients present too late, not out of fear, but out of ignorance. Massive public education programmes in Australia (spearheaded by Queensland) and in the US have led to earlier presentation in those countries and are now being implemented in the UK.

The late Alexander Breslow, the pathologist, showed an inverse relationship between tumour thickness and survival so that the more superficial the lesion at the time of excision, the better the prognosis. The Breslow thickness is measured in millimetres from the granular cell layer of the epidermis to the deepest tumour cells in the dermis. He showed 100% survival in tumours less than 0.76mm, but only 50% 5-year survival in those greater than 3.5mm thick. Data from the Scottish melanoma group on the chances of five-year survival related to Breslow thickness are given in Figure 9.26.

▲ **Fig. 9.25** *Superficial spreading malignant melanoma. Note the varied colours and thickening indicating vertical growth.*

FIVE-YEAR SURVIVAL RELATED TO BRESLOW THICKNESS	
Breslow thickness (mm)	5-year survival rate (%)
<1.5	93
1.5–3.5	67
>3.5	37

▲ **Fig. 9.26** *Breslow thickness. Five-year survival rates are related to the Breslow thickness of malignant melanomas.*

Similarly, Clark related survival to depth of infiltration of the dermis (Fig. 9.27). He showed that levels 1 and 2 have a good prognosis, and that 3 to 5 have an increasingly poor one.

It has become clear that the growth characteristics and hence prognosis of the different types of melanoma vary. Thus lentigo maligna, superficial spreading and acral lentiginous melanoma spread horizontally initially and only subsequently invade vertically. Thus the prognosis is excellent in lentigo maligna which remains *in situ* for many years and in the superficial spreading malignant melanoma during its horizontal spreading phase before vertical invasion occurs. In contrast, the nodular malignant melanoma, which has no horizontal phase but grows vertically from the start, has a much poorer outlook. Prognosis is also determined by the site of the lesion, being much worse on the back (possibly because it is less visible) than on the leg. Females also fare much better than males.

Most malignant melanomas develop *de novo* in skin that was previously normal. However about 20% can be shown histologically to be associated with a pre-existent naevus (although this does not always correlate well with the patient's recollection of such a mole). As most Caucasians have 20 or more moles, prophylactic removal is neither warranted nor practical, nor cosmetically acceptable. However, there are certain predisposing conditions. The first two are discussed in Chapter 7.

(1) Bathing trunk naevus syndrome
(2) Congenital melanocytic naevi
(3) Dysplastic naevus syndrome (Familial atypical mole malignant melanoma syndrome — FAMMM).

CLARK'S LEVELS	
Level	Depth of infiltration of the dermis
1	Confined to the epidermis (*in situ*)
2	Infiltration of the papillary dermis
3	Infiltration to the junction of the papillary with the reticular dermis
4	Infiltration of the reticular dermis
5	Infiltration of the subcutaneous fat

▲ **Fig. 9.27** *Clark's levels. Prognosis is good for levels 1 and 2 but increasingly poor for 3 to 5.*

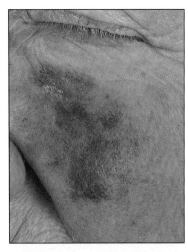

◀ **Fig. 9.30** *Lentigo maligna (Hutchinson's freckle). The lesion is irregular in outline and colour. It is flat and therefore confined in this case to the epidermis and is premalignant.*

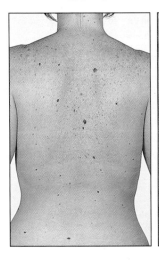

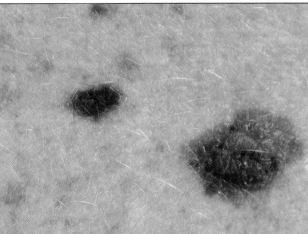

◀ **Figs 9.28 & 9.29** *Dysplastic naevus syndrome. The patients often have a lot of large ugly moles (left). On closer examination (right) the moles have irregular margins and are larger than ordinary moles.*

This is a recently recognized condition, in which patients have large numbers of atypical moles. Patients and their families are at increased risk of developing malignant melanoma. The naevi develop in the first or second decade and are much larger than usual, being 1 or 2 cm in size. They have atypical features of slightly irregular margins (Figs 9.28 & 9.29) and slightly irregular pigmentation. They are not obviously malignant melanomata, but on the other hand they are not quite as regular as ordinary moles. The diagnosis is made histologically. These naevi are very sensitive to solar irradiation.

Subtypes of cutaneous malignant melanoma

Lentigo maligna melanoma

Diagnostic features
- Most commonly on the face or neck.
- Most commonly in elderly patients.
- Very slow initial horizontal growth phase.
- Signs of chronic solar exposure.
- Easily visible and yet invariably diagnosed late.

Clinical features
The lesion occurs on the face, usually the cheeks, nose, temple, or forehead. It appears as a flat, pigmented lesion which gradually enlarges. The colours within the lesion vary from light tan to brown or black, sometimes with patches of red, blue, grey or white (Fig. 9.30). The margin is irregular, being notched or indented. Eventually, when invasion through the basement membrane into the dermis occurs, part of the lesion becomes thickened and eventually nodular (Fig. 9.31).

Superficial spreading malignant melanoma

Diagnostic features
- Young adults.
- Females predominate.
- Legs (females) and trunk (males) are the most common sites.
- Irregular outline and distribution of pigment.
- Nodule formation later.

Clinical features
The lesion begins as a flat patch of pigmentation which becomes just palpable (Fig. 9.32). It spreads out laterally and horizontally, has an irregular outline, often notched and indented, and has an uneven distribution of pigment and colours within it. There are various shades of brown (Fig. 9.33) often mixed with black and foci of red, blue and purple. The

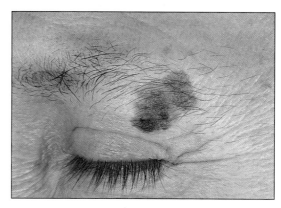

▲ **Fig. 9.32** *Superficial spreading malignant melanoma. It is astonishing that this lesion was neglected in such a visible site; it was diagnosed incidentally by the family doctor.*

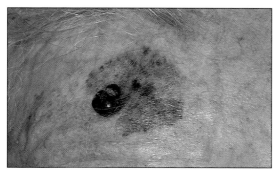

▲ **Fig. 9.31** *Lentigo maligna melanoma. Eventually invasion occurs and part of the lesion becomes thickened and in this case nodular.*

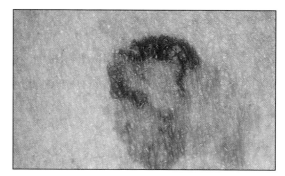

▲ **Fig. 9.33** *Superficial spreading malignant melanoma. The lesion is irregular in outline and consists of many different colours ranging from light tan to brown, grey and black.*

prognosis is excellent during this horizontal growth phase but diminishes with increasing Breslow thickness, as it thickens and becomes nodular (Fig. 9.34).

Acral lentiginous (palmar plantar mucosal) malignant melanoma

Diagnostic features
- Palms, soles, mucosae or subungual.
- Most common in Orientals and Negroes.
- Irregular, flat patch of pigmentation.
- Early development of nodular change.

Clinical features

The clinical features are similar initially to those of lentigo maligna, but invasion and nodule formation occurs early and consequently metastasis does so too. The lesion may occur under the nail, in which case there is usually a flat, irregular patch spreading onto the adjacent skin which begins to distort and split the nail as it becomes thickened (Fig. 9.35).

Nodular malignant melanoma

Diagnostic features
- Often bleeds.
- A nodule.
- May be ulcerated.
- Predominantly black, but often with a little thin eccentric margin of brown.

Clinical features

The patient notices the rapid growth of the lesion and often comments that it has bled. It is the malignant melanoma which is most likely to have given rise to this symptom. It is raised, nodular and in the later stages sometimes ulcerated. The outline may (Fig. 9.36) or may not be irregular. It may be predominantly black with little flecks of brown at the margins (Fig. 9.37). However it can be purple or red/brown with very little pigmentary change, although usually there is a tell-tale little rim of brown to one side of the lesion. It is not always an easy malignant melanoma to diagnose with confidence.

Differential diagnosis of malignant melanoma

The commonest diagnostic problems are seborrhoeic warts, pigmented melanocytic naevi, dermatofibromata, pigmented basal cell carcinoma, blue naevi, epidermal naevi and trauma.

All of these have been dealt with elsewhere except trauma. A commonly misdiagnosed condition is the *black heel syndrome* (Fig. 9.38). This occurs during vigorous exercise such as playing squash. It is due to haemorrhage into the stratum corneum secondary to shearing of the papillary capillaries. It is sometimes mistaken for a malignant melanoma but paring of the lesion with a scalpel blade reveals flecks of the blood in the skin.

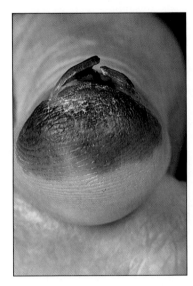

◀**Fig. 9.35** *Subungual malignant melanoma. There are various shades of pigment on the skin beyond the nail, with nodule formation under the nail causing it to split.*

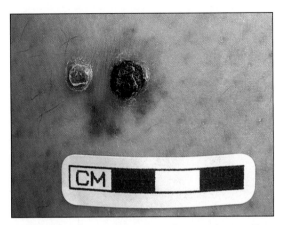

▲**Fig. 9.34** *Superficial spreading malignant melanoma. Two nodules indicating vertical growth have formed within the patch. This stage should not be allowed to happen. Note the notched outline.*

Management of malignant melanoma

Despite the fact that the lentigo maligna is visible on the face it is often quite sizeable at presentation, such that surgical excision and repair of the defect is technically complex. Since the malignant potential of the lentigo maligna is low, and the patient is often elderly and infirm, and not suitable for general anaesthesia, many physicians observe them at regular intervals, intervening only if part of the lesion becomes raised denoting the development of a lentigo maligna melanoma. Others, however, advocate surgery, radiotherapy or cryotherapy at an early stage.

Surgery is the only successful treatment for the other types of melanoma. In the horizontal stage the lesion can usually be excised and primarily repaired. If vertical invasion has occurred then surgical intervention is traditionally more aggressive with wide excision and grafting. This however is quite arbitrary for there is no good evidence that wide excisions are life-saving. It is quite probable that 'lumpectomy' will be all that is required in future, since radical excisions clearly have no effect if the lesion has already metastasized. At this time, until the controversy has been finally resolved, it is probably reasonable policy to excise the melanoma with a 1cm clearance for every (clinically) estimated millimetre of its depth. Amputation of the digit is required for malignant melanoma of the nail bed.

If the lymph nodes are clinically involved, they should be removed, but sadly there is no successful treatment for metastatic disease at the present time. In such instances, the patient should be referred to centres specializing in its management. Perfusion of isolated limbs with cytotoxic drugs is used for axillary or inguinal lymph node involvement, and various regimens of combined chemotherapy for widespread metastatic disease. However, it cannot be said that any one drug has been shown to have been of great benefit in treating this disease.

The most important goal in the management of malignant melanoma is widespread education regarding the dangers of ultraviolet light and sunburn, and regarding the features of malignancy, so that its incidence can be reduced and the diagnosis can be made early by patients and doctors.

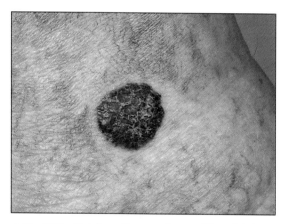

▲ **Fig. 9.36** *Nodular malignant melanoma. The nodule is black with an irregular outline and slight pale halo. It was present on the leg, the commonest site in women.*

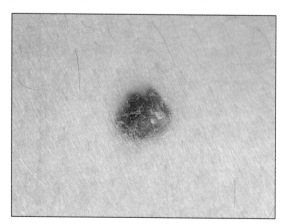

▲ **Fig. 9.37** *Nodular malignant melanoma. The nodule is black with a slight brown rim; it was only 1.1mm in Breslow thickness so the prognosis is good.*

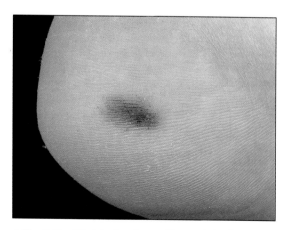

▲ **Fig. 9.38** *Black heel syndrome. Characteristic minute black dots due to haemorrhage at the edge of the bleeding into the skin.*

10 BACTERIAL INFECTIONS OF THE SKIN

INTRODUCTION

If the integument is intact and the host is immuno-competent, it is difficult to produce infection of the skin even experimentally. The relative dryness of the skin, natural antibacterial substances in sebum and the resident microflora limit colonization of the skin by potential pathogens. The resident organisms include *Propionibacterium acnes* (an anaerobic diphtheroid), aerobic diphtheroids, *Staphylococcus epidermidis*, a small number of anaerobic staphylococci and, in moist areas, Gram-negative bacilli. They only become pathogens if given the opportunity, for example around indwelling catheters or prosthetic valves.

The majority of primary pyodermas are secondary to *Staphylococcus aureus* or group A streptococci. They are common invaders of eczematous or traumatized skin. Staphylococci may also colonize the skin either transiently or, in certain sites such as the nose, more permanently as part of the carrier state. They may produce toxins such as the exfoliating toxin responsible for the staphylococcal scalded skin syndrome, or the pyrogenic exotoxin which causes the *toxic shock syndrome*. The latter occurs particularly in association with septic abortion and has been described in menstruating women using super-absorbent tampons. Fever, toxic erythema, multisystem involvement and circulatory collapse result.

Staphylococci are primarily transferred via the hands from nasal carriers and this is important in hospitals and nurseries. Host factors, especially immunosuppression and topical and systemic steroids, increase susceptibility to infection. The widespread emergence of staphylococcal resistance to antibiotics has become a major problem in therapy.

Essentially, all group A streptococci are haemolytic and can be identified in the laboratory by their sensitivity to bacitracin. They cause primary pyodermas and may spread via the lymphatics to produce lymphangitis (see Fig. 11.16) and suppurative lymphadenitis, and via the bloodstream to produce bacteraemia as do staphylococci. Other groups are much more likely to be secondary invaders. Non-suppurative allergic sequelae such as acute rheumatic fever, acute glomerulonephritis and erythema nodosum are limited to Lancefield group A, hence their importance and the need to treat them. Strains of pharyngeal group A streptococci may also produce erythrogenic toxins which result in scarlet fever or, more commonly, a milder illness and toxic erythema which results in a widespread desquamation particularly of the extremities. Streptococci are responsive to penicillin or, for those allergic to penicillin, erythromycin.

IMPETIGO

Definition
An acute, contagious and superficial infection of the skin, due either to *Staphylococcus aureus* or a beta-haemolytic streptococcus or both.

Diagnostic features
- Blisters which break easily.
- Golden crusts.
- Rapid spread.
- Often on the face.

Aetiology
The disorder is common in the young. It is contagious and outbreaks occur in institutions such as nurseries and boarding schools. The infected individual is otherwise healthy but sometimes there is a predisposing factor such as insect bites, head lice or trauma. A pre-existing skin disorder such as eczema may make the skin more vulnerable to secondary bacterial infection, in which case the term 'impetiginized' is used.

Clinical features
The patient or patient's parent invariably remarks that the lesions commence as blisters. In some cases the blisters remain for a couple of days, with yellow pus clearly visible within. Subsequently the blisters rupture and the purulent exudate dries forming golden coloured crusts (see Fig. 1.14). In other cases the blisters are transient and the crusts are the most apparent feature, although remnants of the blistering process may be seen at the margin (Fig. 10.1). The lesions are polycyclic or circinate in morphology and

may occur anywhere on the skin especially the face (Fig. 10.2). If the infection occurs more deeply a shallow ulcer occurs under the crust (Fig. 10.3) and the condition is known as *ecthyma*. This is more common in the tropics and often occurs on the lower limbs secondary to insect bites.

An uncommon complication is the *staphylococcal scalded skin syndrome* (Lyell's disease). This is a disorder of infancy and childhood and is usually contracted from other members of the family or school, who have ordinary impetigo. It is due to an epidermolytic exotoxin, usually from a group 2 staphylococcal infection, phage-type 71. The epidermis is split between the granular and squamous layers by the toxin. The child is ill and complains of burning of the skin. There is a diffuse erythema. Large sheets of skin separate away (Fig. 10.4) leaving behind tender, red raw and oozing erosions.

Occasionally 3 weeks after infection with a nephritogenic strain of streptococcus, nephritis may occur. This is becoming uncommon as socioeconomic conditions improve.

Management

The condition is rarely misdiagnosed, although herpes simplex, particularly primary attacks, is occasionally misdiagnosed as impetigo and vice versa.

Treatment with the appropriate antibiotic is effective. Although topical antibiotics may be used, systemic antibiotics for 5 days are more efficient and the eruption is usually cleared within 24 hours. Streptococci are responsive to penicillin (or erythromycin for those allergic to penicillin), but many staphylococcal strains are resistant and erythromycin or flucloxacillin is the preferred drug.

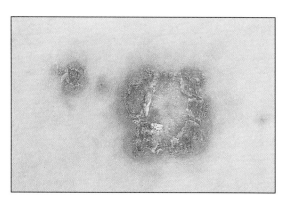

▲**Fig. 10.1** *Impetigo. The remnants of the blistering process are seen at the margin of the lesion and yellow crusting centrally.*

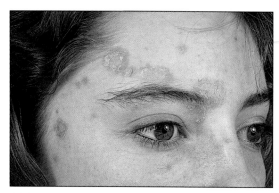

▲**Fig. 10.2** *Impetigo. The face is commonly affected. The eruption spreads rapidly.*

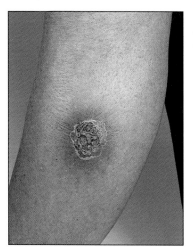

◀**Fig. 10.3** *Ecthyma. Adherent yellow crusts surrounded by erythema occur with an ulcer underneath. The lower limbs are a common site often secondary to insect bites.*

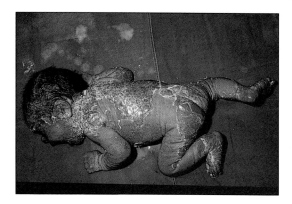

▲**Fig. 10.4** *Staphylococcal scalded skin syndrome. The skin is tender and diffusely red. Large sheets of skin separate away leaving raw oozing erosions.*

FOLLICULITIS

This term may be used to describe any inflammatory disorder of the hair follicle, but in this chapter only those disorders from which pathogenic bacteria are recovered are described.

Staphylococcal or streptococcal folliculitis (Bockhart's impetigo)
Definition
An acute painful, pustular eruption of hair follicles caused either by *Staphylococcus aureus* or streptococci, or both.

> **Diagnostic features**
> - Painful yellow pustules.
> - Surrounded by erythema.
> - Central hair in the pustule.
> - Limbs.
> - Often secondary to topical steroids.

Aetiology
It is caused by the above organisms affecting the outermost part of the hair follicle canal. It may occur *de novo* but it has become particularly common in eczematous or psoriatic patients being treated with potent steroids, particularly under polythene occlusion.

Clinical features
This condition occurs more commonly in the hirsute. Small, painful, distinct, yellow pustules surrounded by erythema are present (Fig. 10.5). In the centre of the pustule, a hair is usually discernible.

Management
The condition responds to erythromycin or flucloxacillin. In patients with underlying skin diseases a topical steroid–antibiotic combination should also be used.

Pseudomonas folliculitis
Definition
An acute pustular eruption of the hair follicles due to *Pseudomonas aeruginosa* contracted from poorly maintained whirlpools or jacuzzis.

> **Diagnostic features**
> - Acute onset.
> - Pustules.
> - Surrounding erythema.
> - Torso and limbs.
> - Exposure to contaminated whirlpools.

Aetiology
Outbreaks of folliculitis due to bathing in contaminated whirlpools have been described in the US since 1975 and are now being reported here. *Pseudomonas aeruginosa* is responsible. Whirlpools are more difficult to maintain than swimming pools, as the chlorine evaporates more easily at high temperatures and with continual agitation of the water; there is also high bather usage per unit volume of water and thus the concentration of organic matter is increased,

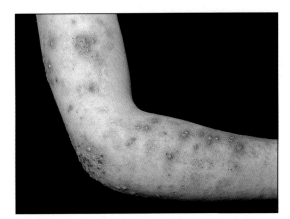

▲**Fig. 10.5** *Folliculitis. Small discrete yellow pustules with erythema surrounding the affected hairs.*

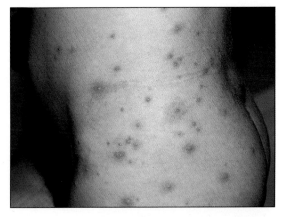

▲**Fig. 10.6** *Pseudomonas folliculitis. Widespread follicular pustules with surrounding erythema may result from using whirlpools contaminated with* Pseudomonas aeruginosa.

encouraging bacterial growth and reducing the chlorine to a less active form.

Clinical features

The patient may or may not feel unwell, with a low-grade fever and lymphadenopathy. Crops of yellow pustules develop in the torso and limbs (Fig. 10.6) 24–48 hours after exposure. Conjunctivitis, otitis externa, mastitis and urinary infections may also occur, requiring antibiotic therapy. The skin condition however is self-limiting and passes within 10 days of exposure.

Management

A swab taken from a pustule should grow *P. aeruginosa* on culture and will often give the clue to the diagnosis if it has not been made already. There is no treatment for the skin eruption and the patient makes a perfect recovery.

FURUNCULOSIS (BOILS)

Definition

An acute abscess of a hair follicle due to infection by *Staphylococcus aureus*.

Diagnostic features
- Painful.
- Red nodules.
- Pustular surface.

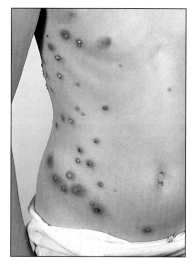

◄ **Fig. 10.7**
Furunculosis. Painful red papules and nodules are present with central pustulation.

Aetiology

The condition differs from folliculitis in that there is a greater degree of inflammation, which spreads away from the hair follicle into the surrounding dermis. The condition is due to *S. aureus*, which is usually also present in the nose, axillae or perineum. It is most common in adolescents and young adults, and the patient is invariably otherwise healthy. A search for diabetes mellitus, although always quoted in textbooks, is commonly fruitless.

Clinical features

A boil is a red, painful nodule, containing pus (Fig. 10.7) which discharges spontaneously and heals with or without scarring (depending on the depth of the lesion), the whole process taking several days. A carbuncle is a collection of boils, such that multiple draining sites occur; in this case, the patient may be quite unwell with a fever.

Management

If the boil is pointing, it may be drained of pus. In cases of multiple boils or in immunocompromised patients a swab should be taken and cultured and the patient started on systemic antibiotics. Erythromycin or flucloxacillin is usually effective, but therapy must be changed if the sensitivities of the cultures indicate resistance. Occasionally, an otherwise healthy patient suffers from recurrent boils. Swabs should be taken from the carrier sites (nose, axillae, scalp and perineum) and positive sites treated accordingly. In severe cases, the whole household should be investigated for a source of the staphylococcus. The patient should take systemic antibiotics for 3 months; in full doses for 2 weeks and then twice daily. The involved carrier sites should be treated with chlorhexidine and neomycin, or other appropriate topical antibiotics. Mupirocin is particularly appropriate since it has no systemic use, and therefore there are no fears regarding resistance. It is useful to add hexachlorophane to the daily bath.

ERYSIPELAS AND CELLULITIS

Definition

An acute infection of the dermis and subcutaneous tissues by *Streptococcus pyogenes*, and occasionally other organisms, which may cause a profound systemic disturbance.

Diagnostic features
- Sudden fever, rigors, vomiting and confusion.
- Unilateral erythema and oedema.
- Face or lower limbs.

Aetiology
The distinction between erysipelas and cellulitis is often not clear clinically, but the teaching is that erysipelas is superficial, involving the dermis and upper subcutaneous tissue, whereas cellulitis may involve the entire subcutaneous tissue. The margins of erysipelas are much more clearly demarcated than those of cellulitis, and streaking lymphangitis is prominent. Erysipelas is almost always due to a group A beta-haemolytic streptococci. Cellulitis is usually caused by *S. pyogenes* but *Staphylococcus aureus* or *Haemophilus influenzae* are occasionally responsible.

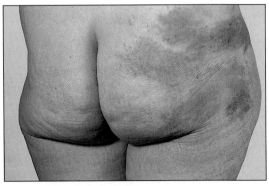

▲ **Fig. 10.8** *Surgical cellulitis. This patient developed recurrent attacks of cellulitis following an inguinal lymph node biopsy.*

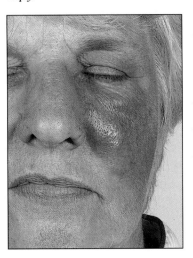

◄ **Fig. 10.9** *Erysipelas. There is unilateral erythema and oedema of the face. The patient is frequently quite ill, has a high fever with rigors and may become confused.*

The disorder may occur at any age, and the under-nourished, alcoholics and those with dysgammaglobu-linaemias are most prone. In clinical practice, however, the patient is often otherwise well and may endure recurrent attacks on the face or lower limbs. These are thought to be due to a lymphatic deficiency, possibly a pre-existing hypoplasia, which does not manifest itself until later on in life but is aggravated by the infection and tends to recur. The point of entry may be a minor abrasion, otitis externa, tinea between the toes, or following surgery (Fig. 10.8). Often there is no obvious cause.

Clinical features
The onset of the condition is abrupt. The patient becomes ill, has a high fever with rigors, and may vomit and become confused and occasionally delirious. Examination reveals a unilateral erythema either on the face (Fig. 10.9) or leg. The area involved is tender, red and usually oedematous, the oedema sometimes leading to blistering and erosions. Streptococcal infections may proceed to nephritis and septicaemia, rendering the condition a medical emergency. When cellulitis affects the leg a number of patients are left with persistent oedema.

Management
The condition responds dramatically to penicillin (erythromycin for those allergic or resistant to penicillin). Some patients however develop recurrent attacks, which can be prevented extremely effectively by a very small (250mg) daily dose of penicillin V or erythromycin for the rest of their lives, a fact which is often not well appreciated. The rationale for this treatment is not understood.

It is important to treat the portal of entry of the organism if it is detectable. For example, in those who have mycologically proven tinea pedis it is worth trying to eradicate the infection with griseofulvin.

ERYTHRASMA

Definition
An intertrigo caused by *Corynebacterium minutissimum*.

Diagnostic features
- Brown discolouration.
- Fine, scaly, wrinkled surface.
- Groin or axillae.

Aetiology

The condition is common in those who come from warm climates. It causes an intertrigo (a skin eruption occurring between two opposing areas of the skin) in the groins, axillae or under the breasts. A warm, humid environment is particularly favourable for the *Corynebacterium*, so it is commonest in hot countries in the flexures, especially of obese individuals. The condition also occurs between the toes.

Clinical features

The condition may be quite asymptomatic or itchy. There is a well-defined, brown discolouration (Fig. 10.10) with a fine, scaly, wrinkled surface, usually in both flexures. Between the toes, however, it is indistinguishable from tinea, for there is scaling, fissuring and maceration.

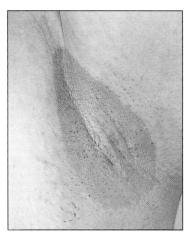

◄**Fig. 10.10** *Erythrasma. A well-defined brown discolouration with a fine scaly wrinkled surface occurs in intertriginous areas.*

Management

The condition fluoresces a very characteristic coral pink colour under a Wood's light (Fig. 10.11) and this is diagnostic. The organism can be seen under the microscope in scrapings of skin treated with potash. The condition responds well to topical imidazoles or sodium fusidate. Erythromycin orally is also effective.

TRICHOMYCOSIS AXILLARIS

Definition

A *Corynebacterium* infection of axillary and pubic hairs.

Aetiology

The condition is most common in young males and is largely due to poor standards of hygiene. The concretions of material found attached to the hair shaft are composed of masses of bacteria belonging to various *Corynebacterium* species.

Clinical features

Yellow collections of matter surround the hairs (Fig. 10.12). They are often an incidental finding not even remarked upon by the patient.

Management

Clipping away the affected hairs is usually enough, but 1% aqueous formalin or benzoic acid compound is effective. Daily washing of the area with soap and water usually prevents recurrences.

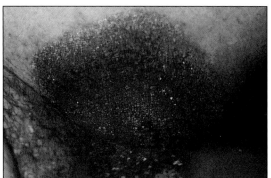

▲**Fig. 10.11** *Erythrasma.* Corynebacterium minutissimum, *which causes erythrasma, fluoresces a coral pink colour under a Wood's light.*

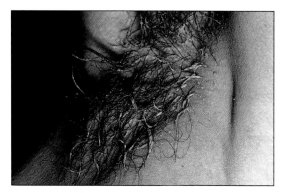

▲**Fig. 10.12** *Trichomycosis axillaris. Yellow concretions of material composed of masses of corynebacteria occur on the axillary hairs, usually in young males who do not wash properly.*

MISCELLANEOUS INFECTIONS AFFECTING THE SKIN

Introduction

The salient cutaneous signs of four important but much less common infectious bacterial diseases are briefly described here.

Tuberculosis of the skin and leprosy are becoming rare in the West but may still be imported. Syphilis and gonorrhoea although quite common are usually recognized early by the patient and treated in genitourinary clinics; but occasionally secondary and other manifestations of syphilis and gonococcaemia occur, and the diagnoses may be suspected from examination of the skin.

Tuberculosis of the skin

Tuberculosis may present in the skin as:

(1) Scrofuloderma. This results from direct extension from an involved lymph node or bone, classically in the neck or axilla.

(2) Lupus vulgaris. This occurs usually on the face as a result of lymphatic or haematogenous spread from a distant focus. It consists of a red brown well-demarcated plaque (Fig. 10.13) which when compressed with a glass slide (diascopy) reveals a brown colour reminiscent of apple jelly. Subsequently the epidermis becomes scaly and atrophic. Skin biopsy should be performed. Granulomas are found in the mid-dermis.

(3) Tuberculosis verrucosa cutis. This results from direct inoculation of the acid-fast bacilli into the skin usually in those handling contaminated material. It is rare.

(4) Fish tank or swimming pool granuloma. This form of direct inoculation, in this case of fish myco-bacteria, is more common. The granulomas — one or several dusky red nodules — occur along the site of lymphatic drainage from the initial point of entry, usually an abrasion on the hand following cleaning out a fish tank in which the fish have died of *M. marinum* or an abrasion received in a contaminated swimming pool.

(5) Tuberculides. These are immunological reactions to a tuberculous focus elsewhere. The most common is *erythema nodosum*, which not only affects the shins but characteristically also the calves (Bazin's disease). Occasionally crops of necrotic indolent papules arise on the extremities, a form known as *papulonecrotic tuberculide*.

Leprosy (Hansen's disease)

This chronic infection due to *Mycobacterium leprae* principally affects the skin and nervous system. The degree of involvement depends on the immunological state of the patient. If resistance is high, the skin lesions are few and neurological damage occurs early (tuberculoid or TT leprosy). If it is low, widespread skin involvement occurs with late nervous tissue damage (lepromatous or LL leprosy). Borderline (BB) and intermediate states BT and BL lie in between.

Tuberculoid leprosy

Skin lesions are few. They are well-defined annular red or hypopigmented patches occurring asymmetrically on the face, buttocks, elbows and knees (Fig. 10.14). The surface of the lesion is dry and scaly, does not sweat and is anaesthetic. The peripheral nerves — especially great auricular, ulnar, radial and peroneal nerves — are usually involved and thickened; sensory loss and motor palsies may occur.

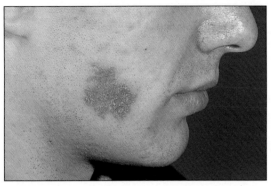

▲ **Fig. 10.13** *Lupus vulgaris. A solitary well-defined red brown plaque occurs, usually on the face. When compressed with a glass slide it has an 'apple jelly' colour.*

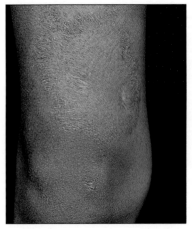

◀ **Fig. 10.14** *Tuberculoid leprosy. A well-defined annular dry anaesthetic patch is present above the knee. Lesions are sparsely and asymmetrically distributed.*

Lepromatous leprosy

Extensive symmetrical, small, red or hypopigmented macules gradually coalesce, with vague ill-defined borders. Anaesthetic plaques and nodules develop later particularly on the cooler areas of the face such as

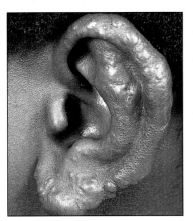

◀**Fig. 10.15**
Lepromatous leprosy. Extensive skin lesions occur. The cooler areas of the face are particularly involved as here with nodular infiltrations of the ears.

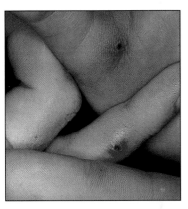

◀**Fig. 10.16**
Gonococcaemia. Discrete haemorrhagic vesiculo-pustules occur sparsely distributed on the extremities.

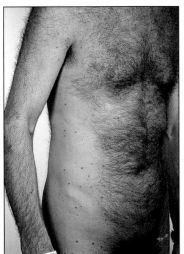

◀**Fig. 10.17**
Secondary syphilis. The rash consists of non itchy macules or papules which are pink initially becoming brown.

the lips, nose and earlobes (Fig. 10.15). Diffuse infiltration results in a leonine appearance. This variety, if untreated, is highly infectious from nasal discharges. Acid-fast bacteria are readily identifiable in skin tissue specimens.

Gonococcaemia

Gonorrhoea is usually diagnosed in its primary stage but in females in particular the discharge may be minimal or not noticed, in which case gonococcaemia may occur. The patient is unwell, has a fever and an arthritis involving one or several joints especially the knee, wrist and ankle. Discrete haemorrhagic vesiculo-pustules occur on the extremities especially the fingers (Fig. 10.16), palms, toes and soles.

Syphilis

The spirochaete *Treponema pallidum* has some features in common with bacteria. The disease is spread sexually although it may be acquired *in utero* or from infected blood products. Syphilis is divided into stages known as primary, secondary, latent and tertiary. The first two are infectious. The primary lesion or *chancre* occurs at the site of inoculation and is a painless ulcer (see Fig. 1.19) with a firm margin. The base is yellow and contains numerous spirochaetes. There is painless regional lymphadenopathy. If untreated it heals completed within 1–3 months.

A *secondary stage* usually ensues a couple of months later. The patient is frequently unwell, feverish, has general lymphadenopathy and other systemic signs. The skin eruption is characteristically non-itchy and widespread (Fig. 10.17); it especially affects the face, genitalia, palms and soles (Fig. 10.18). Initially it is

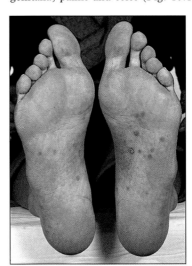

◀**Fig. 10.18**
Secondary syphilis. The soles and palms are usually involved.

macular and pink (roseolar) and gradually becomes papular and more widespread. There is a tendency to cropping of the lesions. The papules may become brown- or copper-coloured or scaly, resembling psoriasis or pityriasis rosea. In the *late stages* the lesions become more infiltrated. In the intertriginous areas, particularly the groin and anus, the papules may become moist and eroded (*condylomata lata*) exuding many treponemes. Oval, slightly raised, sometimes eroded patches occur in the mucous membranes. Hair loss is common. The patient may recover completely at this time or subsequently relapse (secondary relapse) with mucous membrane, genitalia and palmar/plantar involvement and then pass into a latent phase. Even during this phase the patient may recover. If not, it proceeds to *cardiovascular and neurosyphilis*, of which *the gumma* is the cutaneous hallmark. Indurated, red/brown papules or nodules result, usually arranged in an annular pattern in an asymmetrical manner. They may have a smooth or scaly psoriasiform surface. The nodules may break down and ulcerate.

11 VIRAL DISORDERS OF THE SKIN

INTRODUCTION

The diagnosis and management of common viral disorders that are referred to the dermatologist are described in detail here. The childhood viral ailments such as chicken pox, measles and rubella, which are familiar to and rarely referred by family practitioners are omitted for reasons of space and because their full description belongs to texts on infectious diseases.

HERPES SIMPLEX

Definition
An acute self-limiting affliction of the skin and mucous membranes, caused by a double-stranded DNA virus. After primary inoculation, recurrences are common.

> **Diagnostic features**
> - Premonitory symptoms of itch or tingling.
> - Grouped vesicles.
> - Surrounding erythema.
> - Progression to crusting.
> - Lasts 10–14 days.

Aetiology
Herpes simplex is a very common contagious muco-cutaneous infection caused by herpesvirus hominis. There are two antigenically different types of herpes simplex virus (HSV-1 and HSV-2). HSV-1 was originally only associated with oral and facial infections. Due to the increasing frequency of oro-genital sex, HSV-1 is now responsible for a number of genital infections. HSV-2 is most common on the genitalia and around the waist. It may be oncogenic, since carcinoma of the cervix is more common in females who have had genital herpes or who have HSV-2 antibodies.

The condition begins as a primary infection which is often subclinical, since many patients suffer recurrences and have herpes antibodies without any memory of a primary attack. In childhood the infection is usually acquired by droplet infection or by direct contact, for example, being kissed by an afflicted parent or friend. Rugby football players are at risk in the scrum ('scrumpox') from contact with another player with active disease. Patients with atopic eczema are particularly vulnerable to the virus.

The primary infection with the type 1 virus is commonly either a gingivostomatitis or widespread eruption on the face. HSV-2 infection usually occurs after sexual activity has begun and is manifested as primary vulvovaginitis or balanitis. This can occasionally occur in childhood, and in such cases child abuse should be suspected.

Following the primary attack, the virus resides in the sensory nerve ganglion which it reaches via the peripheral nerves. Recurrences occur in some individuals and not in others and vary in frequency, often decreasing with time. The factors governing the behaviour of the virus are not fully elucidated. However, ultraviolet light, mild upper respiratory tract infections, local trauma, menstruation and stress are precipitating factors. Patients with lobar pneumonia, meningococcal infections or malaria, if they are herpes simplex antibody-positive, commonly develop lesions (the so-called 'fever blisters') even if they have never had a clinical herpes infection before. Prior infection with type 1 virus does not protect against HSV-2 virus infections.

Clinical features
Primary infection
The onset is sudden with grouped macules which rapidly become painful vesicles which erode and form crusts. The eruption is extensive (see Figs 11.1 & 11.2): the lips, face and inside of the mouth (gingivostomatitis) may be involved in HSV-1 infections. The patient is uncomfortable and unwell, and may find it impossible to eat satisfactorily. In HSV-2 infections the genitalia are extensively involved, and urinary retention may be a complication. The patient is usually feverish and regional lymphadenopathy is present.

Recurrent herpes simplex
The lesion begins with a tingling or discomfort in the

skin, followed by a cluster of lesions which evolve rapidly from a macule to a papule to a vesicle surrounded by erythema. The vesicles are the hallmark of the disorder. The vesicles coalesce and become dry and scab. They heal usually without scarring, although post-inflammatory hyperpigmentation may be present. The attack lasts from 5 to 10 days. The diagnosis can usually be made from the history, even if the patient does not have an active eruption to examine.

The infection can occur anywhere on the integument, a fact which is not always appreciated, so that the condition may be confidently diagnosed on the face, but the same eruption on the buttock may be quite baffling. The genital form (Fig. 11.3) has become increasingly frequent since changes in moral attitudes in the 1960s. Females may have an infection limited to the cervix and therefore experience no symptoms, so that the disease is unwittingly transmitted.

Complications

(1) Herpesphobia. The disease in the main is of no consequence, but its effect on the individual varies. On the face it is temporarily and tiresomely disfiguring but on the genitalia it can give rise to enormous distress and anxiety. The publicity which the disease has received has transformed its importance, so that it has a significant morbidity.

(2) Maternal genital infection and delivery. The newborn infant has no natural immunity to herpes simplex and is therefore at risk of systemic infection if maternal genital infection coincides with delivery (Fig. 11.4). Caesarian section may then be advisable, if smears from the birth channel are positive.

(3) Kaposi's varicelliform eruption (Chapter 3).

(4) Disseminated herpes simplex infection. The immunosuppressed are at risk of widespread infection. These include those with leukaemias or congenital or acquired immune deficiencies, and those on immunosuppressive drugs.

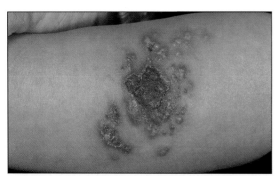

▲ **Fig. 11.1** *Herpes simplex. Grouped vesicles surrounded by erythema are followed by crusting, as seen on this infant's arm.*

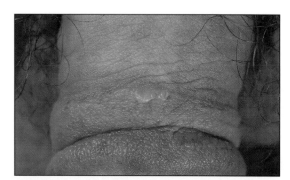

▲ **Fig. 11.3** *Herpes simplex. Grouped vesicles occur on the genitalia from sexual contact.*

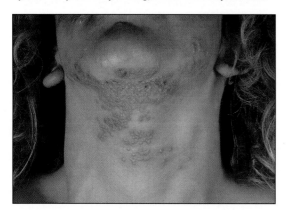

▲ **Fig. 11.2** *Herpes simplex. This young woman contracted an extensive primary herpetic attack from her boyfriend.*

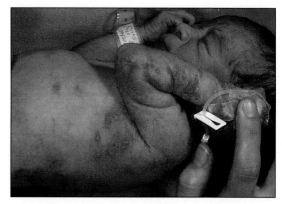

▲ **Fig. 11.4** *Neonatal herpes simplex. Widespread vesicles surrounded by erythema are present. Type 2 herpes simplex was cultured from his mother's birth canal.*

(5) Herpetic whitlow. This is no more than a primary infection occurring on a finger. Medical and dental personnel are particularly at risk, for they may unwittingly inoculate the virus from an infected patient onto the finger. Dentists should defer treatment of patients with active oral lesions if possible.

(6) Kerato-conjunctivitis. Involvement of the eye leads to a purulent conjunctivitis and corneal ulceration. The surrounding skin may be involved showing vesicles and oedema. Blindness is a complication and antiviral agents are gratifyingly effective if prescribed in the early stages.

(7) Erythema multiforme. A small group of individuals suffer from recurrent attacks of erythema multiforme precipitated by herpes simplex.

Management

The diagnosis may be confirmed by taking a swab for culture of the virus. In hospital the virus may be visualized in vesicle fluid under the electron microscope.

Although idoxuridine in dimethylsulphoxide and numerous proprietary preparations have been used over the years, the treatment of minor and major disease has been revolutionized by acyclovir. Acyclovir is an acyclic analogue of deoxyguanosine, one of the nucleotides of DNA. It is a specific substrate for thymidine kinase which is only present in herpesvirus-infected cells so that the virus takes up the acyclovir and viral DNA synthesis is inhibited. It has low clinical toxicity (headaches, nausea, vomiting or diarrhoea). It is not mutagenic, carcinogenic or teratogenic at therapeutic doses, although it is at very high non-therapeutic doses in animals. It decreases viral shedding time and consequently increases healing.

(1) Topical acyclovir. Acyclovir is available as a 5% cream and should be applied immediately the premonitory symptoms of itching are felt. It should be applied five times daily for 5 days and is a suitable treatment for minor recurrent herpes simplex. It does not prevent further attacks, but it does tend to abort attacks.

(2) Systemic therapy. Oral acyclovir, 200mg five times daily for 5 days or intravenous acyclovir is indicated for: (i) severe primary infections, (ii) eczema herpeticum, (iii) disseminated herpes simplex, (iv) herpes simplex in immunosuppressed patients, and (v) frequent recurrences. It is for the last group that it is most difficult to choose systemic treatment. There are some individuals who seem to be rarely free of attacks, especially of genital disease. Prophylactic continuous oral acyclovir (200mg three times daily) is

effective at preventing recurrences, but on stopping the drug the disorder recurs, often in a rebound manner. Although the long-term hazards of continuous therapy (development of viral resistance, carcinogenicity, etc.) are unknown, the psychiatric morbidity arising due to recurrences may be so great in some patients that a long-term approach may be warranted. The drug at present is expensive.

(3) Prevention of transmission. Patients should be warned that the condition is contagious and that they should avoid close physical contact. Condoms may reduce genital spread but abstinence during an attack is wiser.

HERPES ZOSTER (SHINGLES)

Definition

A painful affliction of cutaneous nerves with the varicella zoster virus. It represents a reactivation of a dormant chickenpox virus, a relatively large double-stranded DNA virus belonging to the herpes group.

> **Diagnostic features**
> - Preceding pain.
> - Vesicles.
> - Unilateral.
> - Distribution of a cutaneous cranial or peripheral nerve.

Aetiology

Herpes zoster is a common infection caused by the same virus that transmits varicella (chickenpox).

The virus lies dormant in the dorsal root or cranial nerve ganglion after a patient recovers from chickenpox, and antibodies are present in the serum. There may be a latent period of several decades before the virus is reactivated and commences to spread along the cutaneous nerve. Antibody titres are high in the acute stage of zoster and even higher during convalescence, which indicates that an amnestic response occurs. There is no convincing evidence that shingles can be contracted from another individual. The reactivation of the virus is a purely personal event, probably precipitated by waning immunological surveillance of the dormant virus. Certainly the immunosuppressed are at risk. Thus patients with leukaemia, lymphoma, multiple myeloma, on systemic steroids or undergoing immunosuppression during organ transplantation frequently develop the disease. Infections such as tuberculosis, syphilis, malaria and acquired immune deficiency syndrome (AIDS) predispose to zoster. Approximately 10% of patients with Hodgkin's disease develop shingles, often in a disseminated form, probably as a result of impaired humoral immunity. Absolute leucopenia correlates with severe systemic involvement.

Live chickenpox virus is present in the lesions of shingles until the scabs have formed. Thus the person who has never had chickenpox can catch it from a patient with shingles, although zoster is less contagious than varicella probably because oropharyngeal lesions are less common.

Although the disease is more common in the elderly, it is by no means restricted to this group. The trigeminal nerve is the most frequent cranial nerve to be involved in zoster and is the most frequent nerve to be involved in the elderly (Fig. 11.5). Overall the thoracic is the most common followed by trigeminal, cervical, lumbar and sacral. Second attacks of zoster are rare (4%).

Clinical features

The first symptom is the abrupt onset of pain or discomfort. Examination reveals an eruption which is limited to one side of the body and corresponds to a dermatome. The condition most commonly affects the nerves between T3 and L3 (Fig. 11.6). Each individual lesion begins as a red macule, which rapidly becomes a vesicle surrounded by erythema (see Fig. 1.33). The vesicle is very characteristic of the eruption. The individual vesicles may become confluent. They evolve over the next 2–3 weeks becoming in turn pustular, haemorrhagic and finally scabbed.

As these scabs fall off, a white scar may result. At any one time during the course of the disease, the actual lesions are at various stages of development and there are usually a few satellite lesions to be found away from the affected dermatome. Secondary bacterial sepsis with either *Staphylococcus aureus* or *Streptococcus pyogenes* is common and there is usually regional lymphadenopathy. The patient is rarely well enough to work, and is best advised to rest at home. For most individuals an attack of shingles is a tiresome interlude of 2–3 weeks during which they feel unwell and uncomfortable, but they make a full recovery with no sequelae. However, there are various complications.

Complications
Involvement of certain dermatomes
(1) **The ophthalmic branch of the trigeminal nerve.** The eye may become involved. The nasociliary ganglion is usually affected so that in these cases the side and tip of the nose will be involved by the eruption (Hutchinson's sign).

(2) **Ramsay Hunt's syndrome.** If the geniculate ganglion is involved, facial palsy may result. The ear is painful and vesicles are present on the pinna and in the external auditory canal.

(3) **Sacral nerve involvement.** Herpes zoster affecting the anogenital region may lead to retention of urine and difficulties with defecation.

(4) **Post-herpetic paralysis.** Paralysis of an upper or lower limb (usually temporary) may occur secondary to disruption of motor nerves involved by the dermatome.

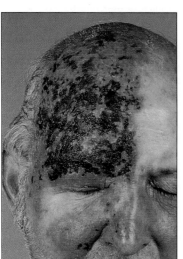

◀**Fig. 11.5** *Herpes zoster. The trigeminal is the most frequent cranial nerve to be involved and the most frequent nerve involved in the elderly.*

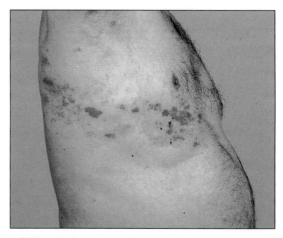

▲**Fig. 11.6** *Herpes zoster. The lesions are vesicles occurring unilaterally in the distribution of a cutaneous nerve.*

Disseminated herpes zoster

This is a serious disorder of the immunosuppressed. The condition begins as classical dermatomal herpes zoster, but vesicles then begin to spread out all over the cutaneous surface, as in chickenpox. Visceral, pulmonary, hepatic and neurological involvement may result and there is a significant mortality.

Post herpetic neuralgia

This is a miserable condition which occurs mainly in the elderly and persists long after the cutaneous eruption has healed. It is very disheartening and responds poorly to analgesics and psychotropic agents.

Management

The virus can usually be identified under the electron microscope but it can also be grown on tissue culture. There are a number of treatments:

(1) **Acyclovir.** Acyclovir 800mg five times daily for 1 week is the treatment of choice for all forms of complicated herpes zoster. It may well be life-saving in the disseminated variety and reduce the incidence of complications that are described above. Acyclovir does not appear to reduce post-herpetic neuralgia but it is very reasonable to give it to any patient over the age of 55. Post-herpetic neuralgia is less troublesome in younger patients, but even in these the drug can be considered.

(2) **Systemic glucocorticosteroids.** These have been advocated in the past as an anti-inflammatory agent for non-immunosuppressed, elderly individuals with herpes zoster. Prednisolone, 40–60mg daily for 2 weeks and with a reduction over the next 3 weeks, is given in an attempt to reduce post-inflammatory neuralgia. Recent trials, however, do not show any convincing evidence that this treatment is effective.

(3) **Topical therapy.** Five per cent acyclovir applied five times daily is gradually replacing 40% idoxuridine in dimethylsulphoxide as a topical treatment.

(4) **Analgesia and bed rest.** Analgesia is essential although it is best to avoid opiates. The benefits of rest at home are often underestimated. The treatment of post-herpetic neuralgia is highly unsatisfactory. However, it is always worth trying amitryptiline or carbamazepine.

(5) **Zoster immune globulin.** Although this is effective at preventing or modifying chickenpox if given early to immunocompromised susceptible individuals (including neonates) exposed to chickenpox it is ineffective at preventing zoster, since patients already have acquired antibody to varicella-zoster virus prior to infection.

MOLLUSCUM CONTAGIOSUM

Definition

A self-limiting mucocutaneous infection caused by a pox virus.

Diagnostic features
- Flesh-coloured.
- Dome-shaped papules.
- Central dimpling (umbilication).

Aetiology

The infection is caused by a large DNA virus of the pox group. It is common in children and young adults and it is contagious. Swimming pools, communal bathing facilities and close contact between children at play are the usual sources. In adults venereal transmission is also well recognized. The incubation period is not known but has been variably estimated at 2 weeks to 6 months.

Clinical features

The lesion is distinctly recognizable. It is an asymptomatic flesh-coloured or dome-shaped papule with a central depression on its surface. This 'umbilication' is the most important diagnostic sign (see Fig. 11.7). The papules vary from a millimetre to a centimetre in size. Multiple lesions are the norm, but sometimes a solitary one occurs and the diagnosis will be missed. The lesions occur anywhere on the body, but particularly on the face (see Fig. 11.8) and neck. Those occurring on the genitalia or lower abdomen are almost invariably contracted during sexual activity. An individual lesion lasts about 2 months but the outbreak resolves spontaneously within a year and rarely returns a second time, thus differing from the wart virus. As the lesion involutes, it may become inflamed or eczematous.

Patients with atopic eczema are more prone to mollusca contagiosa and often have widespread lesions, particularly if they are mistaken for eczema by the patient, parent or clinician and treated inappropriately with topical steroids which favour dissemination of the lesions.

Management

Multiple lesions are easy to diagnose. The umbilication is characteristic. Solitary lesions may not be suspected if the tell-tale depression in the surface of the lesion is missed; but it will not be missed by the pathologist, for it has a characteristic histology of a mass of homogenous, round bodies in the epidermis. These so-called mollusca bodies can also be viewed by squeezing the lesion onto a microscope slide, adding potash, and viewing under the microscope.

Since the lesions involute spontaneously and treatment with liquid nitrogen is not appreciated by children, some dermatologists leave lesions untreated but this is probably unsatisfactory as they remain a source of infection and most parents will press for treatment. The lesions can also be pierced with a cocktail stick dipped in iodine, which brings about their involution over a few days.

In adults with genital lesions, liquid nitrogen is the treatment of choice, and the patient and partners should also be screened for other sexually transmitted diseases.

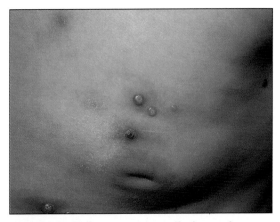

▲**Fig. 11.7** *Molluscum contagiosum. Erythema and eczema may surround the 'umbilicated' dome-shaped papule as it involutes.*

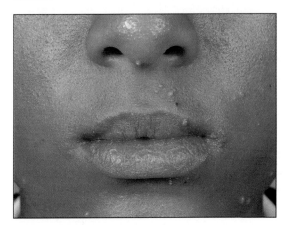

▲**Fig. 11.8** *Mollusca contagiosa. Widespread infections may occur, often on the face.*

WARTS

Definition

A very common papilloma virus infection of the skin or mucous membranes.

Aetiology

Warts are caused by a human papilloma virus (HPV). The incubation period is not exactly known, but in virus inoculation experiments an average of 4 months (range 1–20 months) has been calculated. It commonly affects children and young adults, the maximum incidence being at between 12 and 16 years of age. It occurs worldwide and the incidence is rising, accounting for 10–25% of skin outpatient attendances and thus occupying a considerable amount of dermatological manpower time.

Modern investigational techniques have confirmed that there are many types of human papilloma virus (HPV). Common mosaic warts are mostly HPV-2, plane warts HPV-3, genital warts HPV-6, and deeply inwardly growing warts of the palms and soles HPV-1.

Some wart viruses have long been recognized to be potentially oncogenic in animals.

It is now clear that malignant transformation in the cervix, vulva and penis is associated with genital warts of the HPV types 16 and 18. The other HPV types are not oncogenic, except for HPV-5 which is associated with a very rare skin disorder, epidermodysplasia verucciformis.

The infectivity of the virus in an individual depends on the viral load and host immunity. Cell-mediated immunity is most important and crops of warts are sometimes particularly florid in patients with Hodgkin's disease and in those taking immunosuppressive agents. Humoral immunity appears to be less important so that patients with multiple myeloma are not particularly prone to them. A previous attack of warts does not convey permanent immunity, nor does one type of wart virus convey immunity against another.

Warts are contagious and more easily spread if there is local trauma to skin or mucous membrane. They are common therefore in institutions where there are communal bathing and changing facilities. Hotel bedrooms, bathrooms and the swimming pool are the most common sources. Anogenital warts are clearly contracted from sexual activity. Children with genital warts present a special problem. Papers by dermatologists in the US and evidence from paediatricians in the UK suggest that a number of these cases may be secondary to sexual abuse.

Warts may be transferred to the lips and mouth through nail biting, or spread on the face through shaving, as part of autoinoculation. They are often seen on opposing toes, and are then known as 'kissing warts'. Certain occupations seem to make the patient more prone to the wart virus — it is particularly common in butchers. It is noticeable that patients with stubborn warts often have associated hyperhidrosis or a tendency to cool or cold peripheries.

Clinical features
Common warts
These are discrete, flesh-coloured papules, with a rough surface. They may be single or multiple and occasionally can be quite large. They are most common on the hands (Fig. 11.9) but may occur anywhere. They are usually relatively easy to treat.

Plane warts
These are flesh-coloured or pigmented, very slightly raised, well-defined, flat-topped lesions (Fig. 11.10). They have a smooth or very slightly roughened surface. They occur anywhere, but particularly on the face, hands and limbs. They are quite frequently misdiagnosed, particularly on the face, where they are liable to be treated with topical steroids, in which case they spread. They often occur in lines corresponding to a scratch or other such trauma (the Koebner phenomenon). Plane warts may be peculiarly persistent.

Plantar warts (verrucae)
These are discrete and only just raised, having a roughened surface. They can occur on the palm but are usually found on the sole, where they penetrate deeply because of the pressure of the body weight and are most difficult to treat. They may be quite painful and can interfere with walking. As they involute, minute haemorrhages occur within them (Figs 11.11 & 11.12) due to thrombosed capillaries. If they are pared with a scalpel, minute bleeding points are apparent, and this helps to differentiate a verruca from a corn (in which the skin becomes more and more normal in appearance as it is pared).

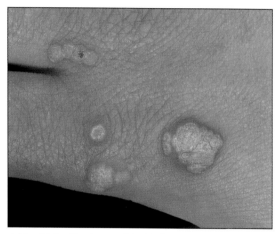

▲ **Fig. 11.9** *Hand warts. Liquid nitrogen is effective but in children is often too painful, and conservative measures are preferred.*

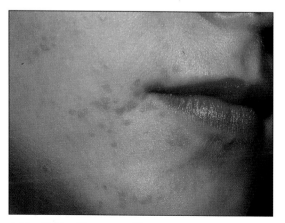

▲ **Fig. 11.10** *Plane warts. The lesions are well-defined, pigmented and very slightly raised. The face is a common site.*

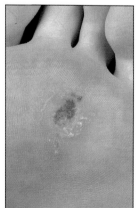
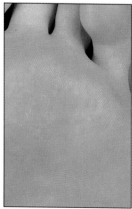

▲ **Figs 11.11 & 11.12** *Involuting warts. As veruccae involute minute thromboses are visible. The warts disappeared without treatment 2 weeks later. (Fig. 11.12).*

Mosaic warts

These are superficially spreading warts forming plaques of roughened skin with individual warts delineated within them (Fig. 11.13). They occur on the soles, heels, palms and around the nails. They last a long time and are particularly resistant to therapy. Fortunately they are rarely painful.

Anogenital warts (condyloma acuminata)

This lesion is soft, pink, filiform and often pedunculated (Fig. 11.14). It has a rough surface. It is found on the penis, scrotum, pubic area and around the vulva and anus, but it may occur within the urethra and vagina, on the cervix and within the anal canal. HPV types 6, 10, 11, 16 and 18 are mainly involved and are associated with vulvar and cervical cancer. HPV-2 has been isolated in a minority of cases, indicating that warts can be transferred from the hands. Genital warts may become quite exuberant, hyperplastic and cauliflower-like during pregnancy. Condyloma acuminata may be spread to the face (Fig. 11.15) from oro-genital contact.

Complications

Warts sometimes become secondarily infected (Fig. 11.16) and painful. Release of the pus with a scalpel relieves the pain immediately. Resolution of the warts often follows.

Diagnosis

Warts are rarely misdiagnosed. However, topical steroids are sometimes misprescribed, either for plane warts when the diagnosis has been missed, or for anal warts when the area has not been properly examined. *Viral warts are uncommon after middle age, so one should beware of such a diagnosis.* The lesion is more likely to be a seborrhoeic wart or a squamous cell carcinoma.

Management

Warts involute spontaneously. Thirty-five per cent have gone within 6 months, 55% within the year and 65% within 2 years. However, the response to treatment does decline with the increasing duration of the wart. Conservative treatment is often the wisest

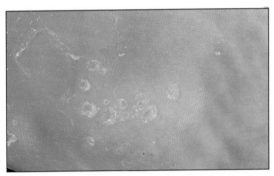

▲ **Fig. 11.13** *Mosaic warts. Well-delineated warts occur in roughened patches on the soles. They are most resistant to therapy but fortunately are rarely painful.*

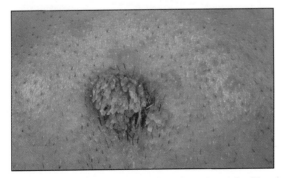

▲ **Fig. 11.15** *Warts. These well-defined papules on the chin, with a rough frond-like surface, were contracted from oro-genital contact.*

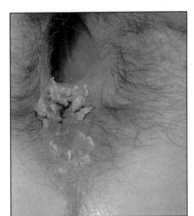

◄ **Fig. 11.14** *Anogenital warts (condyloma acuminata). Soft filiform pink pedunculated lesions are present.*

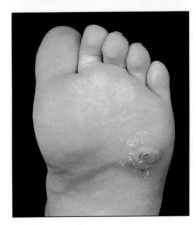

◄ **Fig. 11.16** *Infected warts. The wart is painful. A yellow swelling, containing pus, surrounds it. Lymphangitis is present.*

course, particularly in children. It is unfair to put them through painful procedures such as liquid nitrogen therapy, which essentially is what the referral to a specialist implies. Most warts need at least 3 months of treatment, so patients must be patient as well as dedicated. A wart may be pronounced cured only when the normal skin creases are restored.

Common warts

(1) **Salicylic acid preparations.** Paints made up of salicylic acid in flexible collodium are suitable, and there are various proprietary preparations. They should be applied accurately to the wart with an orange stick or a child's paintbrush as it is not necessary to spread them onto the surrounding skin. Ointment preparations are preferable as paints will spread and burn the skin.

(2) **Liquid nitrogen.** This is an efficient and usually effective treatment although somewhat uncomfortable. Children vary in how well they will tolerate it and occasionally adolescents will faint after treatment, so it is always advisable to treat such patients lying down. Liquid nitrogen causes an inflammatory response after an application of 15 seconds. Erythema results around the wart and subsequently oedema underneath it, which hopefully will result in blistering. The wart usually falls off within 2 weeks, as the blister breaks. If the lesion is overtreated, a painful haemorrhage into the blister sometimes occurs (blood blister). This is very painful but instantaneous relief is achieved by making a small nick with a scalpel into the blister and allowing release of the tension. A single application may be successful, but often a repeat course of treatment with longer application times is necessary.

(3) **Cautery.** If liquid nitrogen is unavailable, cautery may be used, but this will require a local anaesthetic limiting its usefulness.

(4) **Surgery.** This is normally unnecessary, but curettage and cautery under local anaesthesia is helpful for single lesions, especially those on the face.

Plane warts

These do not respond well to topical preparations and on the limbs are often best ignored as they eventually disappear spontaneously. For facial lesions however, freezing techniques such as liquid nitrogen — used accurately by an experienced practitioner for a short exposure — is often effective.

Patients with pigmented skins should be warned of the real hazard of post-inflammatory pigmentation, which may take months to clear.

Plantar warts (verrucae)

(1) **Topical preparations.** There are a number of these based on salicylic acid or in combination with lactic acid, podophyllin, glutaraldehyde and formaldehyde; they are available in liquid, gel, paint and ointment forms. These treatments are suitable for common warts, verrucae and mosaic warts, and each practitioner has his favourites. If they are to be effective, however, it must be impressed upon the patient that they are to be used regularly and conscientiously for several weeks.

I have found salicylic acid (either 20% or 40%) impregnated into a plaster useful. A piece is cut out from the plaster and shaped to the size of the verruca, applied, taped down and left on for 12–24 hours. The area is then pared or pummiced, and then a fresh plaster reapplied. This technique ensures a constant release of the acid into the wart.

All these agents act as keratolytics and are obviously a second-best treatment, but this will remain the case until effective antiviral therapy is available.

(2) **Liquid nitrogen.** Applications have to be longer (30–60 seconds) than for hand warts because the verruca is so deep. The treatment is painful, particularly shortly after it has been completed, as the cryotherapy causes inflammation. Redness, blistering and haemorrhage may result. The application should be repeated every 3 weeks and the patient can use a home-based remedy, such as salicylic acid plasters, in the meantime. Many treatments are often required.

(3) **Cautery.** This employs the same principle as liquid nitrogen but whereas a patient can usually tolerate the intense cold of liquid nitrogen, the heat of cautery normally requires a local anaesthetic, so that cryotherapy is more convenient.

(4) **Surgery.** Although surgery is contraindicated for multiple lesions, the best treatment for a single lesion is surgery. The local anaesthetic is painful and one must assess one's patient with care. Surgery is efficient when compared with multiple treatment with liquid nitrogen. A general anaesthetic is rarely if ever indicated.

A fine incision is made around the border of the verruca with a scalpel, allowing access to and purchase for the curette. The wart is scraped away, the bleeding base is cauterized and then curetted once more before final cauterization. No sutures are required, the procedure only takes 5 minutes and the wound heals within 2–3 weeks. The patient must be forewarned that the area may be uncomfortable for a few days.

Mosaic warts

These are the most difficult of all warts to treat successfully.

(1) **Topical preparations.** The same remedies as have been described previously for common warts are applicable. However, a useful form of treatment is formalin, either in a soak or ointment form.

Formalin, in a 3–10% solution, is put into a saucer. The patient puts a fine film of vaseline around the verrucae to protect the normal skin and then soaks the affected area in the formalin for 10 minutes daily. It is a simple and good treatment. It should be noted that formalin is a desiccant, so that it may dry out the skin, particularly on the heel. Occasionally allergic contact dermatitis does occur, which is no bad thing as this may vanquish the warts. Indeed, contact allergens such as dinitrochlorobenzene have been used to treat stubborn warts successfully. Alternatively, 10% formalin may be incorporated into propylene glycol vehicles such as Unguentum Merck. It is absorbed well into the warts and can be rubbed in with a cotton wool bud daily.

(2) **Liquid nitrogen and cautery.** These are used as described previously.

(3) **Surgery.** This is contraindicated. The warts are usually much too extensive for surgery to be practical and the recurrence rate is unacceptably high.

Anogenital warts

Genital warts are spread sexually, so patients should be examined and investigated for other sexually transmissable diseases as well. Proctoscopy is indicated in patients with anal warts and a speculum examination and cervical smear is important in females. Most patients are best referred to a genito-urinary clinic.

(1) **Podophyllum resin.** This is a cytotoxic resin which has been used mainly for genital warts, but it has to be used with care because it is irritant to normal skin. It must be applied accurately to the lesions, allowed to dry and then washed off within 4 hours. It is probably best applied by the doctor rather than by the patient, except perhaps for lesions on the penis. Application of a protective film of vaseline around the warts, prior to the use of podophyllin is recommended. Podophyllin should not be used in pregnancy or for large masses of vascular warts, because the drug is toxic and may be absorbed (it is not sensible to use it on the hands of children, even in combination with salicylic acid, since they might ingest the material). It has been suggested that it is a carcinogen, which is of some concern since certain types of genital warts, viz. HPV-16 and -18, are potentially oncogenic themselves so that the two could act as co-carcinogens.

(2) **Fifty per cent trichloracetic acid.** If podophyllum resin is contraindicated or has failed, trichloracetic acid applied once every 2 weeks may be tried. It does not need to be washed off. If it is accidentally spilt onto normal skin it can be neutralized by sodium bicarbonate.

(3) **Surgery.** Genital warts may be profuse, especially around the anus and then surgery is indicated. Thomson's strip technique is used, the warts being infiltrated with a solution of 1:300,000 adrenaline and normal saline. The swelling permits them to be visualized individually, allowing them to be snipped away with scissors, the bleeding being controlled with light diathermy (in order to avoid scarring).

CORNS

Warts rarely cause any problem with diagnosis, corns on the feet being the only exception, and although not anything to do with virus disorders of the skin they are described here for the sake of convenience.

Definition

A localized hyperkeratosis of the skin over a bony prominence, usually on the feet but sometimes on the hands, induced by repeated trauma to the skin.

Aetiology

Corns are localized callosities. Callosities are simply thickened areas of skin manifested histologically as hyperkeratosis and are a response of the skin to continual rubbing and friction. They may be self-induced by children or anxious adults picking or gnawing away at the skin on the side of a knuckle or a finger as part of a habit tic. They may be occupational, such as those seen on the hands in manual workers. Most commonly they are seen on the feet, caused by ill-fitting footwear worn over a long period of time in response to the dictates of fashion.

Clinical features

A corn is a localized, tender, thickened area of skin, with a central core over a bony prominence, usually the metatarsal phalangeal joint (Fig. 11.17). It may be differentiated from a verruca by paring as the deeper skin begins to appear more and more normal. Tiny bleeding points appear when a wart is pared. Corns are tender on direct pressure but not when squeezed between the finger and thumb. Exactly the opposite applies with a wart.

A soft corn is the term used to describe the appearance of a callosity occurring on the medial aspect of the fifth toe resulting from friction between that toe and its neighbour (Fig. 11.18). This is also due to tight-fitting shoes, but because of occlusion of the area the skin becomes macerated and white and is often mistaken for tinea.

Management

Corns are best managed by chiropodists. Attention to footwear and the use of metatarsal foot supports are very important. The corns themselves can be treated by salicylic acid plasters, paring and sometimes by excision and curettage.

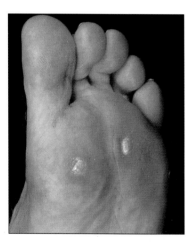

◀ **Fig. 11.17**
Corns. Corns occur over bony prominences and are a response of the skin to friction.

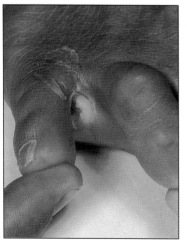

◀ **Fig. 11.18**
Soft corn. Friction due to tight-fitting shoes has resulted in a macerated corn between the fourth and fifth toe.

ORF

Definition

A viral disorder of the skin transmitted from contact with infected sheep or goats.

Diagnostic features
- Single or multiple papulovesicles.
- Lymphangitis, regional adenopathy and fever.
- On the finger most commonly.
- Contact with infected animals.

Aetiology

Orf is caused by a pox virus that can survive for long periods on inanimate matter such as fences and feeding troughs, and which infects particularly newborn lambs and goats. The pustular dermatosis occurs around the mouth and nose ('scabby mouth') of the animals and those tending them, for example by feeding orphaned lambs by bottle, are most at risk.

Clinical features

The condition occurs most commonly on the index finger. It has various stages, which heal uneventfully in 35 days. It begins as a red papule, which proceeds to become a nodule, with a red centre, white middle and red periphery (the 'target' stage) (Fig. 11.19). The surface begins to weep and then crust with black dots and then little papillomas on its surface. The crust becomes very thick and subsequently falls off. Regional lymphadenopathy, lymphangitis and a short-lived fever are common. Toxic erythema or erythema multiforme occasionally accompany the infection.

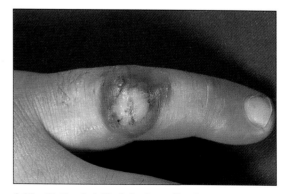

▲ **Fig. 11.19** *Orf. The lesion is usually solitary and on a finger is often contracted from infected lambs. In the 'target' stage the nodule is red centrally and has a white middle and red periphery.*

Management

There is no specific remedy, but secondary bacterial infection may require systemic antibiotics.

HAND, FOOT AND MOUTH DISEASE

Definition

A short-lived coxsackie virus infection resulting in vesicles on the hands and feet and in the mouth.

> **Diagnostic features**
> • Oval, turbid vesicles.
> • Hands and feet.
> • Erosions in the mouth.

Aetiology

The condition occurs in epidemics. There is a 3-day incubation after the coxsackie virus (usually A16 strain) has entered the buccal mucosa and small intestine. It travels to regional lymph nodes and a viraemia ensues.

Clinical features

The oval slightly yellow vesicles surrounded by erythema (Fig. 11.20) sparsely distributed on the hands and feet are characteristic. The vesicles break easily in

the mouth and erosions result. There is a mild systemic disturbance. The condition lasts 7 days.

Management

There is no specific remedy. The condition does not recur.

ACQUIRED IMMUNE DEFICIENCY SYNDROME

This syndrome is caused by a human immunodeficiency virus (HIV) which is often referred to as the human T-cell lymphotrophic virus III (HTLV-III). It is a retrovirus which is largely transmitted by infected homosexuals or infected blood products or needles (haemophiliacs and drug addicts have been especially at risk).

The patient is particularly prone to opportunistic infections (especially *Pneumocystis carinii*, cytomegalovirus, *Aspergillus*, *Candida* and *Cryptococcus*) as a result of immune deficiency. Lymphadenopathy, malaise, fever, weight loss and neurological disorders are other features. The cutaneous signs are similar to those of Kaposi's sarcoma and consist of deep red or purple papules, plaques or nodules (Fig. 11.21) anywhere on the skin but particularly on the head and neck.

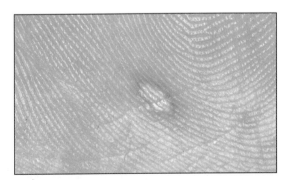

▲**Fig. 11.20** *Hand, foot and mouth disease. Oval white or slightly yellow vesicles are sparsely distributed on the hands and feet.*

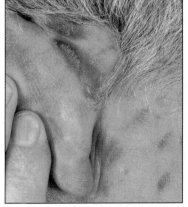

◄**Fig. 11.21** *AIDS. Purple papules, nodules or plaques which are similar to the skin lesions of Kaposi's sarcoma occur particularly on the head and neck.*

12 FUNGAL DISORDERS OF THE SKIN

INTRODUCTION

The very common superficial fungal infections of the skin are described here. Deep fungal infections, such as blastomycosis or coccidiomycosis are rare and therefore their description is omitted.

CANDIDOSIS (CANDIDIASIS)

Introduction

Candidosis is a common infection of the mouth, genitalia, flexures and nails. It is usually caused by *Candida albicans*. This is an oval yeast in its commensal state but in its pathogenic state it divides by budding and produces pseudohyphae.

Eighty percent of normal individuals harbour the yeast as a commensal in the oropharynx, gastrointestinal tract or vagina. It is rarely found on normal skin, except in occluded intertriginous sites. Indeed it is not possible to produce candidosis experimentally on normal skin without occlusion, which increases the local moisture and temperature, providing ideal conditions for incubating the yeast. Candidosis thrives when the stratum corneum is damaged, for example where two apposing folds of skin rub together in the flexures in the obese, or in the mouth under an ill-fitting denture.

Candidosis is more common at the extremes of age and during pregnancy or the menses. Certain systemic disorders predispose to it, for example diabetes mellitus, Cushing's disease, uraemia and malignant disease. Immunodeficiency — humoral and, more especially, cell-mediated (which is the major fault in the rare disease of chronic mucocutaneous candidosis) — is a frequent cause. Neutropenic patients are particularly vulnerable because phagocytosis of candidal organisms depends on functioning polymorphonuclear leucocytes and macrophages.

Candida is a great opportunist and makes the most of iatrogenic opportunities. Broad spectrum antibiotics eradicate the microbial flora which compete with *Candida* for nutrients so that the *Candida* may flourish. Systemic and topical steroids are immunosuppressive and favour the overgrowth of *Candida*.

Indwelling urinary and vascular catheters and intravenous drug abusers provide opportunities for systemic candidosis.

Factors favouring candidosis
(1) Occlusion.
(2) Damage to the stratum corneum.
(3) Immunosuppression.
(4) Neutropenia.
(5) Endocrinopathies, for example diabetes mellitus, Cushing's disease.
(6) Uraemia and malignant disease.
(7) Extremes of age, menses and pregnancy.
(8) Iatrogenic factors, for example antibiotics, oral contraceptives, steroids.

Oral candidosis (syn. thrush)
Definition
An infection of the mouth by the yeast *Candida albicans*.

Diagnostic features
- Pustules which can be easily scraped away.
- Red, raw, bleeding base.

Aetiology
The condition is common in the neonatal period, when immunological defence systems are poorly developed, and is contracted from the mother during

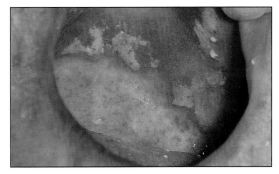

▲ **Fig. 12.1** *Oral candidosis. Confluent white or cream-coloured pustules may easily be scraped off leaving a red raw base.*

vaginal delivery. It is common in very sick and immunosuppressed adults. The condition also occurs in otherwise healthy individuals, who are edentulous and neglect their oral and denture hygiene.

Clinical features

The infant may be in distress or present with feeding difficulties, whereas the adult complains of a sore mouth. On examination there are well-defined white or cream-coloured pustules which occur on the palate (see Fig. 12.1), tongue, buccal mucous membranes or gums. The lesions are easily scraped away with a spatula leaving behind a red, raw, bleeding base.

Differential diagnosis

The condition is rarely misdiagnosed although lichen planus (see Fig. 6.12) is sometimes mistaken for thrush. However, a swab from a pustule and growth of the organism on culture permits identification.

Angular cheilitis
Definition

A red scaly and often raw condition occurring at the angles of the mouth due to *Candida albicans*.

> **Diagnostic features**
> * Erythema, scaling, rawness and cracking.
> * Sides of the mouth.
> * Distortion of the angles of the mouth.
> * Associated with ill-fitting dentures.

Aetiology

Although classically described in the malnourished, in Western societies the condition is seen more frequently in patients who are either edentulous or wear dentures that do not fit properly and are not cleaned adequately. The conformation of the mouth becomes

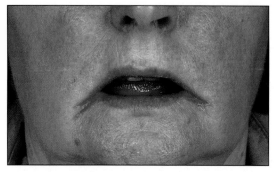

▲ **Fig. 12.2** *Angular cheilitis. Red and raw fissures occur, particularly in those with ill-fitting dentures, which distort the contours of the mouth.*

distorted and sags, such that the upper lip tends to overhang the lower, and a groove forms at the corners of the mouth. Saliva trickles imperceptibly down the fold, which becomes moist and provides a perfect habitat for *C. albicans* to flourish. The patient often sleeps with the denture in position at night and cleans the denture infrequently, or not at all. The denture traumatizes the gums and palate, facilitating the entry of organisms. The condition can also be produced by *Staphylococcus aureus* and sometimes both organisms coexist.

Clinical features

The angles of the mouth are sore, raw and fissured with adjacent erythema and slight scaling, with associated downturning of the corners of the mouth (Fig. 12.2). If the patient is wearing a denture there may be thrush present underneath it.

Genital candidosis

Candida vulvovaginitis
Definition

An infection with *Candida albicans* usually originating in the vagina which may spread to the vulva.

> **Diagnostic features**
> * Irritation.
> * Abundant thick cream-coloured discharge.
> * Erythema and oedema.
> * Maceration and satellite pustules on the skin.

Aetiology

This is a very common infection in young, otherwise healthy women, often precipitated by broad spectrum antibiotics, oral contraceptive therapy (particularly if prescribed together) or pregnancy. In addition, tight-fitting clothing (for example fashionable jeans) produces an occluded warm and moist environment which compounds the problem. Candidal vulvovaginitis can be a presentation of diabetes mellitus in middle-aged, often overweight females, so that it is mandatory to test for glycosuria.

Clinical features

The condition is itchy and sore. A thick, abundant, cream-coloured discharge occurs with associated vaginal erythema and oedema. If the vaginitis is neglected, the adjoining skin becomes involved and an intertrigo results.

Candida balanitis
Definition
An infection of the glans penis with *Candida albicans*.

Diagnostic features
- Yellow pustules.
- Erythema and oedema of glans penis.
- Often uncircumcised.

Aetiology
Candida balanitis is usually acquired from a sexual partner who has active disease. It is much more common in the uncircumcised as the prepuce provides an ideal occluded microenvironment in which the yeast may flourish.

Clinical features
The glans may be red and swollen with yellow pustules, but sometimes the physical signs are much less marked, and the patient complains of tiny pustules which rupture within a few hours.

Candida intertrigo
Definition
An infection with *Candida albicans* occurring between two apposing folds of skin.

Diagnostic features
- Flexures.
- Corpulent individuals.
- Pustules surrounded by erythema.
- Maceration.
- Raw denuded skin.

Aetiology
Intertrigo is a dermatological term indicating an eruption occurring between two apposing skin surfaces.

Thus axillae, groins, submammary regions, and folds secondary to obesity are the most common sites. However the nail folds (see chronic paronychia — later) and the skin between the fingers are also intertriginous sites and infection occurs in those who get their hands wet a lot. Although other skin disorders may occur in these areas, for example seborrhoeic eczema and psoriasis, they are ideal sites for candidosis since they are warm, moist and subject to friction.

Clinical features
The lesions begin as pustules surrounded by erythema (Fig. 12.3). The pustules become confluent and break, leaving behind red, raw skin (Fig. 12.4). The outer margins of the eruption are often macerated, so that the skin appears white, thickened and sodden. Satellite lesions are characteristic and consist of fresh pustules away from the central, red, raw core of the rash. When the condition occurs between the finger webs it is known as *erosio interdigitale*. The pustules break easily leaving a raw erosion surrounded by maceration (Fig. 12.5).

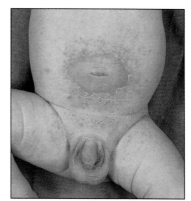

◀ **Fig. 12.4** *Candida intertrigo. A raw erythema is present around the umbilicus, with satellite pustules surrounded by erythema away from the main body of the eruption.*

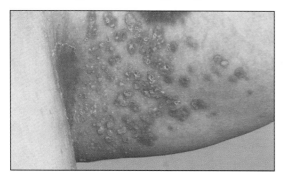

▲ **Fig. 12.3** *Candida intertrigo. The lesions begin as red pustules which become confluent and break, resulting in red raw skin.*

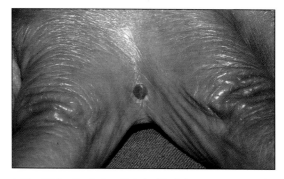

▲ **Fig. 12.5** *Erosio interdigitale. The lesion starts as a pustule which breaks leaving a raw area surrounded by maceration.*

Management of candidosis

A swab should be taken for microscopy, and for culture to confirm the diagnosis, if possible. The urine should be tested for glucose.

Oral candidosis and angular cheilitis

Oral candidosis can usually be remedied with an anti-*Candida* agent in lozenge, pastille, gel or suspension form. Examples are nystatin oral suspension, amphotericin lozenges or oral suspension and miconazole nitrate oral gel. Oral hygiene is of the utmost importance when nursing an ill patient who cannot clean his mouth and teeth properly. Patients with angular cheilitis should be told not to sleep with the denture in the mouth and should be taught to sterilize it overnight. Faulty dentures should be corrected by the dentist. Antimicrobials alone are often not effective for cheilitis because the inflammation will not respond. This is one of the few occasions for polypharmacy, that is, a combination product containing an anti-inflammatory, an anti-fungal and, often, an antibacterial agent such as: nystatin, hydrocortisone and benzalkonium; nystatin, hydrocortisone and chlorhexidine; clioquinol and hydrocortisone; miconazole and hydrocortisone. A facelift is sometimes necessary in severe cases to correct the groove at the angles of the mouth.

Genital candidosis

Genital candidosis may be treated with nystatin or imidazole creams and, in females, pessaries. Precipitating causes — antibiotics, oral contraceptives, partner infection and diabetes — should be remedied.

Candida intertrigo

Candida intertrigo responds to creams or ointments. Combination with hydrocortisone, and sometimes an anti-bacterial, is often necessary. Old-fashioned preparations such as Castellani's paint (0.4% magenta, 4% phenol with resorsinol, acetone, industrial methylated spirits and water) or 0.5% aqueous gentian violet are very helpful in severe cases.

Drugs used in management of candidosis

Nystatin is a polyene antibiotic. It is too toxic to use parenterally but is effective topically. Its disadvantage is that it is yellow and can stain clothing. It can be taken orally, because it is not absorbed, and so is used to sterilize the gut in recurrent cases. Amphotericin B, another polyene antibiotic, is used in a similar manner to nystatin. Both are ineffective against other superficial fungi but amphotericin is used systemically for deep mycotic infections.

The imidazoles are pleasant and easy to use and have a broad spectrum, being also effective against tinea and pityriasis versicolor. In addition, an effective oral imidazole, ketoconazole, is available for severe cases. A drug-induced hepatitis occasionally occurs, especially in those who abuse alcohol, even after 1–2 weeks of therapy. Liver function tests are advisable before and during treatment. Since it blocks ergosteroid synthesis, reduction in libido, gynaecomastia and hypoadrenalism occasionally occurs. Itraconazole, a new oral triazole, is also effective.

PITYRIASIS VERSICOLOR

Definition

A superficial yeast infection mainly of the torso. The yeast, which is ordinarily a commensal, becomes pathogenic in warm, humid conditions.

Diagnostic features
- Macules of various shapes and sizes.
- Brown or off-white (versicolor).
- Fine scales (pityriasis).
- Trunk.
- Asymmetrical.
- Young adults.

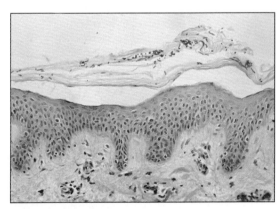

▲ **Fig. 12.6** *Pityriasis versicolor. The fungus lives in the stratum corneum and the pseudohyphae are stained purple with periodic acid Schiff (PAS).*

Aetiology

Pityriasis versicolor is caused by the unicellular yeasts *Pityriasis orbiculare* and *P. ovale*, which are commensals of the skin. They become pathogenic by budding and producing filaments known as pseudohyphae (in this state, the organism is sometimes known as malassezia furfur). The yeast is lipophilic and requires the mature sebaceous gland for growth, so that the condition is rarely seen in the West before puberty but is a common disorder of young adults. The yeast is an opportunist, and growth in the stratum corneum (Fig. 12.6) is encouraged by an increase in environmental temperature and humidity; thus many patients notice that the condition begins after a summer vacation. It is a disorder of the healthy, but the immunosuppressed are at risk. Topical glucocorticosteroids account for many of the widespread cases as the fungus thrives if these are mistakenly prescribed (Figs 12.7 & 12.8). The fungus is of a low infectivity and it is unusual for the disorder to be transmitted to another person.

Clinical features

The condition is insidious in onset and asymptomatic, taking months to become sufficiently widespread to be noticed by any but the most fastidious patients. Most patients present with patches on their skin that do not tan properly, and recognize that there is something wrong with the pigmentation. The condition starts as a macule, which sometimes surrounds the orifice of a hair follicle. Since the fungus invades the stratum corneum, the condition is scaly although this may not be immediately obvious. It can be highlighted by scraping the surface with a blunt scalpel — many fine scales (pityriasis) can be seen on the blade — this sign disappears after treatment.

The colour of the lesions varies. In coloured individuals, the macules may be darker or lighter than the surrounding normal skin in any one individual (Fig. 12.9). In an untanned Caucasian, the lesions are brown or fawn-coloured (Fig. 12.7); however, if a suntan is acquired, the lesions appear pale in comparison to the surrounding tanned skin (Fig. 12.10).

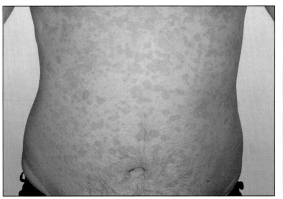

◀**Figs 12.7 & 12.8** *Pityriasis versicolor. Fawn-coloured macules (Fig. 12.8) are characteristic and may become extensive if mistreated with topical steroids.*

▲ **Fig. 12.9** *Pityriasis versicolor. Hyperpigmented macules are present on this West Indian's skin. Scaling, if not visible, may be demonstrated by scraping the skin with a blunt scalpel.*

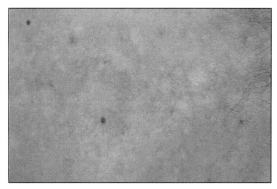

▲ **Fig. 12.10** *Pityriasis versicolor. The lesions may be hypopigmented rather than fawn-coloured or be a mixture of both.*

This is partly because the melanocytes are shielded from ultraviolet radiation by the diseased skin, but there is also evidence that the melanocytes are temporarily damaged by dicarboxylic acids produced by the fungus. Indeed, in treated individuals who are suntanned, the patches may still appear an off-white colour, and it is *often misdiagnosed as incurable vitiligo* (Fig. 12.11); repigmentation may take many months. Pityriasis versicolor may be distinguished from vitiligo, a symmetrical condition, because of its truncal distribution and the asymmetry of the patches.

The macules grow and coalesce, and various shapes and sizes are achieved in an asymmetrical distribution. The condition occurs primarily on the front of the chest, neck and back. The limbs are rarely affected except in extensive cases where topical steroids have been erroneously prescribed. It is very unusual for the face to be involved, despite the fact that it is liberally supplied with the lipid substrate favoured by the organism in the sebaceous glands.

Management

The fungus is easy to demonstrate under the microscope. The lesion is scraped with a blunt scalpel, and the scales are put onto a microscope slide. Thirty per cent potassium hydroxide is added, and thick-walled, spherical yeasts with pseudohyphae can be visualized. Since the yeast takes up certain ink stains, the best preparations are made by adding equal parts of Parker's blue-black ink to the potassium hydroxide, so that the blue ink highlights the organism (Fig. 12.12). The diagnosis can also be established by examining the skin under a Wood's light: the affected areas fluoresce a yellow colour.

The condition is gratifyingly simple to treat, but a certain amount of explanation is required about the pseudovitiliginous state and the possibility of recurrences. All treatments must be performed thoroughly, because clearly if one patch is left behind untreated it proceeds to spread again. It is useful to have a partner treat the back, whilst the patient treats the front. The commonly used treatments are:

(1) **Half-strength Whitfield's ointment.** This is 3% salicylic acid, 6% benzoic acid, 64% cocois oil in soft paraffin. Irritation is a common side-effect and to a large extent the ointment has been superceded by the imidazoles.

(2) **Imidazoles.** These are all effective topically and should be applied once daily for 3 weeks. They are available over-the-counter.

(3) **Selenium sulphide shampoo.** Selenium sulphide is an effective remedy, and is used for widespread cases. It is applied once a week for 8 weeks, but must be washed off 4–5 hours after application, to avoid irritation. It is an effective treatment, but some patients do not like the smell.

(4) **Oral therapy.** *The condition does not respond to griseofulvin* and for this reason the alternative name 'tinea versicolor' should be abandoned, for it gives a false impression. Pityriasis versicolor does respond to ketoconazole 200mg daily or itraconazole 100mg daily, for 5 days. Since there are adequate topical measures for treating this disease, oral agents are usually unnecessary.

Response to treatment

Death of the fungus occurs within 3–4 weeks of thorough treatment. However in those with pronounced hypopigmentation, although the scaling (the sign of the active disease) disappears, white areas remain. The melanocytes do recover and start producing pigment once again, but it may take many months and

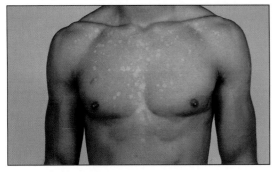

▲ **Fig. 12.11** *Pityriasis versicolor. In some patients a pseudo vitiliginous state results from temporary damage to the melanocytes by the fungus.*

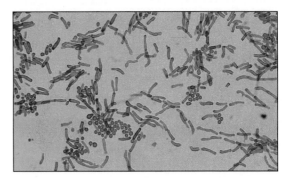

▲ **Fig. 12.12** *Pityriasis versicolor. Potassium hydroxide (30%) in equal parts with Parker's blue-black ink stains the pseudohyphae and spherical yeasts in skin scrapings quite clearly.*

there is no way of speeding up the repigmentation. Recurrences occur in a minority, partly due to inadequate treatment, which may not be entirely the patient's fault. Examination of a treated patient under a Wood's light often shows yellow fluorescence in parts that look macroscopically normal. There is also a group of patients who get frequent recurrences (these are invariably sun worshippers) which lead to the resurgence of the original precipitating factors.

TINEA (RINGWORM)

Introduction

Tinea is caused by a superficial fungus which colonizes keratin; that is, hair, nails and the outermost layer of the skin. It does not ordinarily penetrate into the living cells. The fungus is a dermatophyte — a multicellular organism characterized by hyphae which matt together to form mycelia. The hyphae (Fig. 12.13) can be visualized on direct microscopy of affected hair, nails or skin scales, if treated with potassium hydroxide. ('Tinea' is derived from the Latin word meaning clothes-moth, which the Romans thought was responsible for the disorder.)

There are three genera of dermatophyte, *Microsporum*, *Epidermophyton* and *Trichophyton*. They can only be identified on the basis of the morphology of their macroconidia (asexual spores), after 3–4 weeks culture on Sabouraud's medium. Thus, although the hallmarks of a fungus infection (hyphae) can be seen within a few minutes on direct microscopy, the individual genus and species can only be identified after culture.

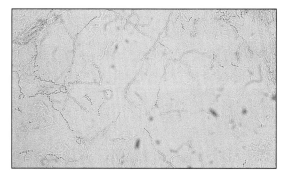

▲ **Fig. 12.13** *Dermatophyte hyphae. The fungal hyphae of tinea may be seen in skin scrapings treated with potassium hydroxide.*

Dermatophytes may be geophilic (soil), zoophilic (animal) or anthropophilic (human) in origin. Geophilic fungi, for example *Microsporum gypseum*, only sporadically infect humans. Animal fungi produce an inflammatory, often suppurative, infection in humans but may be clinically silent in animals. Infection may arise from direct contact or indirectly via clothing or other inanimate materials contaminated with infected animal hair. The exposed parts, viz. scalp, beard, face and arms, are most usually affected. Animal ringworms produce so much inflammation that second attacks are rare. Thus American troops in Vietnam were severely disabled and incapacitated by animal species of *Trichophyton mentagrophytes*, whereas their South Vietnamese comrades were not, presumably because they had acquired immunity as children. Human infections are relatively non-inflammatory, tend to involve covered areas (for example, feet and groin) and are often well-tolerated by the host (especially in the case of *Trichophyton rubrum*).

Host factors are important. Impaired cell-mediated immunity predisposes to these infections. Children are susceptible to scalp ringworm whereas adults are not. Negro children are particularly prone to epidemic human forms. Males have a higher incidence of tinea, probably because females have less exposure to sporting facilities and institutions where tinea is rife.

Tinea infections only occur following damage to the stratum corneum. This probably explains why tinea pedis is a disorder of the shod and not those who go barefoot. The occlusion increases the local temperature and hydration of the skin, leading to impaired barrier function. Thus shoes made of non-porous materials are associated with an increased incidence of infection. Tinea cruris and pedis are common throughout the world. They are caused by anthropophilic fungi only, particularly *Epidermophyton floccosum*, *Trichophyton rubrum* and *T. mentagrophytes* var. *interdigitale*. They are most prevalent in the tropics, because the warm, humid conditions promote growth. *Trichophyton rubrum* was imported into the UK by troops who served in the East during World War II.

Institutions, public changing facilities, including hotel bathrooms, sports centres and swimming pools are the most common sources. The incidence at swimming pools and shower rooms could be reduced if these areas were cleaned and hosed down more often. Males appear to be affected more than females, partly because of greater exposure to sports facilities, and possibly because they wear more occlusive footwear throughout the year and the scrotum occludes the skin in contact with the thigh. They are also less scrupulous about sharing towels and sports clothing. The fungus may be inoculated via the feet or from sitting on contaminated benches. The condition is extremely common, affecting at least 10% of the population at any one time.

Certain fungi have a restricted geographic location, for example *T. soudanense*, in Central and West Africa, but as society becomes more cosmopolitan this situation is changing. For example *Microsporum audouinii*, which was the commonest cause of scalp ringworm in the US and still is in the UK, has been displaced in the US by *T. tonsurans*, probably imported by Mexican and Puerto Rican immigrants.

Although all dermatophytes have a strong affinity for keratin there are differences in their preferences: for example, *T. rubrum* seldom infects hair, and *E. floccosum* rarely infects hair and never the nails.

Fungal disorders are eminently treatable, and it is always a pity when they are misdiagnosed, invariably meaning that they will be inappropriately treated with topical steroids, causing the situation to deteriorate. The term ringworm is a most unfortunate one, because it is a poor description of most of the clinical types of tinea, other than tinea corporis. It also implies that if an eruption has annular features it will be labelled as ringworm. Perversely, more lesions which are ring-shaped are not ringworm than the reverse.

Tinea infections are conventionally described under the sites involved, although *T. rubrum* is described on its own in view of its special characteristics. Treatment of ringworm with topical steroids has produced a condition of its own, known as 'tinea incognito', in which the usual physical signs of inflammation are either masked or modified.

Tinea capitis
Definition
An infection in children of the scalp hairs and skin with dermatophytes, anthropophilic or zoophilic, which can invade either the inner or outer part of the hair shaft.

Diagnostic features
- Children.
- Patchy hair loss.
- Animal ringworm produces florid inflammation.
- Human ringworm is well-tolerated with little inflammation.

Aetiology
Scalp ringworm is more common in the lower socio-economic groups and in conditions of overcrowding and poor personal hygiene. It can be transmitted by shared brushes, combs, caps and pillow cases. Some species are ubiquitous but others have a relatively limited geographical distribution. Tinea infections are rare after puberty, probably because after this stage sebum contains saturated fatty acids which are hostile to the fungus. Certainly this factor has been capitalized on with regard to treatment. Undecenoic acid, a fatty acid, is an effective topical treatment. Interestingly, hair oils are inhibitory, and races which use them routinely are far less prone.

The pattern of eruption is determined by the source of infection and the mode of invasion of the hair. Human infections produce quite minor degrees of erythema and scaling (Fig. 12.14) but animal infections induce considerable inflammation because the host resistance is usually high (Fig. 12.15). This may result in a boggy mass of inflamed and purulent skin, known as a *kerion*. Certain fungi invade the outer root sheath of the hair (ectothrix), giving the hair a rather dull appearance and causing it to break off above the scalp surface. Other fungi invade the inner hair shaft (endothrix), producing more pronounced damage such that the hairs are broken off close to the surface of the scalp.

Scalp ringworm infections are traditionally classified as ectothrix and endothrix infections, kerion and favus respectively. Only *Microsporum* and *Trichophyton* genera are responsible.

The most common infections of the scalp in this country are *Microsporum canis* and *M. audouinii*, the

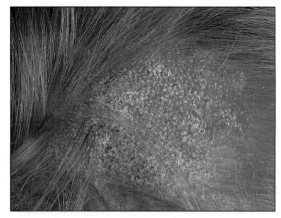

▲ **Fig. 12.14** *Tinea capitis. The condition affects children. In anthropophilic infections there are patches of hair loss with minimal scaling.*

former zoophilic (originating either in a puppy or kitten) and the latter anthropophilic. The fungus invades the stratum corneum of the scalp first and then the outer root sheath of the hair, coating it with spores. This fluoresces bright green under the Wood's light (Fig. 12.16), which is a rapid means of screening children for *Microsporum* infection.

The anthropophilic species of the *Trichophyton* genus rarely cause tinea capitis, but animal fungi do, in particular *T. veruccosum* and *T. mentagrophytes* var *granulare*. Both infect cattle and horses, and the latter infects rodents, so that a pet may be the source. These species of fungus do not fluoresce under the Wood's light.

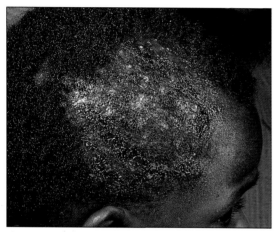

▲ **Fig. 12.15** *Tinea capitis. There is acute inflammation and pustulation associated with the patchy hair loss (kerion). Zoophilic infections are usually responsible.*

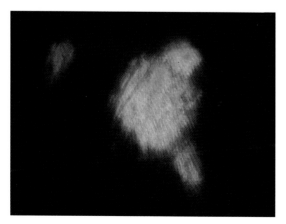

▲ **Fig. 12.16** *Wood's light fluorescence.* Microsporum *hair infections fluoresce green under a Wood's light.*

Endothrix infections are all anthropophilic and are not endemic in the UK. They are *T. soudanense* (Africa), *T. violaceum* (Mediterranean, Central Europe, Russia, North Africa), *T. tonsurans* or *sulphureum* (worldwide, but especially North and Middle America) and *T. schoenleinii* (Middle East, Eastern Europe, Mediterranean and South Africa). The clue to the diagnosis will be that the child has recently been abroad, alerting the practitioner to take scrapings.

Clinical features

There are one or more patches of alopecia. The non-inflammatory epidemic human species, *M. audouinii*, produces scaling with minimal inflammation of the scalp. It starts as a small, red papule surrounding the hair shaft and spreads centrifugally producing well-demarcated patches which may spread from the occiput onto the posterior neck. The affected hairs are grey and lustreless due to a coating of spores and break off just above the level of the scalp.

The inflammatory species of soil or animal origin (*M. canis*, *T. veruccosum*, etc.) produce a pustular folliculitis which may develop into a kerion which is an inflammatory boggy mass studded with broken hairs and oozing purulent material from the follicular orifices. This condition is itchy and sometimes painful; occasionally there is fever and lymphadenopathy.

Endothrix infections so destroy the hair shaft that it is so brittle that it breaks off at the level of the scalp. Black dots, representing the remains of the hairs, are seen with minimal scaling.

Diagnosis

Hair and scales from the affected areas of the scalp should be taken and sent to the laboratory. The fungus may be seen under the microscope in these specimens after they have been treated with potash, but some experience is required. The best way to collect specimens is to brush the scalp and hair vigorously, and to impress the bristles of the brush (for example a tooth brush) into a Sabouraud's plate straight away; but collection of hairs clipped close to the scalp, with plenty of scales, is also satisfactory.

Under the Wood's light, both *Microsporum* species fluoresce a brilliant green. *Microsporum audouinii* is highly contagious and will spread from one child to another at school, so the Community Physician should be notified. Wood's light can be used to screen a class of children, thus controlling a potential epidemic.

The disease is no longer the scourge that it was. Prior to the introduction of griseofulvin in 1959, the condition was a chronic one, which would not be likely to clear until puberty. X-ray epilation of affected hairs was the only effective treatment. Regrettably, in the early days of treatment, many children were over-irradiated and permanent rather than temporary loss of hair resulted secondary to scarring. Some of these patients are still alive and are now at risk of developing malignant tumours of the skin in the previously irradiated areas (Fig. 12.17).

Tinea corporis
Definition
An infection of glabrous (smooth) skin which may be caused by any of the dermatophytes.

> **Diagnostic features**
> - Annular, red scaly patches.
> - Most activity at the periphery of the lesion.
> - Tendency to central healing and post-inflammatory pigmentation.
> - Asymmetrical patches.

Clinical features
The ringworm fungus tends to move outwards in the skin almost as if it were seeking fresh pasture. Thus the lesion is annular and well-defined (Fig. 12.18). The margin is most active and is the important area to examine carefully. It is slightly raised, red and scaly but if the source is an animal, may be quite inflamed (Fig. 12.19) and even pustular (Fig. 12.20). Centrally, there is a tendency to healing and post-inflammatory hyperpigmentation. The patches may be single or multiple, are scattered asymmetrically, and may occur anywhere on the body but particularly on the trunk and limbs.

Two sites commonly cause diagnostic problems and these are the face (Fig. 12.21), including the beard area, and under a watchstrap (Fig. 12.22), the latter being often diagnosed as metal sensitivity and treated with steroids. In both instances the clinical features are the same as when tinea corporis occurs elsewhere, with activity at the periphery of the eruption

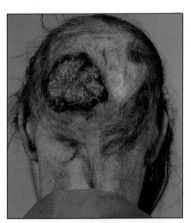

◀ **Fig. 12.17** *Squamous cell carcinoma. Prior to griseofulvin, X-irradiation was used to effect epilation of the infected hairs. Occasionally permanent alopecia and subsequently carcinoma results.*

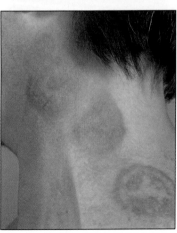

◀ **Fig. 12.18** *Tinea corporis. Ringworm may be distinguished from other annular disorders by a tendency to activity at the margin and central healing.*

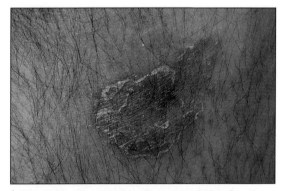

▲ **Fig. 12.19** *Tinea corporis. The margin of this inflamed animal tinea is raised, red and scaly with central healing.*

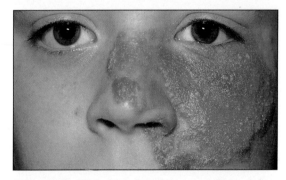

▲ **Fig. 12.20** *Tinea facei. Animal ringworm infections induce an acute inflammatory reaction on the skin. Note the pustulation and the crusted margin with a tendency to central healing.*

and an asymmetrical eruption alerting the practitioner to the correct diagnosis. Tinea on the face, if it is due to an animal source, is often inflammatory and misdiagnosed as herpes simplex or impetigo. The less inflamed varieties, usually from an anthropophilic source are sometimes misdiagnosed as eczema and treated with topical steroids, so it is always worth examining all the skin when faced with a difficult diagnosis. The presence of fungus between the toes or in the groin may raise the suspicion of tinea corporis.

Differential diagnosis

The name of ringworm is misused so often, that it is appropriate to consider other annular eruptions which are frequently mistaken for tinea.

(1) Discoid eczema. The redness and scaling occurs uniformly across the lesion and there is no central healing or preferential peripheral activity.

(2) The herald patch of pityriasis rosea. The lesion is pink throughout, but does have a collarette of scale towards but not at the periphery.

(3) Granuloma annulare. The pathology of this condition is in the dermis and there is no epidermal component, which means that there will be no scaling.

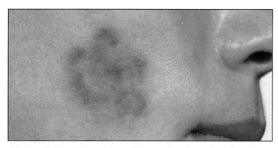

▲ **Fig. 12.21** *Tinea facei. This may be misdiagnosed and treated with steroids. The margin, however, is raised and red with central healing.*

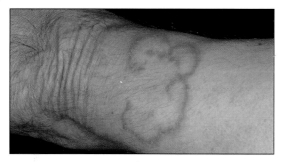

▲ **Fig. 12.22** *Tinea corporis. Occlusion favours the growth of fungal disorders. Tinea under a watchstrap is often misdiagnosed as eczema.*

Tinea cruris (Dhobi itch)
Definition
An infection of the groin by an anthropophilic dermatophyte. It may be secondary to chronic tinea pedis.

Diagnostic features
- Males, mainly.
- Pruritic, red, scaly margin.
- Tends to move down the inner thigh and spare the scrotum.
- May be present in the toe webs, on the feet, and in the toenails.
- Scrapings are positive for hyphae.

Clinical features
The condition is itchy. It is red and scaly, particularly at the margin, which is very slightly raised. The fungus spreads asymmetrically on both sides of the inner thighs downwards (Figs 12.23 & 12.24) away from the genitocrural folds so that the scrotum is rarely involved. In widespread cases, the fungus will spread onto the buttocks. The advancing well-defined border with a tendency to central clearing and post-inflammatory pigmentation are all important signs. If

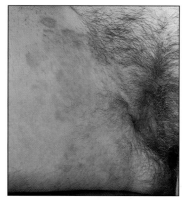

◀ **Fig. 12.23**
Tinea cruris. The periphery of the eruption is raised, scaly and red with post-inflammatory pigmentation in the ring.

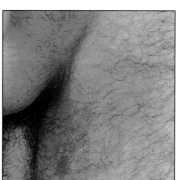

◀ **Fig. 12.24**
Tinea cruris. The eruption spreads away from the groin down the inner thigh. The margin is scaly and raised.

the patient has been treated with topical steroids up to the time of the consultation, the edge may be non-existent and then appear just as a diffuse erythema or scaling, whereas if treatment has been abandoned for a few days, the edge may be quite inflamed and pustular. If powerful steroids have been used for a long time, atrophy and striae result.

Diagnosis

Scrapings are all important for diagnosis. Even if the practitioner does not feel confident in examining scrapings or have time to examine them himself, he can send them to the laboratory. Other organisms such as *Candida albicans* or erythrasma may be present, and indeed the eruption may not be an infection at all but may be psoriasis or seborrhoeic eczema. The feet and toenails should be examined, because this may be the source of the infection.

Tinea pedis
Definition

A fungal infection of the skin of the feet and sometimes the toenails.

> ### Diagnostic features
> - Scaling and/or maceration between the toes (chronic eruptions).
> - Crescentic scaling on the soles of the feet (chronic eruptions).
> - Unilateral vesicles (acute eruptions).
> - Asymmetry.
> - Sometimes toenail involvement.

Clinical features

The condition begins in the toe webs. There is maceration, peeling and erythema (Fig. 12.25), usually in the lateral toe webs, which may spread to involve the undersurface of the toes and soles but rarely the dorsa of the feet. The condition is pruritic but may be sore if the eruption is fissured. It is usually asymmetrical, one foot being more involved than the other, which distinguishes it from endogenous disorders such as psoriasis. The condition may behave in the following ways.

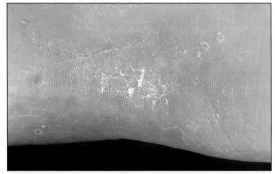

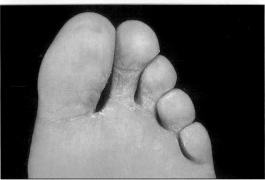

▲ **Figs 12.26 & 12.27** *Tinea pedis. Crescentic scales occur on the soles of the feet (Fig. 12.26) especially on the undersurface of the toes (Fig. 12.27).*

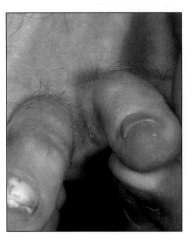

◀ **Fig. 12.25** *Tinea pedis and unguium. There is scaling, maceration and fissuring between the toes and thickening and discoloration of the nail.*

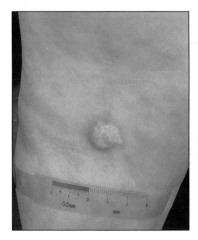

◀ **Fig. 12.28** *Acute tinea pedis. Vesicles and bullae occur on one sole, often with secondary sepsis. Fungal hyphae are found in the roof of the blisters.*

(1) Chronic tinea pedis. The skin is dry and powdery with some peeling and with the production of crescentic scales (Figs 12.26 & 12.27). It is insidious in its evolution. It is usually due to *T. rubrum*, which does not produce much host response. Frequently the nails are involved.

(2) Acute tinea pedis. Vesicles (Fig. 12.28) develop which coalesce and form frank blisters. The eruption is usually unilateral (which distinguishes it from a pompholyx) and is most commonly caused by *T. mentagrophytes* var. *interdigitale*. A lymphangitis with lymphadenopathy may occur.

(3) Tinea pedis and steroids. If tinea pedis is misappropriately treated with topical steroids, it spreads onto the dorsa of the feet, producing an eruption with an active, slightly raised, scaly margin.

Although not common, a bilateral, symmetrical, vesicular pompholyx may develop on the palms of the hands, as a result of a severe fungus infection on the foot. No fungi are isolated from the skin of the hands, and it is considered to be a secondary allergic reaction to the fungus, sometimes known as an Id phenomenon. The condition responds to treatment of the fungus on the foot.

Trichophyton rubrum hand infections

Diagnostic features
- One hand only involved.
- Dry and scaly.
- Powdery filling-in of skin creases.
- Not all nails involved.
- Both feet and toenails may be involved.
- Only responds to griseofulvin or ketoconazole.

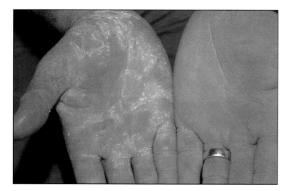

▲ **Fig. 12.29** *Tinea manuum.* T. rubrum *infections affect one hand only. There is scaling particularly in the skin creases and the nails are usually involved.*

Clinical features

Trichophyton rubrum is now the commonest dermatophyte infection. The feet, toe webs, toenails and groin are its favourite haunts. When it affects one hand it does so without ever spreading to the other one (Fig. 12.29), despite both feet being involved. This bizarre phenomenon has not been satisfactorily explained. The palmar or plantar skin feels very dry and there is a powdery filling-in of the skin creases. In addition there are crescentic peeling scales. The toenails are invariably involved at an earlier stage. The finger nails become involved later but in an asymmetrical manner.

Tinea incognito

This title refers to a tinea infection which has been mistreated with topical steroids (Figs 12.30 & 12.31). Topical steroids are powerful anti-inflammatory drugs so that the usual physical signs of inflammation at the margin of the fungal eruption are modified and may

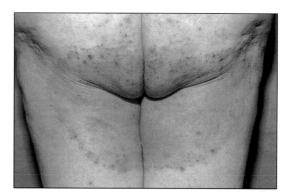

▲ **Fig. 12.30** *Tinea incognito. If tinea is treated with topical steroids the inflammatory and immune response is suppressed. The margin however is well-defined and raised.*

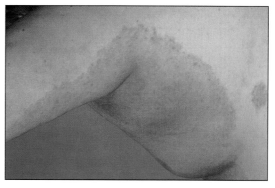

▲ **Fig. 12.31** *Tinea incognito. Most of the eruption is red or hyperpigmented without scaling but the margin is well-defined and raised. Skin scrapings revealed masses of hyphae.*

be barely discernible. There may, however, be an area which has not been treated with the topical steroid, such that the normal physical signs of fungal infection are present, and the correct diagnosis can be more easily made. Alternatively, the topical steroids may result in a pustular reaction. The observant patient often remarks that the condition seems to be getting worse despite the treatment, and this should suggest the correct diagnosis.

Management of tinea

The diagnosis may be established by scraping the skin with a blunt scalpel and taking clippings from the nails if they are involved. In acute tinea pedis it is useful to remove the skin of the roof of a blister with a pair of scissors. These specimens may be treated with potash (potassium hydroxide) and examined for hyphae under a microscope or sent by post to the laboratory for culture.

Topical therapies

There are various topical remedies. Half strength Whitfield's ointment and undecenoic acid ointment are cheap and useful. Tolnaftate is relatively expensive but commonly used. The imidazoles are now the most commonly used. Castellani's paint with or without the magenta is useful for acute tinea between the toes. Potassium permanganate (1:10,000) soaks are extremely useful for the acute vesicular tinea pedis. The foot is soaked for 10 minutes once or twice a day, then dried and an imidazole cream applied. The patient should be warned that it stains the skin and nails brown temporarily.

In tinea capitis topical therapy is of little avail on its own, although it is useful to clip away the affected hairs and shampoo frequently.

A common error is to treat tinea, especially in the groin, with a combined steroid, antibacterial/antifungal drug. Most of these, for example Tri-Adcortyl (Mycolog, US) contain nystatin as the antifungal, but this is only effective against *Candida* and has no effect against tinea. The preparation therefore only worsens the situation because of its steroid effect. There is a tendency to use combined imidazoles/hydrocortisone preparations in the groin: the imidazole is effective against tinea, but this is in danger of being counter-balanced by the steroid. There is no need for steroid combinations even in very inflammatory ringworm, for it responds admirably to griseofulvin. However, if there is doubt about the diagnosis, one of these preparations is permissible until the results of the scrapings are available.

Systemic therapies

Topical therapies are not always effective. The indications for systemic therapy are: (1) acute infections, (2) scalp infections, (3) nail infections, (4) *Trichophyton rubrum* infections, and (5) tinea incognito.

The drugs which are available are:

(1) Griseofulvin. This drug has been available since 1959 and has a long and established safety record. The most common minor side-effects are headache and nausea, although the headache tends to disappear despite continuing treatment. It is occasionally a photosensitizer, and occasionally causes a fixed drug eruption. Griseofulvin is not recommended for use in pregnancy.

All species respond to griseofulvin, but the drug is ineffective against *Candida* and pityriasis versicolor. The paediatric dose is 125 mg three times daily in an elixir form if necessary, and the adult dose is 0.5–1 g a day. Treatment for 4–6 weeks is sufficient for tinea of the groin, body, scalp and feet. The minimum time required to eradicate the fungus from the hand and finger nails is 5 months. Treatment of tinea pedis and toenails is not so satisfactory, particularly in those with poor peripheral circulation. The drug is required for at least 18 months to eradicate it from the toenails and often for 2 years. Even then it cannot be guaranteed that the nails will completely clear. Thus the treatment should only be offered to those who are likely to be obsessional in taking the drug and it is probably best to reserve it for younger individuals.

In tinea capitis microcrystalline griseofulvin, 125 mg three times daily in tablet or elixir form for 6 weeks, is the treatment of choice. Therapy should be supervised and the parent required to bring the medication at each visit, to ensure that it is being given to the child. The success of therapy can be monitored with a Wood's lamp, the green fluorescence disappearing as the affected hairs are eradicated. The child with a zoophilic infection can attend school, since infectivity of an animal infection from human to human is low. The infected animal can be treated with griseofulvin if this is deemed worthwhile. The child with a human infection (*M. audouinii*), should probably remain at home until therapy has been established.

(2) Ketoconazole. This is an alternative therapy to griseofulvin if the patient cannot tolerate the latter.

(3) Itraconazole. This is a new oral triazole. It works in a similar way to the imidazoles. It is active against candida, pityriasis versicolor and tinea. Clinical trials suggest that it may be more effective than griseofulvin in tinea. It is contraindicated in pregnancy and liver disease and long-term side-effects are unknown.

13 INFESTATIONS OF THE SKIN

INTRODUCTION

The common infestations giving rise to irritation of the skin, pediculosis, scabies and insect bites, are discussed. Three unusual disorders transmitted by insects or parasites — leishmaniasis, larva migrans and Lyme disease — are mentioned briefly because they may be acquired on vacation abroad and Lyme disease is becoming more common in the UK.

PEDICULOSIS

Definition
An infestation of the skin with a blood sucking insect, which causes considerable irritation.

Introduction
There are two species of louse which are specifically ectoparasitic on man. *Phthirus pubis* (the crab louse) and *Pediculus humanus*. The latter may affect the head (pediculosis capitis) or body (pediculosis corporis). Both are elongated in shape and have slight anatomical differences, *P. pubis* being shorter and as broad as it is long. *Pediculus humanus* is quite mobile but *P. pubis* does not move far (its name is derived from the crab-like claws on its legs with which it grasps the pubic hair and where it prefers to remain). Lice have six legs and are wingless. Unlike the acarus, no immunity develops in the human to louse species, so repeated infestations may occur.

Pediculosis capitis

Diagnostic features
- Intense irritation of the scalp.
- Red grouped papules on the neck.
- Mobile pediculi.
- Nits attached to hair shafts.

Aetiology
This infestation of the scalp occurs particularly in schoolchildren, and occasionally in adults. It is remarkably common at present, having been particularly prevalent during World War 2 and then rare by 1960.

Transmission is by shared caps, brushes and combs, and the general physical contact between children and their parents and teachers.

Clinical features
The condition is itchy and the lice are obvious to the naked eye (Fig. 13.1) when they move. The eggs, which are known as 'nits', are attached to the shafts of the hairs. Small itchy papules occur on the nape of the neck particularly (see Fig. 13.2), but also on the wrists from bites by the lice.

If the diagnosis is missed, secondary bacterial infection may supervene, with matting and crusting of the hair and lymphadenopathy. The child may be quite unwell at this stage.

Management
The diagnosis is usually obvious. However, a louse may be picked off with forceps or attached to sellotape and visualized under the microscope for more definite identification. The eggs may be distinguished from dandruff because they are firmly attached to the hairs. If an affected hair is cut off and examined microscopically, the oval egg capsule is visibly attached to the hair shaft.

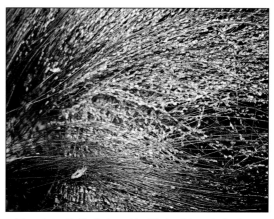

▲ **Fig. 13.1** *Pediculosis capitis. The head louse is clearly visible together with masses of nits attached to the shafts of the hairs.*

Because resistance to gamma benzene hexachloride has been reported, 0.5% malathion is now used. If this fails then 0.5% carbaryl is also effective. The lotion is applied to the scalp and left on for 12 hours. The ova and insects are killed within 2 hours with one application. Alcohol-based lotions may sting; all the lotions smell. A shampoo is available but must be applied on three occasions with three clear days in between. The nits should be removed with a fine-toothed comb. It is important that other members of the family and the rest of the children at the school be examined, otherwise reinfestation will occur.

Pediculosis corporis

Diagnostic features
- Intense irritation of all the skin.
- Widespread excoriations.
- Often secondary sepsis.
- Pediculi and nits mainly in the clothes and not on the skin.

Aetiology
This is a disorder of the unfortunate, and is rare in normal circumstances. It occurs under disaster conditions where there is chaos, overcrowding and a breakdown in hygiene. Under these circumstances, the body louse may transmit rickettsia and result in typhus, trench or relapsing fevers. Vagrants are frequently affected because they acquire the infestation from other inhabitants and from shared bedding in temporary, unsatisfactory accommodation. This louse is not found on the skin, although it sucks blood and feeds off the patient. It lives and breeds in the clothing and bed clothing.

Clinical features
There is intense pruritus in the areas of the skin closest to the clothes such as the shoulders, neck, breasts, and around the buttocks, and examination reveals urticated papules and widespread excoriations, sometimes leading to sepsis. As a result of continual scratching, the skin becomes pigmented, thickened, dry and scaly.

Management
The diagnosis is sometimes missed because the doctor fails to examine the clothing; the louse particularly favours the seams of the underclothes.

Theoretically the patient will recover if he is separated from his infested clothing, although the body is usually treated with gamma benzene hexachloride in the same way as for scabies. The patient must be provided with a fresh set of clothing whilst his own is fumigated with DDT (I have seen patients put on their old clothes after treatment in a casualty department, which clearly is a complete waste of time). This is usually all that is needed, although occasionally systemic antibiotics may be necessary for associated sepsis. Sometimes a mild steroid is helpful after treatment, if eczematization has occurred.

Pediculosis pubis

Diagnostic features
- Pubic irritation.
- Slow-moving pediculi.
- Nits attached to hairs.
- Other regions may be involved.

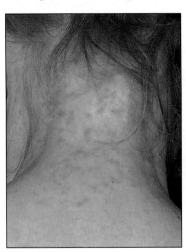

◀ **Fig. 13.2** *Pediculosis capitis. Urticated papules occur on the back of the neck.*

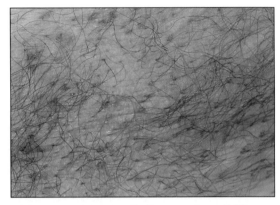

▲ **Fig. 13.3** *Pediculosis pubis. Brown specks are visible amongst the hairs which on closer inspection may be seen to move.*

Aetiology

The crab louse (*Phthirus pubis*) is usually transmitted sexually, but clearly may be contracted by wearing borrowed infected clothing.

Clinical features

The crab louse is found primarily in the pubic hair (Fig. 13.3) but it may spread, especially in a hirsute individual, to the limbs, chest, axillae, and even eyebrows or eyelashes, but never as far as the scalp. It is intensely itchy and the crab louse and its eggs are readily visible.

Management

The diagnosis is rarely missed provided the condition is considered and the patient is examined.

Gamma benzene hexachloride should be applied thoroughly to all the affected areas, and washed off 24 hours later. The application should be repeated 10 days later to destroy any lice which may have hatched out in the interim. It is not necessary to shave the pubic hair. The underclothing can be disinfected with DDT.

INSECT BITES

Definition

A cutaneous reaction to a biting or stinging arthropod, usually causing itching and sometimes acting as a vector of disease.

> **Diagnostic features**
> - Itchy.
> - Urticated papules, sometimes with central punctum, often excoriated.
> - Sometimes blisters.
> - Occur in groups.
> - Asymmetrical.
> - Often one member only of the family affected.

Aetiology

The problem occurs worldwide, the sources varying with location and so a knowledge of local arthropod behaviour is essential. The most common sources are:

(1) **Domestic pets.** Dogs and cats carry fleas, sarcoptic mange (animal scabies) and *Cheyletiella*, another arthropod. It is sometimes difficult to persuade owners that their pet which 'never goes out' or 'is ever so clean' is responsible: brushings from the animal should be sent to the laboratory, to convince the patient. Of course the offending animal may not be the patient's own, but that of a friend whose home is visited periodically.

(2) **Birds.** Birds, especially pigeons, may carry mites or fleas, and the house should be examined to see whether there are nests on the window ledges, under the eaves or in the attic. The insects gain entry into the home via open windows.

(3) **The garden.** Foxes and hedgehogs carry fleas and it is not unusual for them to frequent suburban gardens. There may be biting insects in gardens, and a particular problem recently in England has been the brown-tailed caterpillar moth which lives off the leaves of trees and may fall on individuals walking below. Pronounced urticarial eruptions occur secondary to the urticating spines of the caterpillar.

(4) **Bedding, furniture and soft furnishings.** Bed bugs live in crevices, in furniture and walls. A recently acquired 'antique' such as a bed may be the source, or the bed in new lodgings. Fleas breed in cracks, crevices, floorboards and soft furnishings, especially if they are dusty and dirty. They particularly enjoy centrally heated houses and fitted carpets. They can survive for months without a meal and will attack new occupants of a house or flat that has lain empty, so it is important to discover whether the previous occupant had kept pets.

(5) **Travel.** Travel abroad is commonplace and may result in exposure to mosquitoes, ticks and sandflies. These may transmit diseases, for example malaria (mosquitoes), rocky mountain spotted fever (ticks) and leishmaniasis (sandflies).

Clinical features

The cardinal symptom is itch. The patient may have initially suspected bites but then have discounted the possibility, as often only one member of the household is affected. This can mislead patient and doctor. The lesions may consist of urticarial wheals, sometimes with a central punctum and often excoriated. Papules and vesicles, and occasionally large blisters (Fig. 13.4), may be present and post-inflammatory pigmentation can occur. The lesions are usually scattered asymmetrically over the body, or concentrated primarily on the lower legs (Fig. 13.5) and ankles. There is often secondary bacterial sepsis, especially in warm climates.

Fleas often produce a group of three or four lesions in a linear arrangement (Fig. 13.6), often referred to as 'breakfast, lunch, tea and dinner'. They particularly attack the lower limbs and especially the ankles.

Women and children are more prone than adult males because trousers are usually preventative. Cats are the usual source and flea collars are not effective deterrents. Fleas are at their most prolific during summer and early autumn.

Cheyletiella are mites which colonize cats, dogs, rabbits, foxes, squirrels and some birds. Dogs are most commonly affected and they are asymptomatic: the animal develops fine scaling rather like dandruff along the mid-line of the back, sometimes with loss of hair. The mites can penetrate clothing to attack man, causing urticarial or papular vesicular eruptions; the distribution usually corresponding to where the animal is held in contact with the human. Lesions are thus found on the lap (lower chest, abdomen, forearms and thighs). The human condition is commoner in the autumn and winter than in the summer (when the animals are out of the house more often).

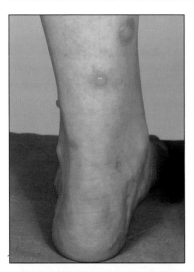

◀**Fig. 13.4**
Insect bites. The lesions may be bullous. The lower legs are a common site for flea bites.

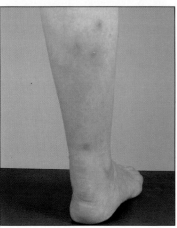

◀**Fig. 13.5**
Insect bites. The lesions are grouped and urticarial, often with a central punctum.

Animals may acquire scabies (sarcoptic mange) and pass it on to humans. Dogs are particularly affected and they suffer from severe pruritis with scaling and loss of hair over the face, ears and elbows. In man there is no incubation period for animal scabies nor are burrows found, unlike human scabies. The eruption is immensely itchy and multiple tiny red papules, appear on parts of the body in contact with the animal, particularly the trunk and limbs.

Bed bugs (cimex lectularius) produce more inflammation than fleas in the human. They shun the light and come out at night, feeding on exposed areas of skin which are not covered by night attire or bedding. The lesions may be quite substantial, red and oedematous, and blood may be found on the bed clothing the following morning, though most patients sleep on unaware of the attack. With recurrent attacks the patient may become quite unwell, with secondary sepsis, fever and lymphadenopathy. The bugs favour substandard dwellings with cracked woodwork, loose skirting boards and peeling wallpaper.

A complication of any insect bite is *papular urticaria*. This condition affects small children predominantly and consists of recurrent attacks each year of insect bites. Most lesions are the result of fresh bites, but some authorities believe that a specific hypersensitivity occurs, leading to urticated lesions not necessarily preceeded by a bite.

Management
The diagnosis can sometimes be difficult to make and, more especially, to prove. One is often faced with a disbelieving patient, so a certain amount of investigation is required. I have found the following measures to be useful:

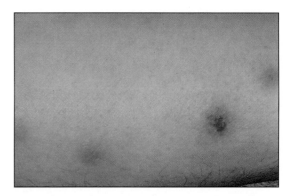

▲**Fig. 13.6** *Insect bites. The oedematous papules are often grouped particularly when due to flea bites and are known as 'breakfast, lunch, tea and dinner'.*

(1) The 'SOS' appointment should be offered. It is useful to examine a patient when the eruption is at its height, when tell-tale urticated papules may be present. It is also easier for the patient to recall exactly where he has been and what he has been doing in the preceeding 48 hours, which may give the clue to the source of the infection.

(2) Examining the pets. Examination of the pet may be helpful. Red brown collections of the faeces from fleas may be found on the animal's coat, or loss of hair and profuse scaling from *Cheyletiella*. Specimens may be collected by standing the animal on a piece of brown paper (shiny side up) and brushing it vigorously. Scurf, hair and scale may then be collected and sent to an entomologist for microscopic examination.

(3) Examining the house. The patient should examine every room and the window sills and eaves for specks which may represent the parasite or its parts, and these should be brought for examination. If the patient has a pet, the pet's bedding and favourite armchair and other haunts should be particularly examined. (It is useful to shake the animal's bedding into a polythene bag so an examination may be made of the debris. The carpet where the animal sleeps can be vacuumed and the contents of the bag examined by an entomologist.) In difficult cases it is useful to call in the Public Health Department.

(4) A biopsy. Insect bites do produce a specific pathology: a diffuse dermal infiltrate consisting of lymphocytes, plasma cells and often prominent numbers of eosinophils. The biopsy also has a therapeutic effect, the patient feeling that something has been done to discover the cause of the condition.

Clearly the source must be identified and treated or the condition will persist. However helpful topical remedies to use during the investigation, and until the source is removed, are:

(1) Crotamiton/hydrocortisone. Proprietary preparations consisting of crotamiton, an antiparasitic drug, in combination with hydrocortisone, which is helpful for its anti-inflammatory effect.

(2) Calamine. Calamine lotion is useful for its antipruritic effect.

(3) Systemic antihistamines. These are useful especially at night.

(4) Systemic antibiotics. These are indicated if sepsis is present.

Occasionally the patient is convinced that she (the condition usually occurs in women) is infested, and yet there is nothing wrong on examination of the skin.

The tiny specimens that she brings consist only of dust and scales of skin. The patient ends up seeing many doctors and calling in pest control agencies who are always baffled by the problem. She is suffering from *delusional parasitophobia*.

SCABIES

Definition
An intensely itchy, contagious eruption caused by infestation with a mite that burrows into the stratum corneum.

> **Diagnostic features**
> - Intense itch.
> - Intimates also affected.
> - Burrows, especially on palms and soles.
> - Papules between the fingers, on the trunk and genitalia.
> - Excoriations and bruising, especially on the legs.

Aetiology
Scabies is an infestation with *Sarcoptes scabiei* an eight-legged mite, the acarus (Fig. 13.7). It is transmitted from one individual to another by prolonged physical, and usually intimate, contact. It cannot be caught from short social contact such as shaking hands. Rarely it is contracted from inanimate objects, as Mellanby showed in his work on scabies during World War II, though he was only able to infect three in a hundred conscientious objectors by having them spend the night in sleeping bags recently vacated by sufferers with the disease. It is therefore most often

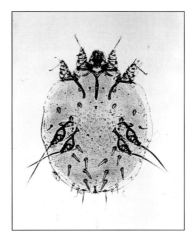

◀ **Fig. 13.7** *Scabies. Scabies is caused by a mite known as the acarus.*

contracted by the promiscuous rather than those in monogamous or celibate states. However, infants and small children are susceptible because they are lovingly handled often and long enough to permit the acarus to travel to their skin from an infected individual. Children spread the disease quite easily between them since they play with each other in a more physical manner than adults do during normal social intercourse.

Having reached a new host the acarus travels in search of a mate or, if female and already gravid, to those areas of skin where the stratum corneum is thickest and easiest to burrow in, particularly on the palms and soles. The female lays two eggs a day for about 2 months. The larvae hatch out in 2 or 4 days and leave the burrow. The nymph moults in 4–6 days and the adult commences the cycle again. The female may be ovigerous within 14 days of being an egg.

An immune response to the acarus develops within a few weeks and the pruritis and papular eruption results. Immunoglobulin levels, particularly IgG and IgM, increase.

Clinical features

The itch begins insidiously on the thighs. It is intermittent but is usually worse after bathing or undressing and in bed. The itch soon intensifies and involves all areas except the face. The condition is contagious so that bed-fellows or other intimates will become similarly affected.

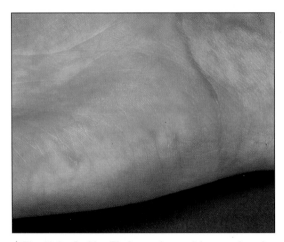

▲**Fig. 13.8** *Scabies. The burrow is a serpiginous track made by the gravid acarus in the stratum corneum, usually where it is thick as on the palms or soles.*

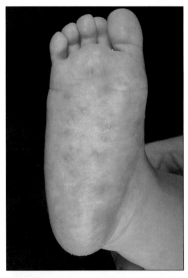

◄**Fig. 13.10** *Scabies. The soles are particularly involved in children with burrows and papulovesicles.*

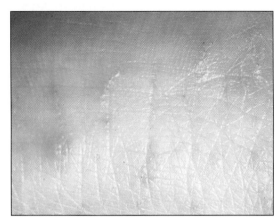

▲**Fig. 13.9** *Scabies. Burrows are usually found on the palms and especially on the thenar eminences.*

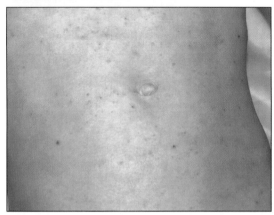

▲**Fig. 13.11** *Scabies. A papular eruption occurs after an incubation period of 4 weeks on the trunk and limbs.*

The finding of a burrow usually on the hands or feet, is diagnostic (Fig. 13.8). It is a serpiginous, linear track a few millimetres long, which is slightly raised, with a black dot visible at one end. An observant patient notices that the burrows are particularly pruritic. The characteristic locations are along the sides of the fingers, on the palms (Fig. 13.9) and around the wrists, although they also occur on the soles and along the sides of the feet, especially in infants (Fig. 13.10).

The burrow is visible early in the disease but there is usually a delay of a few weeks before symptoms arise. These are a result of an allergic reaction to the presence of the mite, and an erythematous papular eruption develops that is often micropapular on the trunk (Fig. 13.11) and is particularly well-visualized by observing the patient from the side in a good light. Papules are also found between the fingers (Figs 13.12 & 13.13), on the elbows, buttocks, fronts of the axillae, around the nipples and on the genitalia. The male genitalia are so frequently involved (Fig. 13.14) that there is an adage that papules on the shaft and glans of the penis and on the scrotum are so characteristic as to be virtually pathognomonic of scabies. In some patients these papules enlarge to become nodules (Fig. 13.15) that may persist for many weeks and remain intermittently itchy despite successful eradication of the infestation.

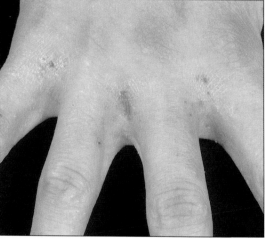

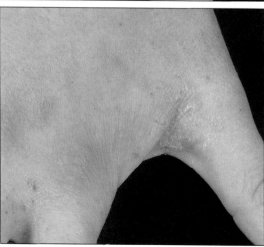

▲ **Figs 13.12 & 13.13** *Scabies. Papules and burrows between the fingers are characteristic and especially over the first dorsal interossei (Fig. 13.13).*

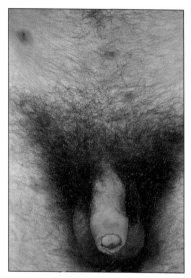

◀**Fig. 13.14** *Scabies. Papules and nodules are common in the pubic area and are virtually always found on the male genitalia.*

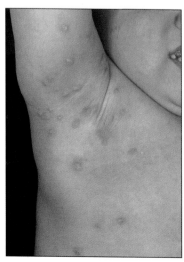

◀**Fig. 13.15** *Scabies. Red brown nodules occur in a minority of patients particularly around the axillae.*

The unpleasant itch leads to widespread excoriations of the skin particularly on the lower limbs. Bruising, secondary to scratching, is often marked, particularly on the thighs of women (Fig. 13.16). A patchy eczema may occur (Fig. 13.17) on the limbs, following scratching the skin. This can be confusing and frequently leads to an erroneous diagnosis and prescription of topical steroids, which permit the mites to flourish because they are immunosuppressive; occasionally extensive infestations (sometimes called 'Norwegian' scabies) result. Most patients, however, on direct questioning will note that topical steroids, although producing momentary relief, make the condition worse.

The physical signs vary greatly between healthy individuals, probably in relation to their personal hygiene. The more frequently the patient bathes the more likely the acarus is to be removed mechanically, thus reducing the load of infestation but not the degree of itch. In these patients there will be fewer burrows, rendering the diagnosis a little more difficult. It is wise to consider the possibility of scabies in any person who complains of irritation, having been previously unafflicted by skin disorders.

Diagnosis

The diagnosis of scabies should be entertained in any patient who is itching, but of course this is a very common symptom and the most usual diseases to be confused with scabies are: eczema, lichen planus, insect bites and prurigo. A burrow should be found and the acarus or her eggs extracted by scraping the burrow with a pin, which the mite conveniently clings to when the roof of her burrow is scraped off. The acarus is only just visible to the naked eye but can be easily visualized under the microscope when placed on a slide with a few drops of potassium hydroxide: this is the ultimate proof of diagnosis. It is often helpful for the patient to see the mite under the microscope as well, in order to appreciate the diagnosis and its treatment.

Management

The disease is eminently treatable but success depends on a certain amount of explanation and follow-up. All the remedies are potential irritants of the skin and may result in a secondary dermatitis and thus confusion. Gamma benzene hexachloride is preferable to benzyl benzoate, which is poorly tolerated. It should be applied after a warm bath to all the skin, excluding the face. It is important to emphasize that all areas should be treated, even those with no visible rash — the soles of the feet, between the toes, the natal cleft and the genitalia are often forgotten. Clearly the treatment will fail if the mite happens to be present on skin which is not treated and this point should be made to the patient. The lotion is left on the skin for 24 hours then washed off and reapplied for a further 24 hours.

Problems of irritant dermatitis arise if further applications are made. However despite exhortations to the contrary, patients frequently do use the treatment several times, largely because *the itch does not subside straight away.* Although the disease is cured by two applications, the allergic response may take up to a month to subside. Thus although the itch lessens considerably and the patient can at last sleep, spasmodic bouts of itching may occur. The patient mistakes this for further disease and reapplies the lotion.

Scratching in scabies induces a partial eczematous response in some patients and treatment may compound this. It is essential therefore to follow up the

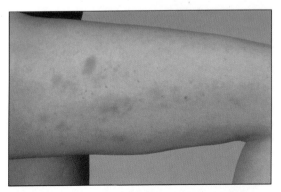

Fig. 13.16 *Scabies. The itching is intense especially at night and bruising as a result of scratching is often prominent especially on the thighs in women.*

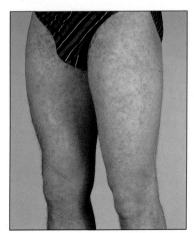

◀**Fig. 13.17** *Scabies. Scabies is exceedingly itchy and eczema develops particularly on the limbs in some patients, leading to an erroneous diagnosis.*

patient after treatment because a topical steroid and an emollient may be required to settle the secondary eczema. Surprisingly scratching rarely produces secondary bacterial infection.

Scabies is a contagious disease and it is imperative to trace and treat contacts. Certainly it is wise to treat the patient's immediate family whether or not they are symptomatic. If a patient is informed that the disease is usually contracted a few weeks prior to the first symptoms he or she may be able to recall the original contact and arrange treatment accordingly.

CUTANEOUS LEISHMANIASIS (ORIENTAL SORE, BAGHDAD BOIL)

The condition results from a bite from a sandfly infected with the protozoan *Leishmania tropica*. It is common in the middle east, the tropics and the subtropics but may occur in Mediterranean countries so it is occasionally encountered in holidaymakers.

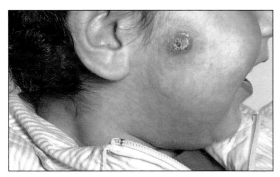

▲ **Fig. 13.18** *Cutaneous leishmaniasis. A firm red nodule, which crusts and ulcerates, results from an infected sandfly bite.*

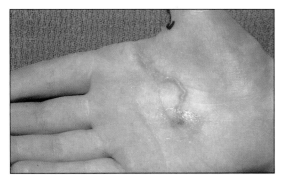

▲ **Fig. 13.19** *Larva migrans. Linear, mobile, serpiginous tracks result from the entry of dog hookworm larvae.*

The lesion is a firm papule or nodule which ulcerates and crusts (Fig. 13.18) and then very slowly heals. *Leishmania* may be found in skin smears or demonstrated as Leishman–Donovan bodies in large histiocytes on skin biopsy.

LARVA MIGRANS

This is caused by hookworm larvae, from the faeces of an infected dog, penetrating bare human skin. It is common in the Caribbean and on the Florida coastline. Anyone walking or sitting on a contaminated beach is at risk. *Ancylostoma braziliense* is the most common hookworm responsible. The site of entry (usually the buttocks or foot) is itchy and the patient subsequently notices a linear mobile serpiginous lesion (Fig. 13.19). The condition responds to topical application of a 10% suspension of thiabendazole.

LYME DISEASE

This is a systemic illness transmitted by tics, infected with the spirochaete *Borrelia burgdorferi*. It was first described in Lyme, Connecticut, but occurs in Europe, with notable outbreaks in the New Forest in England. Small mammals and deer are the main reservoir for the infection. *Erythema chronicum migrans*, an annular erythema (Fig. 13.20) expanding outwards from the papule of the tic bite, is followed by a constitutional upset with fever, arthralgia, myalgia and headache. If it is not treated with tetracycline neurological, cardiac and arthritic sequelae may occur.

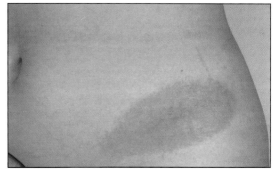

▲ **Fig. 13.20** *Lyme disease. An annular erythema spreads out from the site of the tic bite after a few days.*

DEVELOPMENTAL DISORDERS OF THE SKIN

INTRODUCTION

Certain inherited disorders that solely affect the skin, such as ichthyosis, keratosis pilaris and Darier's disease, and that are likely to present to the family practitioner for diagnosis and treatment are described here. Others, which have cutaneous manifestations in association with systemic abnormalities, such as tuberous sclerosis, Ehlers–Danlos and pseudoxanthoma elasticum, are omitted because they are well described in general medical texts.

ICHTHYOSIS AND DISORDERS OF DESQUAMATION

Introduction

The term 'ichthyosis' refers to a group of disorders which are usually present at birth and are characterized by a chronic generalized, and in the common varieties non-inflammatory, scaling of the skin. The fundamental defect is a failure to shed (desquamate) the skin properly. Thus in the commonest type, ichthyosis vulgaris, although the stratum corneum (the outermost layer of the skin) is formed at a normal rate, the bonds which bind the corneocytes (the cells of the stratum corneum) together fail to loosen so that when desquamation takes place collections of corneocytes (so-called lamellae) separate together instead of individually.

The corneocytes are built of proteins and connected to each other by a lipid material. It appears that the key to understanding this set of disorders will lie in the unravelling of their lipid and protein biochemistry. It is already known that dry skin may be produced in humans by lipid-lowering drugs, such as clofazimine, and in experimental animals by essential fatty acid deficiency. Also enzyme deficiencies, involving lipid metabolism, may produce ichthyosis. Thus in *Refsum's disease*, which is a rare disorder of ichthyosis (similar clinically but not histologically to ichthyosis vulgaris) associated with cerebellar ataxia, peripheral neuropathy and retinitis pigmentosa, there is a failure to catabolise phytanic acid. The latter is a fatty acid found in green vegetables which accumulates and displaces unsaturated fatty acids such as linoleic acid from tissue lipids.

Recently it has been shown that the cause of recessive X-linked ichthyosis is a steroid sulphatase deficiency that causes an accumulation of its substrate, cholesterol sulphate, in the skin and serum. X-linked ichthyosis is an uncommon disorder that only affects males. Their mothers have a placental steroid sulphatase deficiency, which results in prolonged labour.

Unfortunately the fundamental defect in ichthyosis vulgaris is less well understood, but may soon be unravelled. The epidermis and stratum corneum are of normal thickness, but the stratum granulosum is absent and the corneocytes are abnormal under the electron microscope. Ichthyosis vulgaris is normally inherited as an autosomal dominant with an estimated incidence of 1 in 250, but very occasionally it may be acquired, in which case it may be secondary to an underlying lymphoma or hypothyroidism.

There have also been advances in the therapy of the ichthyoses. The retinoids, and in particular etretinate, are lipid raising agents which have been shown to have profound effects in correcting ichthyosis. They are of great importance in the management of the rare, extremely unpleasant forms of ichthyosis, but are not indicated in the disorders which are described in this chapter, for the risk:benefit ratio is unacceptable. Other less toxic retinoids are in the process of being developed.

Xeroderma (xerosis)
Definition
A persistent, generalized, scaling of the skin without inflammation, giving the impression of dryness.

> **Diagnostic features**
> - Generalized fine scaling.
> - Skin feels dry and rough.
> - Often accompanied by eczema.

Clinical features
The skin looks and feels dry (Fig. 14.1), although there is no real evidence to suggest that the abnormal stratum corneum contains less water than normal.

Virtually all the skin is affected, including the flexures. It commonly accompanies atopic eczema and is probably part of the eczematous process. Others may have it without ever having eczema, but often they have an atopic family history. The disorder becomes troublesome at low ambient temperatures with low relative humidity and improves in the warmer months. The effect of winter on this type of skin is profound and leads to deterioration of any eczema present and also to an eczematous condition known as 'winter itch' (Fig. 14.2). Although winter itch was first described in the US, particularly along the north-eastern seaboard, it is now becoming more common in the UK as central heating, which reduces the relative humidity, becomes commonplace. The cold weather, coupled with wind which is responsible for the chill factor, dries out the skin, which becomes itchy. 'Chapping' is a form of xerosis which can occur in virtually anyone, given the right atmospheric circumstances.

Ichthyosis vulgaris
Definition
An autosomal dominantly inherited disorder resulting in widespread scaling of the skin.

Diagnostic features
- Small fine white scales.
- Rough surface.
- Extensor surfaces of limbs and trunk.
- Sparing of flexures.

Clinical features
The disorder is usually present at birth, with the entire skin feeling dry and rough. On examination small, fine, white scales are found (Fig. 14.3), particularly on the extensor surfaces of the limbs and on the trunk. Larger, more adherent, scales are found on the fronts of the shins. In some individuals, the follicular orifices on the upper outer arms and thighs

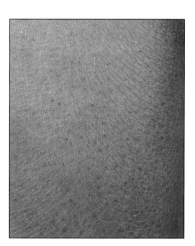

◀ Fig. 14.1
Xerosis. The skin feels dry and rough and is scaly. Xerosis is frequently associated with atopic eczema.

▲ **Fig. 14.3** *Ichthyosis vulgaris. The skin is dry and rough. Small fine scales are present, especially on the extensor surfaces.*

◀ Fig. 14.2
Winter itch. Eczema may complicate xerosis in the winter and may give rise to pruritus.

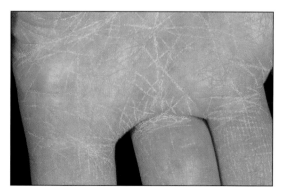

▲ **Fig. 14.4** *Ichthyosis vulgaris. The palms and soles may be involved. The skin is dry and rough, especially in the creases. Cracking of the skin occurs in the cold.*

are plugged with keratin, forming spines, so that keratosis pilaris occurs with it. There is a characteristic sparing of the flexures, especially of the knees and elbows. The palmar and plantar skin creases are often exaggerated (Fig. 14.4) and frequently there is hyperkeratosis. There is often associated atopic eczema. The condition is worse in winter and improves in summer, sometimes virtually clearing in warm humid climates. It may improve in adult life but deteriorate once again in old age.

X-linked ichthyosis vulgaris
Definition
An uncommon recessive disorder occurring in males, resulting in universal involvement of the skin with large dark scales.

Diagnostic features
- Large dark scales.
- Present at birth, in males only.
- No association with atopy.
- Life-long affliction.
- Steroid sulphatase deficiency.

Clinical features
These boys are occasionally born encased in a collodion like membrane, or more usually with large dark scales involving all the skin, including the flexures, unlike ichthyosis vulgaris of the dominant type. The skin gives a general false impression of dirtiness (Fig. 14.5). It may be quite severe. Occasionally corneal abnormalities and cryptorchidism are present.

Keratosis pilaris
Definition
A common disorder of keratinization affecting the hair follicles which appear plugged. It is most prominent on the extensor surfaces of the proximal parts of the limbs.

Diagnostic features
- Horny plugs on the outer aspects of upper arms and thighs.
- Does not respond to topical steroids.
- Almost physiological in adolescents.
- Other types are inherited and persistent.

Aetiology
The condition is extremely common. Probably 50% of adolescents have it temporarily, when it is regarded as being physiological. Others have the tendency from childhood, when it is probably dominantly inherited, and it persists into adult life. It can also occur in association with the dominant form of ichthyosis vulgaris. It can be seen as a consequence of systemic steroid therapy in Cushing's syndrome, and also in gross nutritional deficiency when it is known as *phrynoderma*.

The orifice of the hair follicle is distended by a keratin plug which may contain a hair. The cause is unknown but all varieties improve in the summer.

Clinical features
Discrete, small, grey, horny, rough papules (Fig. 14.6) develop around hair follicles on the posterolateral aspects of the upper arms and thighs, although

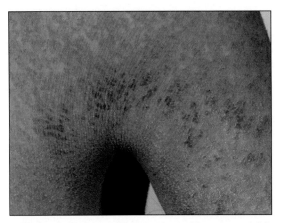

▲ **Fig. 14.5** *X-linked ichthyosis vulgaris. The corneocytes fail to separate from each other and shed individually so that large dark scales form.*

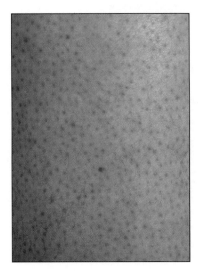

◄ **Fig. 14.6** *Keratosis pilaris. Discrete small rough papules occur around the hair follicles, often with surrounding erythema on the extensor surfaces of the upper arms and thighs.*

the buttocks and forearms may be involved. There may be erythema surrounding the horny plugs. The lesions are asymptomatic, other than being rather unpleasant to feel.

Palmar-plantar keratoderma

Definition
A pronounced thickening of the skin of the palms and soles.

> ### Diagnostic features
> - Thickened palmar and plantar skin.
> - Diffuse, punctate or linear.
> - Occasionally other ectodermal defects are present.

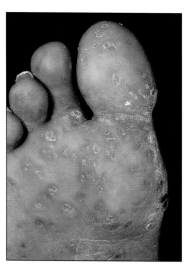

◄ **Fig. 14.7**
Punctate keratoderma. Punctate forms of keratoderma occur particularly in Negroes.

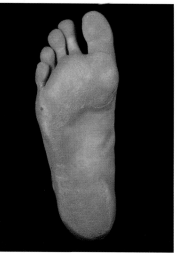

◄ **Fig. 14.8**
Palmar-plantar keratoderma. The skin is markedly thickened and often has a somewhat yellow colour. The keratoderma is symmetrical.

Aetiology
The stratum corneum of the palms and soles is markedly thickened histologically but the rest of the epidermis is normal. There are a number of varieties, all of which persist throughout life and are of unknown cause. These may be associated with other ectodermal defects, for example of the teeth (*Papillon–Lefèvre*) or nails (*Pachyonychia congenita*). The common 'diffuse' type affects the whole palm and sole. There is a rare inherited type occurring late in life in association with carcinoma of the oesophagus, which is known as *tylosis*.

Sometimes the condition affects only part of the palms and soles and is punctate (Fig. 14.7) or linear, especially in Negroes.

Clinical features
The eruption is symmetrical and very well-defined, ending abruptly at the sides of the hands and fingers or feet. The skin is excessively thick and often a slightly yellow colour (Fig. 14.8). It feels rough, tends to crack and becomes painful, especially in the winter months.

Management of ichthyosis and related disorders
At present the major goal of therapy is to increase the water content of the stratum corneum because its pliability and suppleness is a function of its water content. Occlusive materials which prevent the evaporation of water are thus the mainstay of treatment. There are various greasy materials available: true fats, waxes, mineral greases and macrogols (Fig. 14.9).

MATERIALS USED IN MANAGEMENT OF ICHTHYOSIS AND RELATED DISORDERS	
fats in fluid form	arachis oil, olive oil
fats in ointment form	lard, wool-fat (lanolin)
solid fats	beeswax, emulsifying wax, cocoa butter
mineral greases	liquid paraffin (mineral oil) paraffin ointment (petrolatum, vaseline) macrogols (polyethylene glycol, e.g. cetomacrogol)

▲ **Fig. 14.9** *Materials used in the management of ichthyosis and related disorders.*

151

Emulsions are commonly used in dermatology. They are a dispersion of two or more immiscible liquid phases, usually aqueous and oily, which are thermodynamically unstable and tend to separate out, so emulsifying agents such as sodium lauryl sulphate are added to improve stability by reducing surface tension. Thus aqueous cream is an example of an oil/water system where oil is dispersed as small droplets in water, being 30% emulsifying ointment with 70% water with chlorocresol as a preservative. Emulsifying ointment itself is 30% emulsifying wax (which contains sodium lauryl sulphate), 20% liquid paraffin and 50% white soft paraffin.

These emollients can be used as moisturizers or soap substitutes and bath additives. Commonly used emollients are:

(1) **Moisturizers** such as aqueous cream, E45 cream and Aquaphor (popular in the US, related to woolfat).

(2) **Soap substitutes and bath additives** such as emulsifying ointment and various preparations based on liquid paraffin. Baths based on a colloidal oat fraction or on soya oil are also favourites.

(3) **Urea-containing preparations.** Creams containing 10% urea.

(4) **Lactic acid preparations.** Emollients containing lactic acid can be useful.

(5) **1% Menthol, 2% Phenol in aqueous cream** is particularly helpful for winter itch.

In general, it is important to emphasize the deleterious effect of excess bathing and washing on dry skin, especially in winter.

Of interest, for the future, are the retinoids such as etretinate, which have been a major advance in the treatment of serious forms of ichthyosis. However they are not indicated for the common forms, because long-term side-effects are not yet known. The drug does increase lipid levels, and it would seem unwise to tolerate a hyperlipidaemic state only for the sake of improving a form of ichthyosis which is a nuisance but not serious. Etretinate is also teratogenic and potentially hepatotoxic.

It is important to note that ichthyotic and xerotic conditions do not respond to topical steroids except when eczema is present, in which case class III are invaluable as, for example, in the treatment of winter itch. The choice of vehicle is important: ointments are most helpful and creams are best avoided since they exacerbate dryness.

DARIER'S DISEASE (KERATOSIS FOLLICULARIS)

Definition
A dominantly inherited disorder of epidermal cell adherence resulting in abnormal keratinization and warty papules on the skin.

Diagnostic features
- Symmetrical, small, firm, red/brown papules.
- Greasy, crusted and warty surface.
- Face, front and back of chest.
- Nail abnormalities.

Aetiology
There is imperfect formation and maturation of the tonofilament–desmosome complex such that the epidermal cells do not adhere together properly. As a result acantholysis and splitting occurs in the epidermis and keratin is formed incorrectly and prematurely.

Clinical features
This condition usually begins in childhood. Symmetrical, small, firm, red/brown papules with a rather greasy, crusted or warty surface occur on the face (especially the forehead and ears), scalp, back, front of the chest (Fig. 14.10) and flexures. The distribution is rather similar to that of seborrhoeic dermatitis. The papules may coalesce into plaques if secondary infection occurs, resulting in malodorous vegetations. Wedge-shaped notches occur in the distal margins of the nails. Pits on the palms are characteristic.

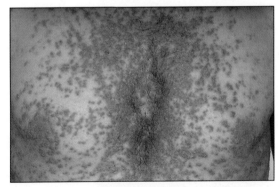

▲**Fig. 14.10** *Darier's disease. A symmetrical profuse eruption of small firm red-brown papules occurs on the front and back of the chest.*

Management

A skin biopsy should be performed to confirm the diagnosis because the histology is diagnostic. The condition is chronic but exacerbations may occur in response to ultraviolet light exposure (which should be avoided) and to sepsis. Secondary bacterial infection should be treated with antibacterials. Class III steroids combined with antibiotics are generally helpful. All retinoids are partially effective and may be necessary. Occasionally herpes simplex (Kaposi's varicelliform eruption) may occur and systemic acyclovir is indicated.

HAILEY–HAILEY DISEASE (BENIGN FAMILIAL CHRONIC PEMPHIGUS)

Definition

A dominantly inherited condition resulting in blisters, erosions, fissures and crusts in areas of skin particularly subject to friction.

Diagnostic features
- Flexures.
- Easily ruptured vesicles.
- Erosions, fissures and crusts.

Aetiology

This is a dominantly inherited disorder which is sometimes associated with Darier's disease. There are abnormalities in the tonofilament–desmosome complex, so that epidermal cells do not bind to each other strongly and are vulnerable in areas of friction. As a result, flaccid blisters, erosions and crusts occur, rather like those seen in pemphigus, which Hailey–

Hailey disease resembles histologically. Immuno-fluorescence however is negative in Hailey–Hailey disease.

Clinical features

It usually commences in adolescence in the axillae, the groins and sometimes the neck. These are areas of skin that are readily traumatized. The vesicles that result rupture easily, so that an appearance of eroded, fissured skin results (Fig. 14.11). The skin tends to crust as it heals.

Management

All patients should be strongly advised to avoid ultraviolet light exposure. Since sepsis may trigger an exacerbation, swabs should be taken and appropriate antibacterial and anti-*Candida* agents prescribed. Class III topical steroids are effective, although it is not known why. In severe cases affected skin in the groins or axillae may be excised and grafted successfully.

EPIDERMOLYSIS BULLOSA

This term covers a number of inherited disorders characterized by a failure of the epidermis to adhere correctly to the dermis, so that the skin blisters easily in response to trivial trauma. The conditions are rare, but they are mentioned here because the severe forms are devastating. They are under intense investigation at present and this has resulted in considerable light being thrown onto the fundamental structure of the skin.

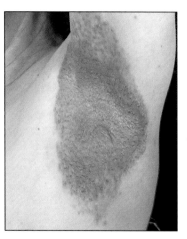

◄ **Fig. 14.11** *Hailey-Hailey disease. In areas subjected to trauma, such as the flexures, vesicles result and subsequently splitting and fissuring of the skin occur.*

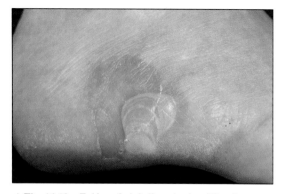

▲ **Fig. 14.12** *Epidermolysis bullosa simplex. Blistering occurs in response to trauma, particularly on the hands and feet, in hot weather.*

The different types may be distinguished by electron microscopy. Abnormalities are found in the fibrils which anchor the basal lamina to the dermis and in the number and nature of the hemidesmosomes. The severe varieties may be diagnosed prenatally by fetal sampling of the skin via a fetoscope and subsequent electron microscopy. The common simplex varieties begin in childhood and the blisters tend to occur mainly on the hands and feet (Fig. 14.12), and they heal without scarring and so constitute an inconvenience only. The other varieties are more serious and are present at birth. In these, the blisters occur on pressure points and result in scarring and milia (dominant *epidermolysis bullosa dystrophica*). Mutilating deformities occur in the recessive variety of epidermolysis bullosa dystrophica (Fig. 14.13). The nails and teeth are also involved. There is no specific treatment but investigation, specialized nursing and genetic counselling are required.

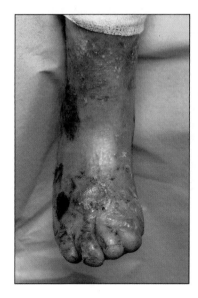

◄**Fig. 14.13** *Recessive dystrophic epidermolysis bullosa. The blisters are followed by erosions which are slow to heal, milia, scarring and deformities especially of the digits.*

REACTIVE DISORDERS OF THE SKIN AND DRUG ERUPTIONS

INTRODUCTION

There are a variety of recognizable patterns occurring on the skin in response to one of several possible noxious agents. They have been given names such as toxic erythema, erythema multiforme and erythema nodosum. They really represent a collection of physical signs, rather than constitute a diagnosis *per se*. The agent which is responsible for them (often a drug) must be discerned if possible. Drugs may also produce certain patterns which are only caused by a drug, for example a fixed drug eruption. They also occasionally simulate a skin disease (lichenoid eruptions) or may exacerbate one (for example psoriasis). This chapter attempts to cover these conditions.

TOXIC ERYTHEMA

Definition
A generalized, red, macular or maculopapular (morbilliform) eruption of the skin.

Diagnostic features
- Widespread.
- Itchy.
- Blotchy redness.

Aetiology
This is one of the commonest abnormal cutaneous patterns. The causes may be:

(1) Drugs. The mechanism of these morbilliform reactions is not known and they do not always recur with rechallenge. There are no laboratory tests to determine which drug is responsible. Any drug may produce this very common clinical picture but the most frequent offenders are:

(a) *Antibiotics.* Penicillin derivatives (such as ampicillin (Figs 15.1 & 15.2) amoxycillin and flucloxacillin) and sulphonamides (particularly septrin) are the most frequently implicated. The rash appears several days (classically 10 days) after commencing treatment, often after the course is finished, which confuses the patient and sometimes the doctor. Ampicillin is the commonest cause, with about 10% of the population reacting in this manner. A hundred per cent of patients with infectious mononucleosis react in this way, so ampicillin should be avoided if that diagnosis is suspected. If it is inadvertently represcribed when the patient has recovered he will probably not develop a second attack of toxic erythema; however the drug should probably be avoided for life. Patients with lymphatic leukaemia are also prone to these types of drug eruptions.

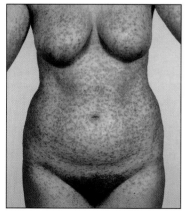
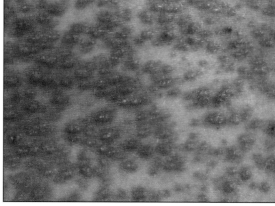

◄Figs 15.1 & 15.2 *Toxic erythema. The eruption is widespread, erythematous and often papular (Fig. 15.2). Drugs, in this case ampicillin, are commonly responsible for these morbilliform patterns.*

(b) *Barbiturates*, especially phenobarbitone.

(c) *Non-steroidal anti-inflammatory drugs* such as phenyl-butazone, fenclofenac and diclofenac.

(d) *Amitryptilline*.

(e) *Radiotherapy*.

(2) Bacteria. The skin eruptions of scarlet fever or the toxic shock syndrome are examples of toxic erythemas. The former is produced by a streptococcal erythrotoxin and the latter by a staphylococcal pyrogenic exotoxin.

(3) Viral infections. The exanthematic and morbilli-form eruptions of rubella and measles are examples of toxic erythema where the evolution, distribution and morphology of the eruption, coupled with the accompanying symptoms and physical signs (for example

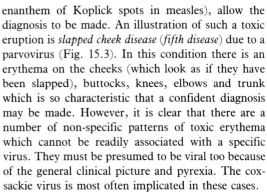

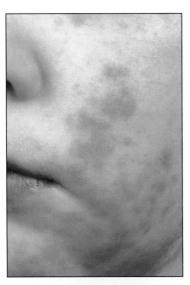

◄**Fig. 15.3**
Fifth disease (slapped cheek disease). A parvovirus causes a toxic erythema at certain sites, especially the cheeks.

enanthem of Koplick spots in measles), allow the diagnosis to be made. An illustration of such a toxic eruption is *slapped cheek disease (fifth disease)* due to a parvovirus (Fig. 15.3). In this condition there is an erythema on the cheeks (which look as if they have been slapped), buttocks, knees, elbows and trunk which is so characteristic that a confident diagnosis may be made. However, it is clear that there are a number of non-specific patterns of toxic erythema which cannot be readily associated with a specific virus. They must be presumed to be viral too because of the general clinical picture and pyrexia. The cox-sackie virus is most often implicated in these cases.

(4) Toxic erythema of the newborn (erythema toxi-cum neonatorum). This is a very common rash which occurs within 48 hours of birth. A blotchy, macular erythema (Fig. 15.4) occurs on the face, trunk and proximal parts of the limbs and clears within 2 days. There is no systemic upset and the cause is completely obscure.

Clinical features

Red macules which may become papular and often morbilliform are the hallmark of the eruption, but since the lesions merge into one another a general impression of a blotchy erythema is given. Practically all the body surface is affected (Fig. 15.5). The eruption often resolves by desquamation. The eruption is usually itchy if due to a drug, and asymptomatic if due to an infection. Fever usually accompanies the latter, and specific symptoms and signs should indicate the source of the latter.

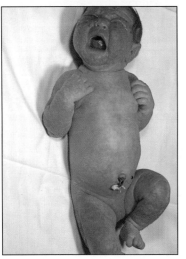

◄**Fig. 15.4**
Toxic erythema of the newborn. A blotchy erythema commonly occurs within the first 48 hours of life, which clears within 2 days. Its cause is unknown.

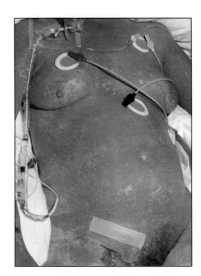

◄**Fig. 15.5**
Toxic erythema. The whole cutaneous surface may be involved so that the patient is erythrodermic.

Management

Management depends on the diagnosis. Bacterial infections are treated with the appropriate antibiotic, viral infections are treated symptomatically, and drug eruptions are managed as follows:

(1) The drug must be discontinued immediately lest an erythroderma results.

(2) The patient should be reassured that the eruption will go away within 8–10 days. If patients know what to expect it is easier for them to tolerate the rash. It is a mistake to assume that the patient will recover straight away.

(3) Prompt relief of the irritation, which is often considerable, may be achieved by the use of: (a) *Calamine*, with or without 1–2% menthol. This is one of the really helpful uses of calamine. It is often used indiscriminately for any itchy eruption and then only serves to mask the physical signs and hinder diagnosis. (b) *Systemic antihistamines*, which are of symptomatic value. (c) *Systemic steroids* occasionally are required, either as a single injection of Synacthen Depot or ACTH, or as oral prednisolone, starting at 30 mg daily and reducing by 5 mg every third day.

(4) If the condition occurs in hospital the general practitioner should be informed and the allergy recorded prominently on the notes.

(5) It is often wise for a patient to wear a 'Medic-Alert' thereafter.

ERYTHEMA MULTIFORME

Definition

A distinctive clinical and histological pattern affecting the skin and, sometimes, mucous membranes.

> ### Diagnostic features
> - Limbs, hand and feet.
> - Symmetrical 'target' lesions and, occasionally, blisters.
> - Mucous membrane ulceration with systemic toxicity (Stevens–Johnson syndrome).

Aetiology

This cutaneous picture is readily identified but not necessarily so easily explained. Histologically there is vasodilatation and oedema in the upper dermis, with a lymphohistiocytic infiltrate surrounding the blood vessels, which is most prominent in the region of the dermo-epidermal junction. This is followed by a varying degree of extravasion of red cells with

destruction of the lower and occasionally the entire epidermis. The pattern is thought to be a manifestation of an immune complex disorder; the commonest known causes are given in Figure 15.6.

Clinical features

By convention three forms of erythema multiforme are differentiated, depending on the degree of damage done to the integument. Not surprisingly, there is overlap between them.

(1) Iris type. This is the commonest pattern. There are symmetrical, essentially round, red or purple lesions occurring on the extremities, particularly on the backs of the hands, palms (Fig. 15.7), forearms, dorsa of the

---

> ### COMMONEST CAUSES OF ERYTHEMA MULTIFORME
>
> Viruses: herpes simplex, vaccinia, infectious mononucleosis, orf, hepatitis B
>
> *Mycoplasma*: primary atypical pneumonia
>
> Fungi: histoplasmosis
>
> Drugs: penicillin, diphenylhydantoin, barbiturates, sulphonamides, rifampicin, phenylbutazone, salicylates
>
> Radiotherapy
>
> Lupus erythematosus, polyarteritis nodosa, Wegener's granulomatosis
>
> Malignant disease

▲ **Fig. 15.6** *The commonest known causes of erythema multiforme.*

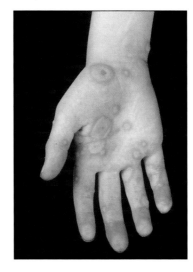

◀ **Fig. 15.7** *Erythema multiforme. The extremities are most frequently involved. The centre of the lesions are more affected than the periphery, simulating a target. The commonest known cause is herpes simplex.*

feet, soles and lower leg. The characteristic feature of these annular lesions is that the central area is more involved than the periphery, being slightly raised and cyanotic, probably because the central area has borne the brunt of the vascular damage. This configuration resembles a target so they are called target lesions (see Fig. 1.30). The disorder is self-limiting and the patient has generally recovered within 3 weeks.

(2) Vesiculobullous type. This is an intermediate between the simple iris type and the Stevens–Johnson syndrome. The degree of damage to the skin is greater and the centre of the target lesion becomes a vesicle or bulla (Fig. 15.8) with less marked changes around the periphery. The eruption is more widespread and the trunk and mucous membranes may be involved too. As the blisters break, raw, painful erosions and ulcers result, particularly in the mouth and nose and on the genitalia.

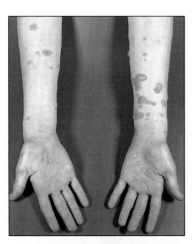

◄**Fig. 15.8**
Erythema multiforme. In more severe forms blistering may occur in the centre of the lesions.

(3) Stevens–Johnson syndrome. This is a rare condition and is included here for the sake of completeness. There is widespread involvement of the skin (although occasionally it is spared) and mucous membranes, with blistering and ulceration. The patient is unwell and febrile, and ulceration in the mouth (Fig. 15.9) may make it impossible to eat. Conjunctival involvement may lead to corneal scarring and blindness, and genital and urethral involvement may be followed by urinary retention. It is a multisystem disorder which may involve the joints, lungs, gastro-intestinal tract and kidneys. There is an appreciable mortality. When it is due to sulphonamides, it usually begins a week or two after ingestion of the drug.

Management

The common iris type is unmistakeable. The blistering types may be confused with bullous pemphigoid, and a skin biopsy for histology and immunofluorescence is invaluable. Immunofluorescence is positive in bullous pemphigoid but not in erythema multiforme.

It is important to attempt to identify and treat the cause. The most common is herpes simplex. A minority of patients get recurrent attacks of erythema multiforme each time they are afflicted with this virus and it is helpful to attempt to limit its precipitants if possible. The herpes simplex should be treated immediately with topical acyclovir and in cases of frequent recurrences oral acyclovir is indicated.

Symptomatic treatment is usually all that is required for mild cases of unknown aetiology because it is a self-limiting condition. However, the Stevens–Johnson syndrome is a serious disorder because of the systemic toxicity. The role of systemic steroids is controversial.

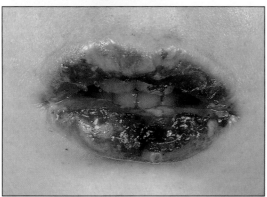

▲**Fig. 15.9** *Erythema multiforme. The condition is known as Stevens–Johnson syndrome if the mucous membranes are involved. Blistering leads to painful ulceration.*

CAUSES OF ERYTHEMA NODOSUM	
streptococci	*Yersinia* infection
tuberculosis	drugs, especially oral
sarcoidosis	contraceptives,
leprosy	sulphonamides,
viruses	penicillin and
infectious mononucleosis	tetracyclines
chlamydiae	radiotherapy
lymphogranuloma venereum	ulcerative colitis
cat scratch disease	Hodgkin's disease

▲**Fig. 15.10** *The causes of erythema nodosum.*

Many will attest to their virtue but a large trial in France of severe cases of Stevens–Johnson's syndrome showed that many patients died from side-effects of the steroids.

ERYTHEMA NODOSUM

Definition
The occurrence of crops of tender red nodules on the lower limbs.

Diagnostic features
- Acute onset.
- Red, tender nodules.
- Lower legs especially shins.

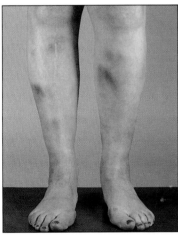

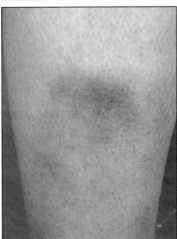

◀**Figs 15.11 & 15.12** *Erythema nodosum. Painful red nodules (Fig. 15.12) occur on the front of the shins. Drugs, streptococci and sarcoidosis are the most common causes in the UK.*

Aetiology
The disorder is relatively common. The particular causes depend on local conditions but in the UK, sarcoidosis, streptococcal infections and drug eruptions are most to blame. A list of causes is given in Figure 15.10.

Pathologically there is a vasculitis particularly involving the deep dermal and subcutaneous vessels and fat (*panniculitis*). In a small group of individuals, usually female, no cause is found; the disorder is then ·chronic and is known as a *nodular vasculitis*.

Clinical features
The onset is acute and the patient complains of painful red nodules, usually on the extensor surfaces of the shins (Figs 15.11 & 15.12) but occasionally on the calves. It is sometimes associated with ankle oedema. More unusually, the thighs and extensor aspects of the upper limbs are affected. The individual lesions last for 1–2 weeks and attain a diameter of 3–4cm. They are bright, red, tender nodules which then go mauve and have no surface change. They occur in crops, the whole attack usually being over within 6 weeks. There is sometimes associated malaise, joint pains and a slight fever.

The nodules do not ulcerate except in *erythema induratum* (Bazin's disease), when nodules on the backs of the calves (Fig. 15.13) are particularly involved, often in middle aged women, in association with active tuberculosis. Sometimes, an identical clinical picture is seen in patients who have no overt signs of tuberculosis but who have an unusually pronounced response to the Mantoux test at 1:10,000 and a past personal/family history of exposure to tuberculosis. Anti-tubercular therapy is often effective.

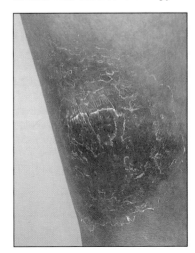

◀**Fig. 15.13** *Erythema induratum. This young Vietnamese woman had painful red ulcerating nodules on her calves and a strongly positive Mantoux test without overt signs of TB. She responded to antituberculosis therapy.*

Management

The clinical picture is readily recognized. Management involves identification and treatment of the cause. A full physical examination is necessary, and a full blood count, ESR, chest X-ray, ASO titre and Mantoux test are all basic investigations. A biopsy may be helpful.

URTICARIA AND ANGIO-OEDEMA

Definition

A condition characterized by transient itchy red swellings of the skin and mucous membranes secondary to the release of histamine and other vasoactive agents.

Diagnostic features
- Itchy and transient.
- Red swellings with central pallor.
- Various sizes and shapes.
- Acute or chronic.

Aetiology

The urticarial wheal is the result of the release of histamine and other vasoactive amines from granules within mast cells which are found in blood vessels. Histologically there is vasodilatation, dermal oedema and a mild perivascular infiltrate of lymphocytes and eosinophils. If the deep dermis and subcutaneous tissues are involved the condition is known as angio-oedema.

Mast cells may degranulate as a result of direct or immunological stimulation. Thus certain drugs (for example morphine, codeine, ethanol, polymyxin B) and bacterial, plant or invertebrate toxins stimulate the mast cells to degranulate directly. IgE on the other hand is responsible for allergic reactions to drugs, serum injections, penicillins in dairy products, foods and inhaled allergens. This immediate or accelerated form of hypersensitivity is due to the reaction between the antigen and IgE molecules fixed to sensitized tissue (skin, respiratory, gastro-intestinal or cardio-vascular) mast cells or circulating basophils. Thus bronchospasm, laryngeal oedema and anaphylactic shock may accompany urticaria. The reaction occurs within minutes or up to 36 hours after exposure. Penicillin is the most common cause.

Immune complex induced urticaria associated with serum sickness, on the other hand, occurs 4–12 days after exposure. The antigen has to remain in the circulation long enough such that when the antibody (IgG or IgM) has been synthesized, circulating antigen–antibody complexes are formed. *Serum sickness* is characterized by fever, urticaria, arthralgia, nephritis, neuritis and hepatitis. Drugs are now more common causes than serum (for example penicillin, sulphonamides, thiouracil, streptomycin, cholecystographic dyes, diphenylhydantoin and aminosalicylic acid).

The anaphylotoxins C3a and C5a derived from the classical and alternative pathway of complement may also act upon mast cells. Mast cell degranulation may be inhibited by agents which raise intracellular cyclic AMP and stimulated by those which raise cyclic GMP.

In acute cases, the cause may be readily determined by both patient and doctor, particularly when drugs or foods are to blame. Only very occasionally is urticaria a manifestation of systemic disease, for example thyrotoxicosis. The urticarial eruptions associated with serum sickness, the prodrome of serum hepatitis and lupus erythematosus are more persistent than in true urticaria and are actually histologically a leuco-cytoclastic vasculitis. In chronic cases, which are arbitrarily defined as attacks of urticaria lasting longer than a couple of months, a cause is rarely elucidated.

Clinical features

Urticaria consists of intensely itchy red swellings (see Fig. 1.13) which last a few hours and then disappear without trace. The swellings resemble the changes which occur after meeting a stinging nettle, so that the disorder is known colloquially as 'hives' or 'nettle rash'. There may be no physical signs when the

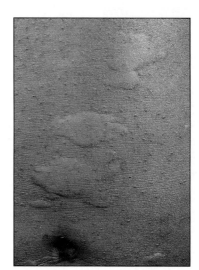

◀ **Fig. 15.14**
Urticaria. Itchy oedematous swellings, which last a few hours and disappear without trace are known as wheals. The erythema may not be obvious in pigmented skins.

patient is examined by the doctor, but the history is usually typical enough for the diagnosis to be made anyway. The patient describes the lesions as blotches, blisters or wheals. They vary in size and shape and are raised and smooth with no surface scale or change (Fig. 15.14). They are red peripherally, with a tendency to central pallor, and are short-lived, lasting only a few hours and fading without trace. The wheals may occur anywhere on the body but especially where clothes are tight (Fig. 15.15), such as under a waistband. They may occur particularly around the eyes and on the lips, genitalia and hands, producing a dramatic effect called angio-oedema. If this affects the tongue and larynx, the disorder becomes life-threatening, due to the possibility of asphyxia. Anaphylaxis and circulatory collapse may then result.

Urticaria, rather like eczema, is a physical sign. There are a number of possible causes which may be classified as follows:

Acute urticaria

This is the most satisfactory type of urticaria in terms of being able to provide an adequate explanation for the malady, although more often than not it is the patient who provides the doctor with the answer. Each time the allergen is ingested the condition reappears and is thus reproducible. However, challenge is inadvisable especially where drugs are suspected because of the danger of anaphylaxis. When a food is implicated, the commonest being shellfish, strawberries or mushrooms, there is sometimes an associated gastro-intestinal upset. The most common causes are given in Figure 15.16.

Physical urticarias

These are very common and the diagnosis can be made from the history.

(1) Dermographism. This simply means that direct pressure on the skin produces urticaria. The patient notes that the skin irritates and linear wheals appear as a result of scratching (Fig. 15.17). It is an exaggerated response of the skin to trauma resulting in the release of histamine and other vasoactive agents from mast cells. The patients, who are often young adults, may have ordinary urticaria as well. The doctor can reproduce the condition by drawing a line on the skin

CAUSES OF ACUTE URTICARIA	
Drugs	Allergic: penicillin, cephalosporins, aspirin, toxoids, animal sera, polypeptide hormones (e.g. insulin), quinidine
	Direct histamine liberators: morphine, codeine
Foods	Fish, nuts, eggs, chocolates, shellfish, tomatoes, pork, strawberries, milk, cheese, spices and yeast
	Dyes and additives, benzoates and tartrazine
Infection	Focal sepsis (e.g. urinary tract), viral (e.g. hepatitis), *Candida*, protozoa
General	Lupus erythematosus, lymphoma, polycythaemia, macroglobulinaemia

▲**Fig. 15.16** *The most common causes of urticaria.*

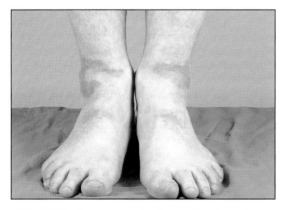

▲**Fig. 15.15** *Pressure urticaria. Pressure (in this case from tight boots) may be entirely responsible for a physical urticaria or aggravate ordinary urticaria.*

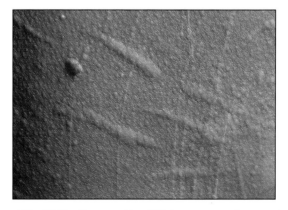

▲**Fig. 15.17** *Dermographism. This is an exaggerated response of the skin to trauma, which is common in young adults. It may persist for years before disappearing spontaneously.*

of the back. The tendency to dermographism ultimately disappears but it may take months or years. Antihistamines are of limited benefit.

(2) **Pressure urticaria.** This is rather a rare condition if seen on its own but it does occur in a minor degree in many patients with ordinary urticaria. The patient remarks upon swellings that are often more painful and itchy after prolonged pressure, for example on the buttocks after sitting for a long time, or on the soles of the feet after standing all day in a shop. The lesions last many hours. It does not respond well to antihistamines but eventually spontaneous recovery occurs.

(3) **Solar, cold and heat urticaria.** These conditions are rather rare but the history leads to the correct diagnosis. The wheals can be reproduced by solar simulating equipment, ice cubes or a test tube of hot water, depending on the physical entity involved. Patients with cold urticaria must be warned against bathing in cold water as this may produce a massive transudation of fluid into the skin, with hypotension, syncope and anaphylactic shock. Drinking cold water may produce swelling of the lips, tongue and pharynx. The condition is acquired in adolescence and is usually self-limiting.

(4) **Aquagenic urticaria.** This is very common indeed. Patients remark that on exposure to water, and particularly after a bath or shower, small itchy wheals develop which last 10–15 minutes. The temperature of the water does not modify the response. It is rather a tiresome complaint which may persist for many years and some patients are quite frustrated by it. There is really no satisfactory treatment. It is occasionally a presenting symptom of polycythaemia.

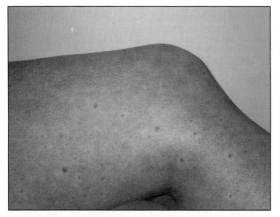

▲**Fig. 15.18** *Cholinergic urticaria. Very small, short-lived red wheals occur in young people, precipitated by such stimuli as exercise, emotion or sweating.*

(5) **Cholinergic urticaria.** This is a common condition again occurring in young people. The lesions are intensely pruritic, red wheals, less than 2mm in diameter (Fig. 15.18), which develop in response to sweating, exercise, emotion and hot foods. It is postulated that an increase in blood temperature triggers a neural reflex which releases acetylcholine from sympathetic nerve endings. Acetylcholine increases intracellular cyclic GMP, activating the mast cells to degranulate. Attacks last only a few minutes. The condition ultimately resolves. Treatment is unsatisfactory, as prophylactic antihistamines do not usually work very well.

Chronic non-allergic urticaria

This is an extremely common disorder characterized by recurrent itchy swellings of the skin, which are controllable with prophylactic antihistamines. It is defined as an urticaria which lasts longer than 6 weeks, for which no obvious cause can be found. The wheals occur sometimes on a daily basis or less frequently. Ultimately it disappears, often to return years later. The patient is otherwise perfectly healthy.

One of the problems with this disease is that it is extremely difficult to explain to a patient who is convinced that it is an allergy, that there is no good evidence for this at present and that we know little about its aetiology. Certainly, the physical signs are identical to those occurring in acute urticaria (in which allergens can be identified), and it is obviously reasonable to extrapolate from this experience. However, most patients have done some 'detection' work of their own in terms of eliminating suspected foods, without success. Most allergists admit to failure, but the disorder is undoubtedly open to elimination diets and alternative medicine. Certainly various ingested materials, such as salicylates, penicillin and indomethacin, may exacerbate the disease and so should be avoided. Some doctors believe that yellow tartrazine dyes and benzoates, which are incorporated as colourings and preservatives in food stuffs, are offenders. Fortunately, these additives are now more readily identifiable by their 'E' numbers on packaging labels, and it may be worth trying to eliminate them from the patient's diet. The problem however is reproducibility. In patients with dermatitis herpetiformis, which is a true allergy to a dietary allergen (gluten), one can 'cure' the disease by withdrawing the substance and cause it to return by introducing it. This is not the case in chronic urticaria.

Chronic non-allergic urticaria is more common in those with a personal or family history of atopy, which gives more weight to an allergic mechanism. Hayfever is clearly precipitated when the Timothy grass pollen count is high, and resolves as it is reduced. Asthmatic attacks may be induced by animal fur. Nothing is so clear-cut with urticaria. In the rare disorder *hereditary angio-oedema* — where there is a deficiency of the esterase inhibitor of the first component of complement, such that the usual brake on the complement cascade is absent — angio-oedema and wheals result. It is theoretically possible that there is something similar wrong with the check mechanism inhibiting the release of histamine in chronic non-allergic urticaria. The disorder may be rather like a burglar alarm which goes off with no burglar present; that is, the allergic system is at fault rather than an allergen being responsible.

Management

The history is most important and the patient usually gives the clue to the cause of an acute urticaria, in which case the cause should be withdrawn. The physical and chronic urticarias too have a characteristic history. Investigations are rather unrewarding. Blood tests, such as a full blood count, ESR, and anti-nuclear factor and SMAC, are usually normal. Skin prick tests are often positive in a non-specific way as part of an atopic diathesis (that is, pollen and animal fur positivity) but elimination of the allergens elicited usually makes little difference.

In chronic cases it is often wise to ask the patient to make a list of the things ingested 24 hours prior to each attack, if only to demonstrate that there appears to be little reason to them. An elimination diet free from preservatives, under the guidance of a dietitian, may be worth trying.

Prophylactic antihistamines are the mainstay of treatment and are very effective indeed. Previously the limiting factor was the hypnotic effect of the older antihistamines. However, the advent of terfenadine and astemizole, which are not soporific, have made all the difference. The drug should be taken in the amount which controls the symptoms, even if this is greater than the manufacturer's recommendations. This appears to be a safe approach with most anti-histamines, although astemizole has recently been reported to have arrhythmic effects in high doses. It is important to take the drugs regularly and prophylactically to control the disease, rather than taking them at the time of the attack, as this makes the condition much easier to bear. They should be taken until the disorder has cleared completely and then tailed off, watching carefully for recurrence of symptoms.

In cases of anaphylaxis, adrenaline 1:1,000 is required. It is either given sub-cutaneously in a dose of 0.5 ml to 1 ml, or intravenously as 0.1 ml over a period of 1 minute. Resuscitation equipment is necessary, including an airway, oxygen, suction apparatus, and equipment for tracheotomy. Other drugs which may be given are injectable antihistamines, such as chlorpheniramine and systemic steroids, viz. hydrocortisone hemisuccinate intravenously or intramuscularly injected. Aminophylline may be necessary.

Occasionally admission to hospital is beneficial. It affords an opportunity to study the effects of elimination diets and allows the patient to rest, and is particularly useful if psychogenic factors are present. These do not cause the disease, but undoubtedly some patients become very distressed, disproportionately to the degree of their affliction. This is sometimes because there are other factors in their lives that are frustrating them and making the urticaria worse. Management of these sources of unhappiness will be of benefit, coupled with encouragement and prophylactic antihistamines.

PURPURA AND VASCULITIS

Introduction

Purpura is a term used to describe a physical sign and is thus not a disease *per se*. The lesions are purple and, unlike erythema, do not blanche on pressure. Flat purpuric lesions less than 1 cm in diameter arc known as petechiae (Fig. 15.19); larger lesions are called

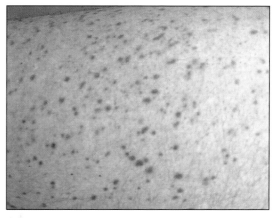

▲ **Fig. 15.19** *Petechiae. Small purpuric macules which do not blanche on pressure are known as petechiae. The lower extremities are most commonly affected in thrombocytopenia.*

ecchymoses (bruises) (Fig. 15.20). Purpura is either due to a disorder of the blood or an abnormality affecting the blood vessels. A simplified scheme is depicted in Figure 15.21. As a general rule non-inflammatory causes produce flat petechiae (for example thrombocytopenia or macroglobulinaemia) or

ecchymoses (for example coagulation defects or solar purpura), whereas vasculitic or embolic disorders produce palpable purpuric lesions (Fig. 15.22; see Fig. 1.24).

The likely cause of the purpuric eruption is sometimes indicated by the site involved (Fig. 15.23).

Diagnostic features
- Purpuric lesions do not blanche on pressure.
- Purple macules (petechiae) may indicate platelet or plasma protein abnormalities.
- Purple patches (ecchymoses) may indicate a coagulation or vessel wall defect.
- Inflammatory palpable purpura may indicate a vasculitis or embolic disorder.

Vasculitis
Introduction
The classification of vasculitis is confused. It has variously been based on clinical features, histology

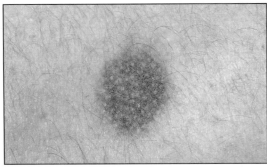

▲ **Fig. 15.20** *Ecchymosis. Extensive bleeding into the skin causes ecchymoses (or bruising). The patient has haemophilia.*

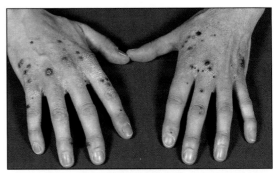

▲ **Fig. 15.22** *Vasculitis. Purpuric and necrotic papules may occur on acral areas such as the hands and feet in disorders such as chilblains or endocarditis.*

CLASSIFICATION OF PURPURA
Blood disorders
Platelet abnormalities
Idiopathic thrombocytopenic purpura
Secondary thrombocytopenia Bone marrow infiltration (e.g. leukaemia or carcinomatosis) Bone marrow arrest (e.g. drugs or irradiation)
Coagulation abnormalities (e.g. haemophilia)
Plasma protein abnormalities (e.g. macroglobulinaemia)
Blood vessel defects
Congenital defects of vessel walls (e.g. Ehlers–Danlos syndrome)
Increased vascular permeability (e.g. scurvy)
Fragility of vessel walls (e.g. solar or steroid)
Damage to vessel walls (e.g. vasculitis or embolic)

▲ **Fig. 15.21** *A simplified classification of purpura.*

SITES OF PURPURA ACCORDING TO CAUSE	
Dependent areas (buttocks and legs)	platelet disorders, macroglobulinaemia, Henoch–Schönlein purpura, meningococcaemia
Acral areas (fingers and toes)	emboli, chilblains vasculitis from infected valves and prostheses
Backs of hands and arms	steroid or solar purpura

▲ **Fig. 15.23** *Sites of purpura according to cause.*

(the size of blood vessel involved and type of infiltrate in the vessel walls) or on immunology. Regrettably the correlation between them is poor and many patients cannot be easily categorized.

Kussmaul first described polyarteritis nodosa which involves large blood vessels. Subsequently Wegener's granulomatosis and cranial arteritis were recognized. Then hypersensitivity reactions to drugs, especially sulphonamides, were defined. These have been shown to be due to immune complexes in small blood vessel walls. Serum sickness and the Arthus reaction are examples of these.

A common cutaneous form is known as a leucocytoclastic vasculitis because of its pathological features. Its distinction from polyarteritis nodosa is that the vessels in the superficial horizontal plexus in the upper third of the dermis are involved in leucocytoclastic vasculitis, whereas the larger vessels in the lower horizontal plexus at the dermal-subcutaneous junction are involved in polyarteritis nodosa. Clinically there is palpable purpura due to increased vascular permeability in both conditions but the latter is also associated with thrombosis and haemorrhagic infarction.

Vasculitis also involves other organs than the skin and most frequently the joints, muscles and kidneys. It may occur as a result of a connective tissue disorder such as lupus erythematosus, a leukaemic process or a drug reaction. There is, however, a rather specific entity known as Henoch–Schönlein purpura which can be recognized as a separate symptom complex with a rather definite outcome, which is described here. Many patients however are not easily classified at all and are known as suffering from allergic vasculitis or cutaneous–systemic vasculitis. This is an immune complex disorder of unknown cause which may involve the skin alone or various organs, including the kidneys, nervous system, lungs, gastrointestinal tract, joints and heart. It can commence at any age, but usually between 30 and 60 years, and may last a few weeks or years with an episodic course. The prognosis depends on the degree of systemic involvement, especially of the kidney.

Henoch–Schönlein purpura
(anaphylactoid purpura, allergic vasculitis)

Definition
A usually short-lived benign leucocytoclastic vasculitis of the skin, kidneys, joints and gastrointestinal tract, usually occurring in children and young adults following an infectious prodrome.

Diagnostic features
- Polymorphic purpuric lesions.
- Buttocks and legs.
- Sometimes renal, joint and gut haemorrhage.
- Children and young adults.
- Often a preceding upper respiratory tract infection.

Aetiology
The disorder is quite common particularly in the spring. It frequently follows an upper respiratory infection. Beta-haemolytic streptococci have been isolated in some cases but not in all. Viral infections may be relevant but no specific virus has been incriminated. Children, especially boys, are affected and the name Henoch–Schönlein purpura is most frequently associated with this. However, an identical condition occurs in adults, known as allergic vasculitis, anaphylactoid purpura or Henoch–Schönlein purpura. The skin may be the only manifestation of the disorder. The condition is usually self-limiting within a month but it may persist longer and a minority suffer recurrences. Prognosis is related to the degree of renal damage if present. A small percentage do develop chronic renal insufficiency.

Clinical features
The eruption is acute. The ankles, legs (Fig. 15.24) and buttocks are primarily affected, but occasionally the arms and abdomen may be. Although purpura is

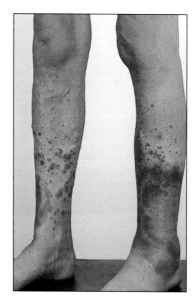

◄Fig. 15.24
Henoch–Schönlein purpura. Palpable purpuric papules or papulovesicles occur on the legs and buttocks.

the hallmark of the eruption, all manner of lesions may be present. These are papules, vesicles, urticarial wheals and bullae leading to necrosis and sometimes ulceration. The lesions occur in crops, but gradually the disorder remits over 3–4 weeks.

There may be a constitutional upset with fever and arthralgia, which often manifests as flitting pains of the ankles, knees, elbows and small joints of the hands. If the gastrointestinal tract is involved, there may be abdominal pain and a bloody diarrhoea. If the renal tract is involved, there may be loin pain, with associated macro- or microscopic haematuria and proteinuria.

Management

The differential diagnosis of leucocytoclastic vasculitis is given in Figure 15.25. Allergic vasculitis is clearly a complicated and variable condition and management depends on the degree of systemic involvement, if any.

A skin biopsy is necessary to confirm the leuco-cytoclastic vasculitis. The urine should be examined for haematuria and proteinuria. If these are positive, full renal testing is indicated, with appropriate treat-ment. If it is possible to identify the cause, in particular a focus of infection, this should be treated. Usually this is not so, and the patient is managed with bed rest and analgesia.

Systemic steroids are sometimes helpful. Predni-solone 35mg daily, with reduction by 5mg on every fourth day, may be given. Longer courses may be necessary. Dapsone is also useful, but its mechanism of action is unknown.

COMMONER CAUSES OF LEUCOCYTOCLASTIC VASCULITIS

Henoch–Schönlein purpura

Cutaneous–systemic angiitis

Connective tissue disorders

Drug eruptions

Lymphoma, leukaemia and carcinoma

Infection: endocarditis, gonococcaemia, meningococcaemia, viral meningitis, hepatitis B, Rocky Mountain spotted fever

▲**Fig. 15.25** *The more common causes of leucocytoclastic vasculitis.*

PITYRIASIS LICHENOIDES CHRONICA

Definition

A chronic erythematosquamous eruption of unknown aetiology affecting predominantly the limbs.

Diagnostic features
- Red macules with an adherent scale.
- Brown papules.
- Symmetrical.
- Inner aspects of limbs.
- Often mistaken for psoriasis or lichen planus.

Aetiology

The disorder affects children and young adults. There are no associated symptoms, although in more acute

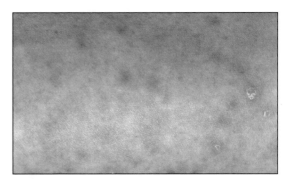

▲**Fig. 15.26** *Pityriasis lichenoides chronica. The lesions are pink papules with an adherent scale which go brown as they resolve.*

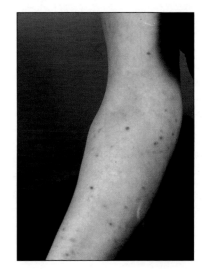

◀**Fig. 15.27** *Pityriasis lichenoides chronica. The lesions occur most profusely in a symmetrical manner on the inner aspects of the limbs.*

cases there may be an antecedent mild fever and malaise. The disorder is thought to be an immune complex disorder because circulating immune complexes are present and immunoglobulins and complement have been found in the blood vessel walls of affected skin. The histology shows a lymphocytic infiltrate surrounding and sometimes involving small blood vessels causing vascular damage. It is possibly initiated by a virus. It is not particularly common but is distinctive enough to be simply diagnosed.

Clinical features

The initial lesion is a purple macule which rapidly becomes a red brown papule which as it flattens develops an adherent scale (Fig. 15.26) and is somewhat pink. The lesions are found predominantly on the inner aspects of the limbs (Fig. 15.27). In the more acute form, crops of oedematous papules which become vesicular and haemorrhagic and subsequently scar occur, and it is often mistaken for chickenpox (*pityriasis lichenoides acuta et varioliformis*).

Management

The disorder is chronic, although it may go into remission after a number of years. It may temporarily disappear with ultraviolet irradiation and occasionally with a 3 week course of erythromycin.

LIGHT ERUPTIONS

Introduction

Terrestrial sunlight extends from 290 to 400nm. The range 290–320nm is known as UVB and 320–400nm as UVA or longwave ultraviolet light. UVB is principally responsible for sunburn and its effects on the ageing process and cutaneous neoplasia have already been dealt with. On the whole, UVA does not produce burning of the skin which is why 'sunbeds' (which deliver UVA) are such a popular means of acquiring a suntan. Its rôle in the induction of skin cancer is more limited than UVB, but it does have a major effect in the ageing process of the skin. UVA passes through window glass whereas UVB is absorbed by the glass and does not.

Photodermatoses may be classified as in Figure 15.28. The porphyrias are errors of metabolism leading to an accumulation of precursors of haem, some of which are photosensitizers that interact with longwave ultraviolet light (UVA) and produce blistering (Fig. 23.10), skin fragility, pigmentation and hirsutism of

light-exposed areas such as the face and backs of the hands. In xeroderma pigmentosum (Fig. 15.29) the skin is acutely sensitive to light due to a deficiency of an enzyme responsible for repair of damaged epidermal DNA, and the process of solar damage and neoplasia is accelerated. The cutaneous eruption of lupus erythematosus most frequently occurs on exposed sites (Fig. 23.13) and relapses of the systemic condition may be precipitated by sunlight. A band of immunoglobulin and complement is found in the basement membrane zone of the skin and ultraviolet may act as the hapten.

Topical medications resulting in photodermatitis have been discussed in chapter 4 (Contact Dermatitis). Systemic drugs are discussed here together with a common reactive condition, the polymorphic light eruption.

CLASSIFICATION OF PHOTODERMATOSES	
Metabolic disease	porphyria, xeroderma pigmentosum, pellagra
Drugs	topical, systemic
Idiopathic	polymorphic light eruption
Disorders aggravated by sunlight	lupus erythematosus, herpes simplex

▲ **Fig. 15.28** *The classification of photodermatoses.*

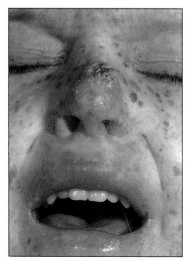

◀**Fig. 15.29** *Xeroderma pigmentosum. Photosensitivity occurs in infancy. Solar lentigines and skin cancer (in this case a squamous cell carcinoma on the nose) develop in childhood.*

Phototoxic reactions

Definition

An erythema of light-exposed areas of the skin and sometimes the fingernails, secondary to the ingestion of a photosensitizing drug.

> **Diagnostic features**
> - An exaggerated sunburn.
> - Sometimes photo-onycholysis.
> - History of drug ingestion.

Aetiology

There are various drugs which regularly produce a phototoxic eruption (Fig. 15.30). Some are always phototoxic, for example psoralens, but usually the effect is idiosyncratic and therefore not predictable in advance in any one individual. The mechanism is not completely understood, although in some patients it seems to be a true delayed hypersensitivity reaction. Factory workers, for example those who manufacture chlorpromazine, may become sensitized and develop phototoxicity on the slightest exposure to light, but most individuals require intense ultraviolet exposure for the condition to manifest itself.

Clinical features

The eruption, which is occasionally eczematous, is most likely to be an exaggerated sunburn which may be followed by blistering. The face (Fig. 15.31) and backs of the hands (Fig. 15.32) are the most frequently involved sites but any exposed areas can be affected. A skier for instance will only have the rash on the exposed parts of the face. There is usually a sharp cut-off at the neck or the 'V' of the neck. The sharply defined pattern of erythema afforded by goggles, glasses or sandals will help to make the diagnosis. A characteristic feature on the face is that the areas under the nose, under the upper eyebrows and under the chin, will be relatively spared, because these areas are shaded.

Management

(1) Stop the drug.
(2) Topical steroids are effective as anti-inflammatory agents. Hydrocortisone cream (2.5%) is indicated for the face and a class III steroid for other sites.

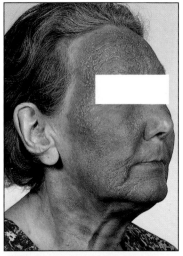

◀**Fig. 15.31** *Phototoxicity. An intense 'sunburn' developed on exposed sites whilst taking a thiazide/amiloride combination (Moduretic). Note the sparing of the skin which had been protected by her hair.*

COMMON PHOTOSENSITIZING DRUGS
Phenothiazines, especially chlorpromazine and promethazine
Tetracyclines, especially demethylchlortetracycline and vibramycin
Sulphonamides
Diuretics, especially thiazides and nalidixic acid
Non-steroidal anti-inflammatory drugs, especially piroxicam and naproxen
Chlorpropamide
Amiodarone
Psoralens
Griseofulvin

▲**Fig. 15.30** *Drugs that commonly produce a phototoxic eruption.*

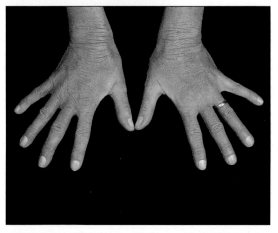

▲**Fig. 15.32** *Phototoxicity. The backs of the hands are involved with erythema and often oedema. This lady had been taking demethychlortetracycline for her acne.*

(3) Systemic steroids are occasionally required: 30–35mg of prednisolone is given and reduced by 5mg every fourth day.

(4) The patient and doctor should record the occurrence.

(5) Some patients would be well-advised to wear a 'Medic-Alert'.

Polymorphic light eruption
Definition
A common sensitivity to ultraviolet light resulting in a pruritic eruption on exposed areas, although usually sparing the face.

> **Diagnostic features**
> - Itchy.
> - Red papules and/or plaques.
> - Develops on sun-exposed areas within 48 hours.
> - The face is usually spared.
> - More frequent in the spring and early summer.

Aetiology
The condition is common in Caucasians although it can occur in pigmented races. It does occur in childhood, but more usually commences in the twenties or thirties; and it is more common in the spring or early summer than it is later in the year. It is thought to be due to the effect of ultraviolet light on an unprotected skin, so that the skin that is pale after the winter is more vulnerable than that which is already tanned,

although this is not true of all patients. Most patients with the condition are sensitive to UVA, some to UVB and a few to both wavelengths. Although it occurs in the UK and northern latitudes it is, not surprisingly, more frequent when the patient goes abroad to a sunny climate. The exact cause of the eruption is unknown.

Clinical features
The onset occurs 24–48 hours after the first sun exposure. The signs and symptoms vary, so that some patients are incapacitated by the eruption whereas others hardly notice it. Red, itchy papules (Fig. 15.33) which may coalesce into plaques, occur on exposed parts, in particular on the backs of the hands, the forearms and the dorsum of the feet, or may be more extensive (Fig. 15.34). The face is usually spared, perhaps because it is continually exposed to ultraviolet and the skin is therefore in some way 'hardened'. The condition persists for about a week even if sun exposure continues and then resolves spontaneously without scarring. It recurs most years but will eventually remit.

Diagnosis
The patient invariably connects the eruption with the sun and calls it 'prickly heat', so the diagnosis presents little problem. However, lupus erythematosus needs to be considered if the condition persists, especially if it is on the face. The polymorphic light eruption may be reproduced experimentally with a solar simulator, but this is an expensive piece of equipment available

▲ **Fig. 15.33** *Polymorphic light eruption. Very itchy red oedematous papules and plaques occur 24–48 hours after exposure to strong sunlight, which persist for about a week.*

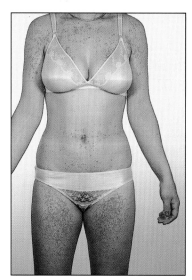

◀**Fig. 15.34** *Polymorphic light eruption. The condition is known colloquially as 'prickly heat'. It consists of very pruritic red papules or plaques on exposed parts, although often the face is spared. This lady had been using a sunbed.*

in relatively few centres. It is the only way, however, that the wavelength responsible in any one individual can be detected.

Management

The immediate management is:

(1) Oral antihistamines.

(2) Topical calamine.

(3) Potent topical steroids although they only have a limited effect.

(4) Systemic steroids. A course commencing at 30mg prednisolone daily, and reduced over the ensuing 10 days is effective.

After such an eruption has occurred many patients will consult the practitioner for advice on how to prevent it. It is clearly unwise to sunbathe, but the condition can occur with ordinary exposure such as walking in the sun. Thus long-sleeved shirts and trousers are advisable, although it is difficult for some patients to accept this, especially as the light eruption will occur through thin material. Broad-spectrum sunscreens are worth trying but, since UVA is often responsible, these are not always satisfactory because the majority of sunscreens do not block out UVA very efficiently. Titanium dioxide is effective, but is often unacceptable, because it is opaque.

More toxic measures for preventing the light eruption are available, but it is a matter of clinical judgement as to whether these are justified. Certainly, if the sensitivity is so severe and the patient so miserable that he has to call out the doctor whilst on vacation, they may be considered. These treatments are:

(1) **Systemic steroids.** Prednisolone, 20mg daily, starting 2 days before the holiday and taken throughout is effective, and it is a worthwhile treatment if there are no contraindications. However, such a treatment should only be used once or, at a maximum, twice a year in severe cases where the patient has tried all other measures.

(2) **Chloroquine.** The eruption may be prevented by 200mg daily, but if this is to become a regular treatment, the potential hazard of ocular toxicity must be assessed. Chloroquine causes various forms of reversible keratitis, but more important can produce an irreversible retinopathy, which may lead to blindness.

(3) **Ultraviolet light.** A course of UVB (E1) prior to the holiday, may accustom the skin to ultraviolet and produce a protective tan, although a polymorphic light eruption may actually occur during this therapy. Equally a course of photochemotherapy (PUVA) may be tried. This is often highly effective, though a polymorphic light eruption may occur during it. Since dermatologists see so many skin disorders resulting from too much cumulative solar exposure, this is a treatment they prescribe with some trepidation and it may be unsuitable for patients with type I or type II skins, as the effects of the ultraviolet irradiation are irreversible.

DRUG ERUPTIONS

Introduction

Drug eruptions are extremely common both in general and hospital practice. It is very important to know what drugs a patient has taken in the weeks preceeding the eruption. It is often not appreciated that an eruption may take a fortnight to appear after the first dose, by which time the patient may have completed the course several days previously and the connection is not realised. This is particularly true of penicillin derivatives. Also, patients do not 'count' as drugs agents which they have purchased from a chemist without prescription (for example laxatives and aspirin), nor drugs that they have been taking for a long time. Although drug eruptions are usually related to a recently prescribed medication, this is not always so. Sometimes fairly intense questioning of the patient is required in order to determine what a patient has ingested.

Probably all drugs can cause an eruption on the skin, but clearly some do so more regularly than others. Antibiotics, for example, are high-rate offenders, whereas a rash due to digoxin must be very uncommon. It sometimes is difficult to know which drug is responsible, because the patient is taking so many, so a list of the top 'offenders' is very helpful (Fig. 15.35). The scene, however, is always changing as new drugs are introduced. In some cases, the risk is already suspected from clinical trials, but this is not always so. It is important that all reactions to new drugs are monitored and reported to the Committee of Safety of Medicines or its equivalent. It is always worthwhile asking the dermatologist to see such cases straight away, because he is in a good position to recognize new causes. There is unfortunately no readily available way of testing for drug reactions. Clearly the definitive test would be to give the patient the drug again, in order to see whether the side-effect was reproducible, but this may be dangerous because anaphylaxis or uncontrollable erythroderma may result.

Drug reactions may result from an allergic or non-immunological mechanism. The risk of immunogenicity is greater if the drug molecule is large and complicated. Small molecular drugs do not produce allergic reactions unless they can form stable covalent bonds with tissue macromolecules, that is act as a hapten. Even if a drug does elicit an immune response (penicillin for example produces antibodies in most patients), only a small number of patients develop a clinical reaction. The route of administration of the drugs modifies the nature of the response. Topical applications produce delayed hypersensitivity contact dermatitis; oral or nasal exposure stimulates the secretory immunoglobulins A and E; and intravenous exposure is most likely to induce anaphylaxis. The ability of the host to metabolize the drug is important. Those who acetylate drugs slowly are much more likely to get a lupus-like syndrome with hydralazine than those who do not. The immunology of allergic cutaneous reactions is not very well understood. The Gel and Coombs hypersensitivity classification has been useful to some extent, but not all rashes can be so classified. However, the urticarial eruption of penicillin is an example of type I immediate hypersensitivity reaction. This is probably the only drug for which it is practical to test sensitivity. Intradermal injection of penicillin produces local wheal and flare within 15 minutes in allergic subjects and RAST testing correlates well with these skin test results. A type II cytotoxic reaction was the explanation underlying the purpura caused by Sedormid, a hypnotic that is no longer available. The antigen (for example Sedormid) attaches to the cell (in this case the platelet) which is destroyed by antibodies and complement resulting in purpura. Type III immune complex hypersensitivity is due to the drug combining with an antibody to form complexes with complement; these are precipitated out in the blood vessels. Erythema nodosum and serum sickness are examples of this. The type IV reaction is that which is seen with topically applied drugs, such as occurs in contact dermatitis.

Non-immunological reactions may be due to an activation of an effector pathway. Thus opiates, polymyxin, D tubocurare and radiocontrast media release mast cell mediators and cause urticaria. Other drugs may activate complement or alter arachidonic acid metabolism, for example aspirin and certain non-steroidal anti-inflammatories, and induce anaphylaxis.

We have already seen that drugs may be responsible for any of the reactive conditons just described, such as toxic erythema, urticaria, erythema multiforme and erythema nodosum. Toxic erythema and urticaria are the commonest patterns, but some drugs may also simulate cutaneous disorders such as lichen planus, acne and psoriasis. The correct diagnosis may be suggested because the eruption is atypical or does not respond to the appropriate therapy for that disease. A list of such mimicry follows. In addition a specific entity, only caused by drugs — a fixed drug eruption — is described.

(1) Acneiform eruptions. (a) Systemic and topical steroids; (b) iodides, including radio-opaque materials, and bromides; (c) ethambutol; (d) isoniazid; (e) anticonvulsants; (f) progesterone.

(2) Psoriasiform eruptions. Beta-blockers occasionally produce these.

(3) Eczematous eruptions. Although contact eczema to topical medicaments is very common, eczematous reactions to systemic agents are rare. However, methyldopa and gold may produce a widespread eczema.

(4) Lichenoid eruptions. Both mepacrine and gold occasionally produce eruptions which simulate lichen planus.

(5) Ichthyosis. Carbamazepine produces a general dryness of the skin, which is followed by an erythroderma. There is usually an accompanying eosinophilia, which helps to establish the diagnosis.

(6) Pemphigus. Captopril and penicillamine may produce pemphigus-like eruptions.

MAIN CAUSES OF DRUG ERUPTIONS	
Antibiotics	penicillin, ampicillin, flucloxacillin, sulphonamides, including co-trimoxazole, trimethoprim, tetracyclines
Non-steroidal anti-inflammatory drugs	phenylbutazone, azapropazone, fenclofenac, salicylates
Diuretics	thiazides, amiloride
CNS drugs	barbiturates, amitryptilline, phenothiazines, carbamezapine
Cardiovascular drugs	beta blockers, amiodarone, methyldopa, captopril
Rheumatological drugs	penicillamine, allopurinol, gold
Miscellaneous	sulphonylureas, sulphasalazine

▲ **Fig. 15.35** *The main causes of drug eruptions.*

(7) Blistering eruptions. Barbiturates may produce blistering on pressure areas, particularly after an overdose when the patient has lain unconscious.

(8) Hair (see later).

(9) Nails (see later).

Fixed drug eruptions

Definition

The occurrence of a skin eruption in an identical site each time a particular drug is ingested.

> **Diagnostic features**
> - Red, brown, oedematous swelling(s).
> - Recurrences in identical site(s).
> - Hand, face, mouth or genitals.
> - Post-inflammatory hyperpigmentation.
> - Laxatives often implicated.

Aetiology

The mechanism for this remarkable phenomenon is quite obscure. The main offenders are: laxatives, especially phenolphthalein; phenacetin; griseofulvin; barbiturates; tetracyclines; and sulphonamides.

Clinical features

The condition is not particularly common but is readily identified. The extraordinary feature is that the disorder recurs in the same site every time the drug is taken. The commonest areas affected are the face, backs of the hands, genitalia, limbs or in the mouth. The lesion develops within a few hours and subsides fairly rapidly once the drug is withdrawn, leaving a fairly characteristic hyperpigmentation of the skin (Fig. 15.36). The lesion may be single or multiple and is well-defined, red/brown, oedematous and occasionally bullous.

Management

The condition resolves if the drug is withdrawn. This seems quite simple but perversely, in a minority of patients, it may be quite difficult because the patient either refuses to accept the explanation or is addicted to the drug, particularly in the case of laxatives. Sometimes the patient is taking so many drugs that it is difficult to elicit which one is the culprit.

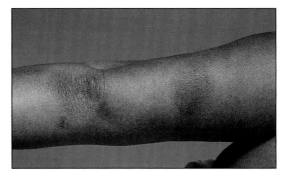

▲**Fig. 15.36** *Fixed drug eruption. A well-defined red or red/brown round oedematous lesion recurs in the same site each time the drug (usually a laxative) is taken; post-inflammatory hyperpigmentation occurs.*

16 SKIN MANIFESTATIONS OF DISORDERED CIRCULATION

INTRODUCTION

Common disorders of circulation are described here. The commonest, which requires careful medical management, is varicose eczema and is described in detail. Vasculitis is discussed in chapter 15.

VARICOSE ECZEMA AND ULCERATION

Definition

A common disorder of the lower limbs resulting from venous hypertension, resulting in eczema (Fig. 16.1) and/or ulceration of the skin.

> **Diagnostic features**
> - Lower legs.
> - Venous hypertension.
> - Eczema.
> - Pigmentation.
> - Atrophie blanche.
> - Fibrosis.
> - Ulceration.

Aetiology

Blood is returned to the heart by three sets of veins — deep, superficial and intercommunicating (perforating) — following contraction of the gastrocnemius and soleus muscles during exercise. Valves prevent the blood from returning downwards. If this system fails in any one of its components, venous hypertension results, causing distention and elongation of the capillary loops. Fibrinogen leaks into the tissues through the widened endothelial pores, and fibrin is laid down in the capillaries forming a 'cuff' which limits the diffusion of oxygen and other nutrients to the skin. In addition, white cells accumulate during periods of immobility and plug the capillaries thus contributing to local ischaemia.

The most common causes of failure of the system are:
(1) Venous thrombosis. Patients are particularly liable to venous thrombosis during any period of prolonged immobility, particularly during surgery, labour or recuperation after a fracture (especially of the hip) or if they are on the contraceptive pill. This causes damage to the valves, to the perforators and obstruction of the veins. The deep venous thrombosis may or may not have been clinically apparent. As techniques for preventing deep venous thrombosis during medical procedures improve, this disorder is becoming less common.

(2) Absent valves. This condition is inherited; usually there is a family history of varicose veins. The valves are absent rather than damaged, and the disorder presents in younger patients.

(3) A compromised muscle pump may result from neuromuscular disease such as poliomyelitis or from disuse atrophy of the muscles themselves, as in patients with severe arthritis.

Clinical features

The disease is common and is more frequent in females who are overweight and from the lower socio-economic groups. It occurs on the gaiter area of the lower leg and particularly around the ankle. The physical signs are:

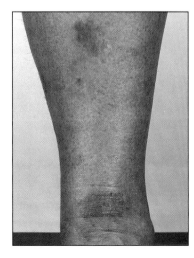

◀ **Fig. 16.1**
Varicose eczema. Patches of eczema occur in association with varicosities and venous hypertension.

173

(1) Pigmentation due to haemosiderin deposition in the tissues following the extravasation of red cells (stasis purpura) and due to melanin deposition following inflammatory change. Discrete brown macules, usually merging into one another and producing diffuse areas of staining, are seen. There is no treatment for the pigmentation.

(2) Eczema is common and the appearance is of patches of redness and scaling (see Fig. 16.1) which itch. The condition responds well to topical glucocorticosteroids and measures designed to reduce venous hypertension. However, a common complication of treatment is *dermatitis medicamentosa* (Fig. 16.2) which is a contact sensitization to topical medica-

ments. The more frequent causes are lanolin, parabens (a preservative), local antibiotics, and anaesthetics and rubber in elastic stockings. Neomycin, soframycin, framycetin and gentamycin are common antibiotic sensitizers and should not be prescribed for varicose eczema or ulceration. Topical tetracycline is usually safe. The diagnosis should be suspected if the varicose eczema or ulcer fails to improve or even deteriorates during treatment. The eczema often becomes acute and in severe cases an autosensitization reaction results. This term implies a reaction of other parts of the skin, particularly the face, neck and arms and around the eyes. The eczema will continue until the offending medicament is discontinued.

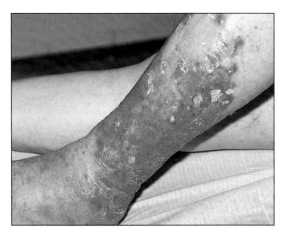

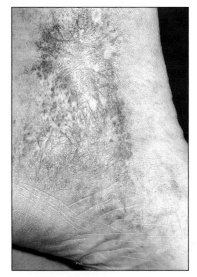

◄**Fig. 16.3** *Venous hypertension. Small white sclerotic plaques (atrophie blanche), haemosiderin pigmentation and tortuous venous dilatation are present.*

▲**Fig. 16.2** *Dermatitis medicamentosa. Varicose eczema and ulceration are particularly prone to contact dermatitis to applied medicaments (neomycin in this patient).*

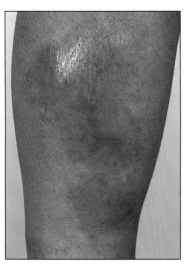

◄**Fig. 16.4** *Cellulitis. Painful erythema and oedema may recur around the varicosities secondary to infection.*

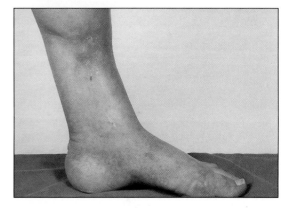

▲**Fig. 16.5** *Lipodermatosclerosis. Chronic venous hypertension, oedema and cellulitis may lead to fibrosis around the ankle, and scleroderma, giving the lower leg the appearance of an inverted champagne bottle.*

(3) Atrophie blanche. This term describes small, white plaques (Fig. 16.3) of sclerosis often with a characteristic red stippling of the surface. It is the end-result of necrosis of the skin and may follow thrombosis in the iliac veins or inferior vena cava.

(4) Oedema is a direct result of venous hypertension which may be made worse by the general medical condition of the patient, for example in cardiac failure. Cellulitis (Fig. 16.4) is an early complication of oedema from which fibrosis may result. Prolonged and neglected oedema leads ultimately to a condition known as *lipodermatosclerosis*, in which the skin feels indurated, woody and rather sclerodermatous. Eventually the leg looks like an inverted champagne bottle, the upper two-thirds of the leg being swollen but the area around the lower third tapered (Fig. 16.5). The fibrosis may lead to fixation of the ankle joint and limitation of the muscle pump, which makes the condition worse.

(5) Ulceration. This is the final physical sign of cutaneous malnutrition and represents breakdown of the epithelium. It is often precipitated in a compromised patient by minor injury or infection. The ulcers vary in shape and size and may be very large indeed (Figs 16.6 & 16.7). The smaller ones are sometimes very painful, the larger ones often being painless. The margin of the ulcer is well-defined but not raised, and the absence of a rolled or heaped up margin differentiates it from basal cell or squamous cell carcinoma. The base of the ulcer varies: some have a yellow slough oozing serum or pus, whereas others are red and haemorrhagic (indicating improved oxygenation of the blood and therefore improved nutrition of the skin, making healing more likely). Venous ulcers occur around the medial and lateral malleoli, whereas ulcers in other sites may be arteriosclerotic in origin. Often both conditions co-exist.

(6) Venous flare. Tortuous dilated veins around the ankles are characteristic of venous hypertension.

(7) Varicosities. These may or may not be present.

Management

It is easy to despair of treating venous ulceration, but it can be a rewarding experience for all concerned if the patient is motivated, and if there is continuity of medical care throughout its often prolonged course. A number of measures help:

(1) Rest and elevation of the leg. Prolonged standing should be prohibited. The patient should be advised to rest the leg as much as possible, with the leg raised 12 inches above the hip to facilitate the venous return. Blocks raising the end of the bed by 9–12 inches are very helpful.

(2) Compression bandages. Bandages which deliver a pressure of 30–50mmHg at the ankle are advisable, to prevent oedema and improve the muscle pump. The patient puts on the bandage first thing in the morning, before getting out of bed and keeps it on until he retires at night.

(3) Exercise. Walking and heel-raising exercises which bring about dorsiflexion and contraction of the calf muscles are required for maintaining the muscle pump.

(4) Diet. Many of the patients are obese and reducing diets are of a great benefit.

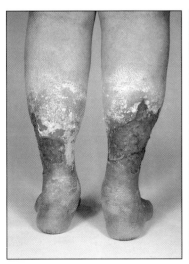
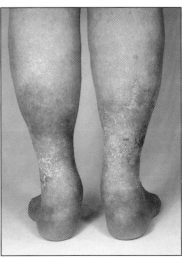

◄**Figs 16.6 & 16.7** *Venous ulceration. Ulceration is the final physical sign of cutaneous malnutrition. Even large ulcers such as these may be healed in outpatient departments with simple remedies (gentian violet and potassium permanganate in this patient), but it takes time (one year in this case; Fig. 16.7).*

(5) General medical condition. Many patients in leg ulcer clinics turn out to have general medical problems such as anaemia, malnutrition, hypertension and heart failure.

(6) Eczema. This may be treated with class III steroids, but not with combination products which contain antibiotics or local anaesthetics, since these will sooner or later sensitize the patient. Steroids delay healing so care should be taken to avoid treating any concomitant ulcer.

(7) Patch tests. These may be very helpful in detecting sensitivities in patients with non-responsive varicose eczema and ulceration.

(8) Infection. Cellulitis should be treated with appropriate systemic antibiotics. However, local infection of the ulcer itself does not respond well to systemic antibiotics and they should not be prescribed unless a beta-haemolytic *Streptococcus* is present. In addition to causing sensitization, topical antibiotics are also responsible for the occurrence of resistant strains of organisms. Measures for cleaning the ulcers, described below, should be adequate for dealing with most forms of infection.

(9) Morale boosting. This is extremely important. Dressings should be performed by the same nurse and supervised by the same doctor, because this gives the patient confidence and motivation. Unfortunately, however, there is a group of patients who have a vested interest in not getting better, because the ulcer guarantees attention from the health centre or hospital.

(10) Measurement. A record should be kept: a quick diagram indicating the length and breadth of the ulcer, and perhaps a polaroid photograph, give real information as to progress.

(11) Local therapy. Granulation tissue is essential to the process of healing. It results in wound contraction and re-epithelialization, which occurs from the periphery and from residual epithelial elements in the ulcer. This can be encouraged by: (a) Removal of the slough and necrotic debris which otherwise impede healing; mechanical debridement with forceps and scissors is much more effective than topical preparations. (b) Cleaning agents. A list of commonly used agents is given in Figure 16.8. Gentian violet may be phased out, as a possible mutagen, although this has never been documented clinically. Half-strength eusol (Edinburgh University Solution: a solution of boric acid and calcium hypochlorite) and eusol in equal parts with paraffin are time-honoured, but experimental data in animals suggests that they may impair the formation of granulation tissue.

(12) Dressings. (a) Absorbent materials: absorbent dressings are necessary for soaking up exudates and providing occlusion and thus a moist environment which increase epithelialization (dry environments lead to scab formation and hinder healing). Paraffin gauze covered by a sterile gauze pad or non-adherent dressings are standard. Newer preparations are carbohydrate polymers consisting of inert hydrophilic microbeads which absorb exudate, for example dextranomer powder or paste. Other polymers include cadexomer iodine, which releases iodine as it absorbs and alginates, which becomes soluble in the presence of sodium ions. Geliperm, an inert polyacrylamide/agar hydrogel, has the advantage of being a transparent moist gel sheet through which the ulcer may be inspected. (b) Bandages. Bandages which contain zinc oxide and coal tar, or zinc paste in combination with calamine, clioquinol or ichthammol, changed once or twice a week are helpful, especially if there is concomitant eczema.

(13) Gravitational syndrome. Lipodermatosclerosis may be painful. It is sometimes relieved by stanozolol 5 mg twice daily or oxerutins 250 mg three times daily. Intralesional triamcinolone is also effective.

(14) Hospitalization. This may be necessary in some patients to enforce rest, elevation of the leg and to provide regular nursing care. It is especially helpful for large ulcers, some small painful ulcers and in the elderly, but it does take its toll in terms of time and expense.

COMMONLY USED CLEANING AGENTS
Eusol
Cetrimide
Chlorhexidine gluconate
Povidone-iodine
Potassium permanganate soaks
Rosaniline dyes (0.5% aqueous gentian violet, carbofuschin and brilliant green)
Oxidizing agents (hydrogen peroxide, benzoyl peroxide 20%)

▲ **Fig. 16.8** *Commonly used cleaning agents.*

(15) Surgery. (a) Varicosities and perforators: consultation with a vascular surgeon regarding injection of varicosities or surgery to perforators is worthwhile, although the long-term effects of surgery are not spectacular. (b) Skin grafting is especially useful for large ulcers, either by the use of pinch grafts (the application of 0.5–1cm pinches of skin taken under local anaesthesia from the thigh) or split skin grafts.

ARTERIAL LEG ULCERS

Definition
Cutaneous malnutrition due to arterial insufficiency leading to ulceration of the skin.

Diagnostic features
- Painful at rest and at night.
- Ulcers on the toes, feet and on the front of the shins.
- Associated skin changes: pallor, dryness, scaliness, atrophy and loss of hair.

Aetiology
Arteriosclerosis is a complex disorder with widespread implications whose description is beyond the scope of this book. Genetic, dietary, and socioeconomic factors, stress, smoking, diabetes mellitus and hypertension are important. The ischaemic leg with ulceration is

discussed here because leg ulceration is a common cutaneous presentation. Although certain features may be helpful in distinguishing arterial from venous ulcers (Fig. 16.9), both types frequently co-exist.

Clinical features
Symptoms
Arterial leg ulcers are frequently painful, particularly when elevated and at night. The patient gets out of bed and walks about in order to obtain relief. Other symptoms of ischaemia are intermittent claudication, coldness, numbness, burning, and paraesthesia secondary to an associated ischaemic neuropathy.

Signs
- The skin is dry, scaly and thin. It feels cool. The colour is pale, cyanosed or that of a blotchy erythema. If the limb is elevated, this pallor is accentuated due to the poor performance against gravity.
- The hair on the lower leg and toes is sparse or absent.
- The toenails are thickened and distorted and the patient may remark that they require cutting less frequently.
- There is increased incidence of fungus infections and, in particular, *Trichophyton rubrum*.
- There are absent or diminished pulses.
- Ulceration results from severe ischaemia. Ulcers are well-defined, punched out and deep, and often have a thick necrotic slough. They occur primarily on the shin (Fig. 16.10), heel, dorsum of the foot or toes, which are quite different sites from those of a venous ulcer.

THE CLINICAL DIFFERENTIATION OF ARTERIAL FROM VENOUS ULCERATION	
Arterial	Venous
Painful	Not usually painful
Toes, heels, shins	Malleoli
Pulses, reduced or absent	Pulses present
Dry, scaly, atrophic, shiny skin	Eczema and pigmentation
Absent hair	Hair present
Nails dystrophic	Normal nails
Pallor, cyanosis, blotchy erythema	No pallor, cyanosis or erythema

▲ **Fig. 16.9** *The clinical differentiation of arterial from venous ulceration.*

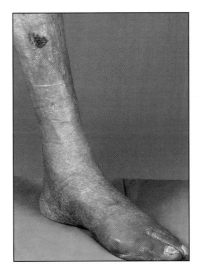

◄**Fig. 16.10** *Arterial insufficiency. The skin is dry, hairless and atrophic. The toes are cyanotic and the nails are dystrophic. The ulcer is on the shin; it is usually painful. The peripheral pulses were absent on examination.*

- The final stage of severe ischaemia is gangrene, when the skin becomes black. The toes are usually affected first.

Differential diagnosis

The major differential diagnosis is from venous ulceration. However, there are a number of conditions that can cause ulcers on the lower limb (Fig. 16.11).

Management

The Doppler ultrasound technique measures the ratio of the ankle to brachial systolic pressure, which obviously should be 1.0 in the normal. A ratio of 0.7 or less indicates arterial disease, and the patient requires referral to a vascular surgeon for arteriographic assessment and consideration of operative techniques, such as lumbar sympathectomy and arterial reconstruction for proximal disease. Associated measures to control diabetes, hypertension, weight and smoking are imperative. Elasticated stockings are contraindicated as they restrict the already compromised blood supply to the leg. Topical remedies are similar to those used for the treatment of venous ulcers but are less effective.

PERNIOSIS (CHILBLAINS)

Definition

Localized inflammatory lesions of the extremities induced by cold.

Diagnostic features

- Itchy or painful.
- Children or young women.
- Winter.
- Dusky red or purple papules.
- Fingers, toes, nose and ears.

DIFFERENTIAL DIAGNOSIS OF ULCERS ON THE LOWER LIMB
Pyoderma gangrenosum
Dysglobulinaemias
Sickle cell and thalassaemia
Basal and squamous cell carcinoma (Fig. 16.12)
Klinefelter's syndrome
Erythema induratum
Necrobiosis lipoidica
Vasculitis (Fig. 16.13)
Pressure (Fig. 16.14)

▲**Fig. 16.11** *Differential diagnosis of ulcers on the lower limbs.*

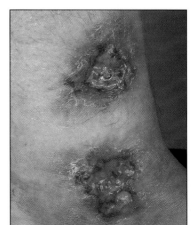

◀**Fig. 16.13** *Vasculitis. This young woman's vasculitis deteriorated and leg ulceration developed. The cyanotic swollen margin is indicative of vasculitis. An identical clinical picture is seen in pyoderma gangrenosum.*

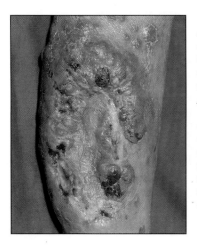

◀**Fig. 16.12** *Squamous cell carcinoma. Occasionally a malignant ulcer of the leg is mistaken for a venous ulcer. The margin however is heaped up in a squamous cell carcinoma and the lesion does not respond to ulcer therapy. A biopsy is indicated.*

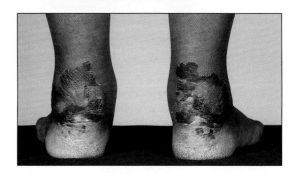

▲**Fig. 16.14** *Pressure sore. This young woman was unconscious and immobile as a result of a barbiturate overdose. The pressure on her heels caused ischaemia and necrosis and ulceration of the skin.*

Aetiology

This is a localized vasculitis occurring in response to cold, which produces an abnormally prolonged vaso-constriction followed by a reactive hyperaemia. It is now less common in the UK, due to improved housing with central heating and double glazing. However, undoubtedly some individuals are more predisposed than others, particularly women, children and also immigrants who are unused to the winters of Northern climates.

Clinical features

The lesions may be very itchy at first and are some-times painful on rewarming. They appear in crops as dusky red or purple swellings (Fig. 16.15) on peri-pherally exposed areas, usually the fingers and toes and occasionally the nose and ears. They sometimes occur on the backs of the thighs, especially in over-weight young women who horse-ride wearing damp tight-fitting jeans.

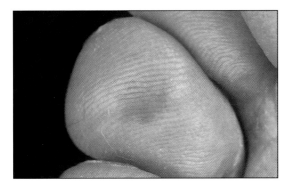

▲ **Fig. 16.15** *Chilblain. Discrete itchy and sometimes painful dusky red or purple swellings occur on peripheral areas such as the toes.*

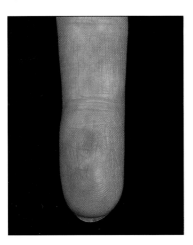

◀ **Fig. 16.16** *Chilblain lupus erythematosus. Painful deep red or purple lesions may occur on the fingers in winter particularly in women with lupus erythematosus.*

Differential diagnosis

(1) Lupus erythematosus. The perniotic lesions (Fig. 16.16) may be more pronounced in this condition and necrosis can occur, but there are also usually other features of lupus erythematosus (such as cuticular haemorrhages and a skin eruption on light-exposed areas) which aid the diagnosis. The antinuclear factor may be positive.

(2) Emboli. Small, cutaneous infarcts of the fingers and toes may result from thrombi from endocarditis, valvular disease, myocardial infarction, atrial fibril-lation or an aneurysm. A careful history and general examination should exclude these.

Management

Basic advice on keeping warm is common sense and essential (it is surprising how some patients fail to grasp the essence of the condition). Thermal under-wear, ensuring the hands and feet are warm well in advance of going out into the cold, and the wearing of fleece-lined gloves or skiing gloves are all advisable. Central heating at home and at work are clearly imperative, but not always possible, and frequently occupations involving working outside, or in cold unheated shops or factories, make the management of this disease difficult. Other treatments that have been tried are:

(1) Ultra-violet light: three times weekly at the begin-ning of the winter, sufficient to produce erythema.

(2) Nifedipine (10mg three times daily) is a calcium antagonist which produces vasodilatation by reducing the vasomotor tone.

DECK CHAIR LEGS

Definition

A common condition of the lower leg resulting from prolonged immobilization.

Diagnostic features

- Lower legs.
- Diffuse erythema.
- Oedema.
- Blistering.

Aetiology

The condition gained its nickname from its description in those rendered homeless during the blitz in London in the Second World War, who passed the night sleeping in deck chairs in the London Underground.

It occurs now in immobile or debilitated patients who lead an armchair existence and sleep in a chair rather than in a bed at night. The lymphatic and venous return is consequently always working against gravity, resulting in oedema and erythema possibly due to a low-grade cellulitis.

Clinical features

The lower limbs are red and swollen and blistering may occur in extreme cases (Fig. 16.17).

Management

Restoration to a normal active life is the goal of treatment, but this is frequently impossible because of accompanying general debility.

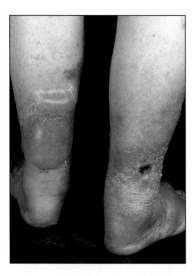

◄ **Fig. 16.17** *Deck chair legs. Prolonged immobilization with the legs dependent, results in red and oedematous legs often with blistering. It is common in those who lead an armchair existence.*

CAUSES OF RAYNAUD'S SYNDROME

Collagen vascular disease, scleroderma, systemic lupus erythematosus, mixed connective tissue disease

Occupational, e.g. pneumatic drills

Neurological disease, e.g. cervical rib

Occlusive arterial disease, Buerger's disease

Immunoglobulin disorders, cryoglobulinaemia, cold agglutinins

Toxins, ergotism, heavy metals, vinyl chloride

▲ **Fig. 16.18** *Causes of Raynaud's syndrome.*

RAYNAUD'S PHENOMENON

Definition

Painful, paroxysmal episodes of pallor and coldness of the fingers and sometimes the toes, followed by cyanosis and reactive hyperaemia, most often precipitated by cold.

Diagnostic features
- White, blue and then red colour changes.
- Fingers.
- In response to cold.
- Painful.

Aetiology

The exact mechanism is not known. Some cases are due to a malfunctioning of the sympathetic nervous system, but circulatory catecholamines, abnormalities of blood viscosity, red cell deformibility, platelet aggregation, or fibrinolysis have been implicated. If there is a known cause (Fig. 16.18) then the disorder is known as Raynaud's syndrome; if not, as Raynaud's disease. Many chronic cases are later found to have systemic sclerosis (see Fig. 23.17).

Clinical features

The patient usually gives an accurate history: that the fingers go white, blue and finally red, in response to immersion of the hands into cold water or in cold weather conditions. The pallor is due to vasoconstriction, the blue colour to subsequent peripheral cyanosis, and the redness to reactive hyperaemia. In severe cases, there may be trophic changes. The skin is tethered and the fingers tapered (sclerodactyly) in these conditions. The nail plates are thinned and ridged. Gangrene is unusual except in those cases associated with scleroderma.

Management

The cause should be identified, if possible, and treated appropriately. Common-sense measures should be taken, such as prohibition of smoking and improvement of local warmth. Battery-heated gloves may prove useful.

Many drug regimens have been tried, including intra-arterial infusion of reserpine, prostaglandin E, prostacyclin and low molecular weight dextran. The latest treatment is nifedipine.

Sympathectomy is worth considering in severe Raynaud's disease.

17 DISORDERS OF THE SEBACEOUS, SWEAT AND APOCRINE GLANDS

INTRODUCTION

Acne and rosacea, although unrelated, are two common diseases which occur primarily on the face. They are occasionally mistreated with topical glucocorticosteroids and the results of this are discussed. A disorder which is confused with acne but is actually self-induced as part of a neurosis is also described. Hyperhidrosis, a common disorder of the sweat glands, and hidradenitis suppurativa, a less common malady of the apocrine glands, are also outlined.

ACNE

Definition
A chronic disorder of the pilosebaceous apparatus resulting in greasiness and a variety of lesions on the face and torso.

> **Diagnostic features**
> - Greasiness.
> - Comedones, milia, papules, pustules, nodules, cysts, scars, keloids and hyperpigmentation.
> - On the face, back and front of chest.

Aetiology
Acne is the commonest reason for a dermatological consultation, other than for warts. It results from an overactivity of the sebaceous gland and a blockage in its duct. The gland is under the control of androgens. It produces sebum which is a mixture of lipids which may be converted into comedogenic and irritant free fatty acids by microorganisms in the gland. These components are considered in more detail.

The sebaceous gland
This gland is found throughout the skin, except on the palms and soles, and is under androgen control. It does not secrete until puberty, apart from a temporary activity during infancy, probably due to adrenal stimulation. The glands are at their largest on the face, neck and front and back of the chest, where they occur in association with hair follicles and share with them a common channel or exit from the skin, which is known as the pilosebaceous duct. Animals require the gland for waterproofing of their fur and perhaps the gland was originally necessary for man, but during the course of evolution it has become something of an inconvenient appendage, like the appendix. Certainly, children seem to do well without active glands.

Sebum
Sebum secretion is undoubtedly increased in acne and it is generally correct to state that the more severe the acne, the greater the production of sebum. However, acne is not a particular feature of certain greasy states such as acromegaly (growth hormone increases the production of sebum) or Parkinson's disease (mechanism unknown). In addition, acne vulgaris usually remits in the early twenties, and yet sebum excretion does not fall precipitously at that time.

The pustules of acne represent a collection of sebum and they are quite sterile, contrary to popular belief. Sebum is formed from the sebaceous gland by a holocrine process, that is the cells of the gland are broken down and completely converted into lipids — glycerides, free fatty acids, wax esters, squalene, cholesterol and its esters. The sebaceous gland is being manufactured all the time, and it probably takes a month to reach maturity, just like other epidermal structures. This may explain why therapy takes this length of time to act. Free fatty acids, the breakdown products of sebum, are irritants and comedogenic: if injected into the skin, they produce a sterile inflammatory response of polymorphs and lymphocytes, which is what occurs if sebum leaks into the skin surrounding the gland.

The function of sebum is unclear. It is known to be fungistatic as far as dermatophytes are concerned, which perhaps explains why ringworm of the scalp is rare after puberty. On the other hand the fungus of pityriasis versicolor is lipophilic and flourishes on sebum and is common after adolescence.

Plugging of the pilosebaceous canal

The comedone or blackhead represents a blockage of the pilosebaceous duct by a keratin plug. This is caused by a failure of the epidermis lining the duct to keratinize properly so that the keratin is not shed correctly. Instead the keratinous squames adhere to one another and, together with sebum and bacteria, block the gland. Certain substances aid the formation of comedones, such as free fatty acids, industrial oils, hair pommades, and brilliantines. As a result of the blockage, the gland distends. If the blockage is superficial, red papules and pustules result. If it is deeper, larger painful papules, cysts and scarring may occur.

Microbiology

Acne is clearly not an infectious disease and it cannot be transmitted from one subject to another. The pilosebaceous duct and the skin surface are however colonized by important microorganisms — *Propionobacterium acnes* (formerly known as *Corynebacterium acnes*), *Staphylococcus epidermis* and the yeast *Pityrosporon ovale* — *P. acnes* being dominant. Although their absolute numbers do not correlate with the severity of the acne, treatments which reduce them improve the disease. The microorganisms probably produce inflammatory mediators which attract inflammatory cells.

Hormones

The sebaceous glands are directly under hormonal control.

(1) **Androgens** are the most important. Sebum excretion at birth is similar to that of adults, but in the period following infancy, through to adolescence, the sebaceous glands are minute and sebum excretion is very low. Acne begins at puberty and indeed heralds adolescence. For this reason, eunuchs do not develop acne unless they are given testosterones. However, it is not known why acne goes into remission after adolescence even though testosterone levels remain the same. It may be that there is target organ overactivity, such that there is increased conversion of testosterone to the more potent dihydrotestosterone by the enzyme 5-alpha-reductase at the androgen receptor of the sebaceous gland. Certainly, there does not seem to be any evidence, in males at any rate, that there is an increased output of testosterone, in that all males are maximally stimulated already. In females, however, studies are conflicting. Target organ overactivity may be the key, and some workers have concluded that circulating androgens are increased. Alternatively, it has been shown in some women that sex hormone binding globulin is reduced and consequently levels of serum-unbound sex hormones are elevated, and these may be responsible. It is not known why the binding globulin should be reduced, or why all the sebaceous glands are not affected by the increased androgen activity at any one time, instead of just a number being affected. Thus acne is a disorder of androgen metabolism, and clearly it can be a feature in women of a virilizing disease, albeit rarely, in which case other signs of virilization will be present.

(2) **Oestrogens** reduce the size of the sebaceous gland. However, high doses such as 50 μg of ethinyloestradiol daily are required in order to produce a therapeutic effect.

(3) **Progesterone** causes water retention with consequent swelling of the epidermis and a resulting blockage of the pilosebaceous ducts. Thus many mature women note their acne is worse premenstrually.

(4) **Thyroxine** stimulates the sebaceous glands so that dry skin is a feature of hypothyroidism.

Mediators of inflammation

The cause of the inflammatory reaction is unknown but *P. acnes*, the major organism involved in acne, is chemotactic for inflammatory cells and produces a prostaglandin-like substance that can activate the classical and alternative pathways of complement.

Clinical features

The physical signs of acne include greasiness, comedones, milia, red papules and pustules (Figs 17.1 & 17.2), occurring sometimes in association with nodules, cysts, scarring (including keloids) and post-inflammatory hyperpigmentation. The lesions occur primarily on the face and trunk.

There are four clinical forms of acne.

Acne vulgaris

This is the common variety of acne. It is one of the first manifestations of adolescence and, as such, is now commencing much earlier than previously so that it is quite usual to see comedones and milia in a 10-year-old. The disorder reaches maximum activity at between 16 and 18 years and then subsides but often does not disappear until the early or mid twenties, a fact which is not generally appreciated by patients. The disorder may be regarded as an almost universal occurrence in some degree during adolescence, so that in some it is purely physiological and can be ignored, whereas in others it represents a disease requiring active treatment. There is enormous variation in what degree of disease patients will tolerate without requesting therapy.

Post-adolescent mature female's acne

This is remarkably common in women in their twenties and thirties who invariably state that they were not troubled by acne in adolescence. The condition usually clears by the middle or late thirties, but not always. It has a characteristic predilection for the muzzle area of the chin (Fig. 17.3) and jaw and results in painful and deep nodules, especially premenstrually. Most patients have low levels of sex hormone binding globulin and the consequent rise in free-circulating testosterone levels is responsible for the acne. Some patients have features of the polycystic ovary syndrome. Some women relate it to either stopping, starting or changing their oral contraceptive, but others have never taken the pill. The more androgenic progestogen-containing pills (levonorgestrel and ethynodiol)

probably aggravate it, whereas the minimally androgenic progestogens (desogestrel and gestodene) combined with ethinyloestradiol may be beneficial.

Infantile acne (milk spots)

This is quite common in early infancy and may be due to transplacental stimulation of the sebaceous glands by adrenal androgens rather than to transfer of maternal androgens via breast milk. The acne occurs predominantly on the cheeks (Fig. 17.4) and passes after a few months. Very occasionally it is a presenting feature of a virilizing tumour or congenital adrenal hyperplasia.

Nodulocystic acne (acne conglobata)

This is an exceedingly unpleasant form of acne. It differs from acne vulgaris in the degree of physical signs, in its chronicity and, until recently, its relative resistance to standard therapy. The condition which usually begins in adolescence, occurs in both sexes but probably more frequently in males.

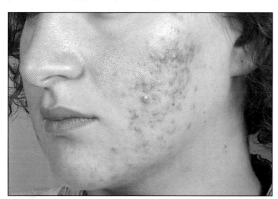

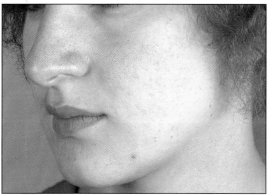

▲ **Figs 17.1 & 17.2** *Acne vulgaris. Deep painful lesions may result in post-inflammatory pigmentation and scarring so that aggressive therapy is required. Minocycline was used here (Fig. 17.2).*

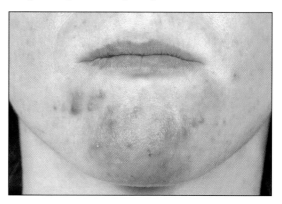

▲ **Fig. 17.3** *Post-adolescent female acne. Papules and pustules occur, particularly on the chin and around the jaw in mature women who often state that they were unaffected by acne as adolescents.*

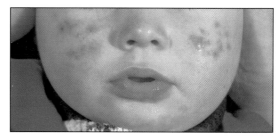

▲ **Fig. 17.4** *Infantile acne. Acne may occur temporarily in the first few months of life probably secondary to transplacental stimulation of the sebaceous glands by adrenal androgens.*

The lesions which distinguish it from acne vulgaris are the deep and painful papules and nodules (Fig. 17.5) that occur and the resulting disfiguring scarring, sometimes with keloid formation (Fig. 17.6). The condition does not remit after adolescence, but frequently persists into early middle age. The face, chest and back may be involved in isolation or together: it is quite startling to examine a patient whose face appears quite normal, only to find severe disease on the back or chest. The treatment of this disease has been revolutionized by 13-cis-retinoic acid.

Factors which affect acne

(1) Climatic conditions. Individuals with a predisposition to acne often become worse in hot, humid and particularly tropical climates. It presented a problem for British troops in the Far East during World War 2, but not for the Americans in Vietnam, probably because those with significant acne were excluded. It can be quite difficult to treat, other than by returning the patient to a temperate zone, although 13-cis-retinoic acid may change this. A variation of this is *Majorca acne*, a condition in which small follicular papules occur mainly on the upper trunk during a holiday in the sun. This may be due to follicular occlusion secondary to epidermal overhydration, possibly exacerbated by suntan oils.

(2) Medicaments. Topical preparations such as hair greases and pommades may aggravate acne. If these preparations spread onto the forehead, the pilosebaceous orifices become occluded and comedones and acne results.

(3) Occlusive circumstances. Acne may be produced by changes in the microenvironment of the skin. Tight-fitting clothes may help to occlude the pilosebaceous ducts, so that those who wear tight jeans may develop acne on the buttocks and thighs. Prolonged sitting in high-backed chairs, particularly if they are made of materials such as plastics, which produce sweating and hydration of the skin, may cause follicular occlusion and acne.

(4) Industrial. Industrial workers may develop acne when exposed to halogenated hydrocarbons (chloracne). An outbreak of this occurred after an industrial accident releasing 2,3,7,8-tetrachlorodibenzodioxin (TCDD) at Seveso in 1976, and resulted in an acute erythema on exposed skin, followed 1–2 months later by a severe acne which lasted for up to 18 months.

(5) Drugs. Halogens may also produce acne when used therapeutically or diagnostically. Thus iodides in cough mixtures, in radiological materials and in the drugs used in the treatment of thyroid disease, and iodine in seaweed if eaten in large amounts, may be responsible. Bromides, although rarely given nowadays, cause acne. Phenobarbitone, troxidone and isoniazid induce acne. Systemic steroids produce a rather characteristic acne situated on the trunk, shoulders and upper arms, with monomorphic, largely pustular, lesions.

Management

It is important to determine from the history the effect of the disorder on the patient's morale, and from the examination the degree of damage being done to the skin. Mild acne may be acceptable to a teenager if his or her peers are similarly affected, but moderate acne may be more difficult to cope with and can sometimes completely interfere with the patient's life. The features to look for during the examination are deep papules (which are usually painful), nodules,

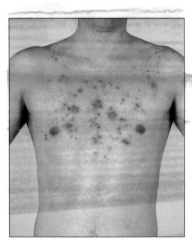

◀ **Fig. 17.5**
Nodulocystic acne. Large inflamed nodules, cysts and scarring occur. 13-cis-retinoic acid has revolutionized treatment.

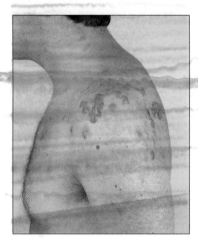

◀ **Fig. 17.6**
Acne keloids. Acne may result in scarring and occasionally keloids especially on the shoulders and front of the chest. This sometimes occurs with minimal acne.

cysts, scarring and post-inflammatory hyperpigment-ation. Post-inflammatory hyperpigmentation (Fig. 17.7) and scarring must be prevented because the former takes a long time to clear and the latter is permanent. These are all indications for energetic systemic therapy (Fig. 17.8).

Topical therapy

This is satisfactory for mild adolescent acne vulgaris and mild acne in pregnancy and as an adjunct to systemic therapy, the face being a more responsive area than the trunk. Topical preparations are largely antibacterial or keratolytic reducing the faulty keratin-ization at the level of the pilosebaceous duct. They are often available in combined formulation and there is justification for this, since there is no single answer to the therapy of acne.

(1) **Benzoyl peroxide** is an effective antibacterial and is also comedolytic. It is sometimes combined with sulphur or other groups of antibacterials. Various strengths (5% and 10%) are available and since it does irritate the skin it is wise to start with the weakest strength, on alternate nights, so that the patient can get used to its effects.

(2) **Retinoic acid.** This is used as a keratolytic, increasing the basal cell mitosis and epithelial turn-over and disrupting the comedones. It causes inflam-mation, which some patients find unacceptable.

(3) **Sulphur, salicylic acid, and resorcinol.** Resorcinol (1,3-dihydroxybenzene), often used in combination with salicylic acid and sulphur, is thought to act as a keratolytic.

(4) **Topical antibiotics.** Benzoyl peroxide is the most commonly used topical antibiotic in the UK. Other topical antibiotics are only just becoming available in the UK although they are widely used in the US, in particular 1% clindamycin. Taken orally, clindamycin may cause pseudomembranous colitis and there have been fears that cases might result from absorption from topical preparations, but these anxieties have not been realized. Bacteriologists have been concerned lest the use of the preparation might lead to clinda-mycin-resistant organisms, but this has not occurred after over a decade of use in the US.

Topical erythromycin and tetracycline are less effective than clindamycin.

Neomycin and chloramphenicol have been avail-able in combination preparations containing sulphur and a weak corticosteroid for some years. However, their use has been criticised for several reasons. It has been suggested that percutaneous absorption could cause systemic toxicity — aplastic anaemia due to topical chloramphenicol, ototoxicity due to topical neomycin — but there is no evidence for this. Nor is there evidence to prove the theory that topical chlor-amphenicol use has increased bacterial resistance to its use orally in the treatment of typhoid. Although neomycin and chloramphenicol are both potential sensitizers of the skin, contact dermatitis to these preparations when used for the treatment of acne is exceedingly rare.

These combination preparations sometimes contain very weak corticosteroids. Although steroids should not be used on their own for acne, they do reduce the inflammatory effects of keratolytics (which some patients find unacceptable) and they are therefore permissible.

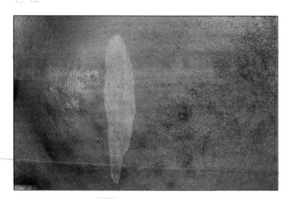

▲ **Fig. 17.7** *Acne vulgaris. Post-inflammatory hyperpigmentation persists for a long time in coloured skins and is an indication for systemic therapy to prevent further damage.*

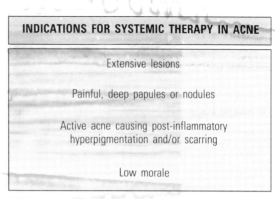

INDICATIONS FOR SYSTEMIC THERAPY IN ACNE
Extensive lesions
Painful, deep papules or nodules
Active acne causing post-inflammatory hyperpigmentation and/or scarring
Low morale

▲ **Fig. 17.8** *Indications for systemic therapy.*

(5) **Ultraviolet light.** Many patients note that their acne is much improved in the summer months. Ultraviolet B is used therapeutically in sufficient doses to produce mild erythema and consequently desquamation of the skin.

Systemic antibiotics

These are the mainstay of therapy. Penicillin orally is quite ineffective, but tetracyclines, erythromycin, trimethoprim, septrin, flucloxacillin and ampicillin are all effective as they concentrate in the pilosebaceous apparatus. They decrease free fatty acid concentrations in sebum, by modifying the action of bacterial lipases. They also reduce the inflammation of acne by inhibiting neutrophil chemotaxis.

Not all antibiotics work in everyone, so the physician must find the antibiotic to suit a particular individual. Neither do the drugs work straightaway, and the patient must be warned not to expect any major improvement for at least a month. Side-effects are not common, probably because smaller doses are used than in conventional antimicrobial therapy.

It is usual to start with a tetracycline such as oxytetracycline, 250mg twice daily. Occasionally higher doses are required. It has to be taken half an hour before food in order to enhance absorption, and must not be taken at the same time as milk products which reduce absorption.

For those patients who cannot tolerate or do not respond to tetracycline, minocycline is, although more expensive, an effective alternative. The dose is 50mg twice daily. It is highly fat-soluble, giving it good tissue penetration, and it has the distinct advantage that it can be taken with food and drink, and with milk. Many dermatologists use it as their antibiotic of choice.

Other alternatives are erythromycin and trimethoprim; the latter probably alone rather than in combination with sulphonamides, in view of risk of hypersensitivity reactions. It is a common mistake to prescribe for only a few weeks. *The drugs must be given for a minimum period of 6 months, but often for longer than this.* There is no such thing as a 'course' of antibiotics for acne as the disorder is a chronic one, and the antibiotics are only controlling it until it has gone into remission.

Hormonal therapy

(1) **High-dose oestrogen therapy.** Oral contraceptives containing 50μg of ethinyloestradiol are of some benefit in the mature woman with a pronounced pre-

menstrual flare of her acne. Conversely, progesterone-containing oral contraceptives may exacerbate this type of acne and should be avoided.

(2) **Combined antiandrogen and oestrogen therapy.** The concept of a drug which limits the conversion of testosterone to the highly potent androgen, dihydrotestosterone, is an appealing one. Dianette, a combination of 2μg cyproterone acetate with 30μg of ethinyloestradiol (not yet available in the US) reduces sebum production. The dose of cyproterone acetate is low and it is sometimes worth combining it with an extra 50 or 100mg of cyproterone from days 5 to 15 of the cycle. The side-effects of the oestrogen are those of oral contraceptives and are well-known. The major side-effect of cyproterone acetate is that it will feminize a male fetus, so it is always combined with an oestrogen to ensure contraception. This approach to therapy is ideal for the female already using an oral contraceptive.

(3) **Systemic retinoid therapy.** The development of 13-cis-retinoic acid has been one of the most important therapeutic advances in dermatology in the 1980s. It was well known that vitamin A was effective in acne, but the side-effects from a therapeutic dose were unacceptable. 13-cis-retinoic acid (Roaccutane) is a potent but less toxic synthetic derivative of vitamin A which influences all the major features of the pathogenesis of acne, it:

- Reduces sebum excretion by 90% within a month.
- Reduces the microorganisms active in acne, particularly *P. acnes*, both at the surface and within the pilosebaceous duct.
- Decreases the plugging of the lining of the duct.
- Reduces inflammation and chemotaxis.

The most impressive feature pathologically is that it shrivels the sebaceous glands to their prepubertal state. It does this not by any hormonal effect but by profoundly influencing epithelial proliferation and differentiation.

This drug is the treatment of choice for nodulocystic acne, for acne that is unresponsive to adequate conventional therapy, and particularly for acne causing scarring. It is given in a dose of 1mg/kg, orally, for 4 months. Like other systemic treatments for acne, it does not work immediately, but an effect should be seen within 6 weeks. Most patients report it to be the best treatment they have ever had, particularly as the condition continues to improve after cessation of therapy. One course is usually sufficient.

All patients develop a dryness of the skin, particularly of the lips (Fig. 17.9), but not severe enough to warrant discontinuing treatment. Similarly, nose-bleeds may occur, but usually only in those who are predisposed to them. Arthralgias and myalgias occasionally occur, especially in adolescents. Headaches can occur, as can benign intracranial hypertension which is a contraindication to its use. Very occasional cases of diffuse interstitial hyperostosis have been described. The drug causes a temporary hyperlipidaemia and as it is metabolized through the liver, it is wise to measure both lipid and liver function prior to therapy.

The most important side-effect is teratogenicity. The drug is only prescribable in the UK by dermatologists, and there have already been a few unplanned pregnancies, but in the US, where its prescription is not restricted, there have been many more. It is unwise to prescribe the drug without concomitant adequate contraception, whether or not the patient is sexually active; so the decision to use the drug in a female must be taken after adequate discussion between herself, her family practitioner and the dermatologist. Contraception should be continued for at least 3 months after cessation of treatment. The drug is expensive.

Other specific therapies

(1) Intralesional triamcinolone. Large inflamed cysts (Fig. 17.10) may be injected with small amounts (less than 0.1ml) of 2.5mg/ml triamcinolone, having first evacuated any material within the cyst. Atrophy may result if the steroid is injected too deeply.

(2) Surgery. Unsightly scars and persistent cysts, when they are no longer inflamed, may be excised. Dermabrasion has not received acclaim in the UK as the results of treatment have been poor. Possibly expertise and dedication to the technique have not been built up in the UK because of variable results. Similar comments may be made about collagen implants.

ACNE EXCORIÉE DES JEUNES FILLES

Definition
A facial disorder secondary to an obsessional and neurotic tendency to interfere with the skin.

Diagnostic features
- Unhappy women.
- Face.
- Excoriations, post-inflammatory hyperpigmentation and scars.
- Virtually untreatable.

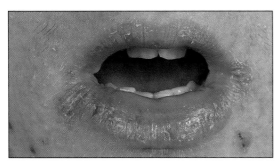

▲ **Fig. 17.9** *Roaccutane cheilitis. 13-cis-retinoic acid profoundly reduces sebum excretion. Dryness of the mucous membranes is a universal side-effect but teratogenicity is the most serious hazard.*

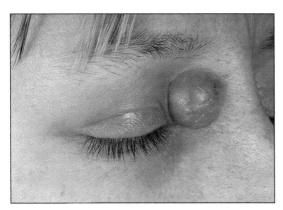

▲ **Fig. 17.10** *Acne cyst. Large inflamed cysts occur in acne conglobata but sometimes occur with minimal acne elsewhere. The lesions can be drained and then injected with triamcinolone.*

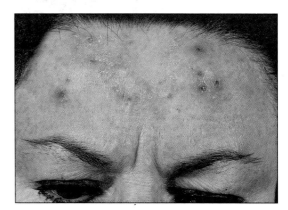

▲ **Fig. 17.11** *Acne excoriée des jeunes filles. This is a chronic neurotic disorder of adult women who admit that they pick and squeeze at their facial skin.*

Aetiology

This disorder is almost exclusively confined to women, who are not always particularly 'jeunes'. Although many individuals pick at and squeeze their spots to a limited extent, women afflicted with this disorder do so in an obsessional and destructive manner. They probably have no real preceding acne at all or, if they do, it is minor. It appears to be a protective device which conceals an emotional failure.

Clinical features

The physical signs are almost exclusively secondary to interference with the skin, such that unsightly excoriations, post-inflammatory hyperpigmentation and scarring result (Fig. 17.11). The face, cheeks, chin and jaw are primarily afflicted.

Management

Although these women freely admit that they pick at their skin, it is virtually impossible to dissuade them from the habit. It may represent a form of defence, perhaps an excuse for inadequate or unhappy lives, but psychiatric assistance is of little avail.

ROSACEA

Definition

A condition characterized by papules and pustules occurring on the face often associated with erythema and flushing.

Diagnostic features
- Papules and pustules.
- Flushing and erythema.
- Cheeks, forehead, nose and/or chin.
- Eyes may be involved.
- Precipitated by alcohol, hot beverages and climatic changes.
- Responds to antibiotics.

Aetiology

The disorder is common, occurs equally in both sexes and appears at any time from the fourth decade onwards. Celts are particularly prone; Negroes rarely get it. The disorder lasts a few months and then goes into remission, although often not permanently. Others have the disease chronically to some degree or another. Histologically there is vascular dilatation and sebaceous gland hyperplasia. The cause is unknown, but there appears to be vasomotor instability, which is apparent clinically from the erythema of the face and a tendency to flush readily. This in turn may be influenced by:

(1) **Diet.** There have been many claims for a gastrointestinal disturbance in rosacea but none have been substantiated. However, many patients note that their rosacea is aggravated by hot drinks and hot, spicy foods. Hot drinks exacerbate rosacea because heat vasodilates the skin, not because of any caffeine content. Any vasodilators, and alcohol is the classic one, can exacerbate the disorder.

(2) **Climate.** Fluctuations in temperature make it worse. Patients note that they tend to flush when they move from a warm environment into the cold and vice versa. Similarly, warm climates aggravate rosacea. It has been proposed that the vasomotor tone of the facial blood vessels is impaired.

(3) **Topical glucocorticosteroids.** These agents have a profoundly deleterious effect in rosacea. In the 1960s and early 1970s there was a widespread erroneous practice in the UK of prescribing powerful topical steroids to treat rosacea. The phenomenon is much less common nowadays, but in certain countries these drugs may be bought over the counter and used indiscriminately by the patients. Alternatively, patients may be given them by well-meaning friends, or use a steroid cream prescribed for another condition. Topical steroids are vasoconstrictors of the skin, so they may appear to be a logical treatment for a disease where vasodilatation is a prominent feature. Indeed the rosacea is often temporarily improved, but deteriorates a short while after cessation of therapy, possibly due to a reactive vasodilation resulting in a rebound phenomenon. Thus the condition flares up every time the patient stops using the steroid and, thinking erroneously that the steroid is helping to control an otherwise deteriorating condition, the patient reapplies the steroid to calm it. A vicious circle develops and a state of pseudoaddiction results.

Although a vasomotor disturbance seems likely as the cause of rosacea, the correct treatment is with antibiotics, which might indicate that a microbiological explanation is called for. As yet, none has been found. A mite, *Demodex folliculorum*, which is a normal inhabitant of the follicular apparatus, has been implicated in the aetiology of rosacea because it can sometimes be found in large numbers in the lesions. However, the numbers do not decline with treatment; so if this organism is relevant, its role at present is obscure.

Clinical features

The condition is unmistakable, but is often misdiagnosed and mismanaged. The patient complains of spots, often with yellow heads, erupting on the face and notes a tendency to flush easily and deterioration if the environmental temperature changes. On examination there are red papules (Fig. 17.12) and yellow pustules but none of the comedones, cysts or scars seen in acne. The cheeks, nose, forehead and chin are often red and surmounted by the spots. This is the classical case of rosacea but there are clinical variants:

- Occasionally only the nose is affected by erythema (Fig. 17.13) with little in the way of spots elsewhere.
- The nose may be afflicted by an exuberant overgrowth of its soft tissues, secondary to sebaceous gland hypertrophy. This condition, which is more

common in males, is known as 'rhinophyma' and may occur without much concomitant rosacea (Fig. 17.14).

- The eyes may also be affected. The patient complains of discomfort, often described as grittiness, in the eyes. Conjunctivitis, blepharitis and keratitis, with ulceration and vascularization of the cornea, may be present.
- Lymphoedema around the eyes may be prominent.

Differential diagnosis

The condition is sometimes confused with acne, and has in the past been called 'acne rosacea', but there is no aetiological resemblance to acne and this term should be dropped. The more obvious distinctions between them are given in Figure 17.15.

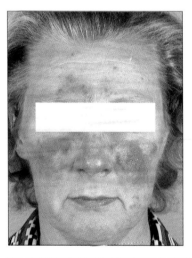

◀Fig. 17.12 *Rosacea. Papules and pustules occur on the forehead, cheeks, nose and chin. Not all these areas may be affected in any one patient.*

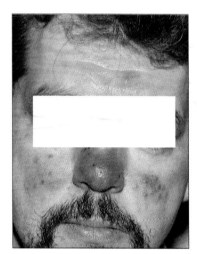

◀Fig. 17.13 *Rosacea. The condition sometimes predominantly affects the nose with few lesions elsewhere.*

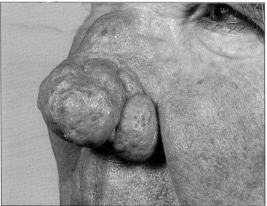

▲**Fig. 17.14** *Rhinophyma. The shape of the nose may change due to sebaceous gland hypertrophy. There may or may not be concomitant rosacea.*

DISTINCTION BETWEEN ACNE AND ROSACEA

Acne	Rosacea
Second and third decade	Later
Greasiness	Flushing and erythema
Comedones, cysts, scars, papules and pustules	Papules and pustules only
Slow response to antibiotics	Rapid response

▲**Fig. 17.15** *Distinction between acne and rosacea.*

Management
This is one of the most gratifying disorders to treat.
(1) **Antibiotics.** Tetracyclines, erythromycin, septrin or metronidazole are all effective. Usually small doses are all that are required, for example oxytetracycline 250mg twice daily. Rosacea responds to therapy within a few days (more quickly than acne). The drugs do have to be taken long-term to maintain control, but lower doses are required than for acne, so patients can be instructed to tailor the dose to give complete control. Thus oxytetracycline daily or on alternate days may be quite sufficient.
(2) **Topical remedies.** None are very effective and rosacea is best managed systemically. Sulphur cream starting at 1% and gradually increasing thereafter, is a time-honoured preparation and is reasonable to consider in pregnancy when tetracyclines in particular are contraindicated, although erythromycin is acceptable after the first trimester if the rosacea is severe.
(3) **Diet.** Many patients have a strong liking for tea or coffee and consume it in large amounts. It is well worthwhile reducing this or adopting the American habit of taking iced tea or coffee. Curries and other spicy cuisine should also be restricted. It is important that alcohol abuse is diagnosed and managed appropriately.
(4) **Topical steroid abuse.** It is essential to discover whether patients are applying topical steroids (Fig. 17.16) because treatment thereafter is so straightforward. The patient is told to stop the drug, and warned that there will be a rebound for 3 or 4 days whilst the antibiotics begin to take effect. If the patient understands that the skin has become 'addicted to the steroid' there is rarely any difficulty in breaking the habit. The rosacea will respond to low doses of antibiotics and will need nothing topically other than perhaps a moisturizer. A total recovery can be expected.

The variants of rosacea may be managed as follows:
(1) **Rhinophyma.** Plastic surgeons are skilled at paring away the hypertrophic sebaceous glands and remodelling the nose in a pleasing manner. Rhinophyma does not respond to antibiotics, but it may be necessary to keep any accompanying rosacea under control with antibiotics.
(2) **Eye complications.** Antibiotics are of benefit, but the ocular changes are complicated and referral to an ophthalmologist is recommended.
(3) **Red nose.** Some patients have erythema of the nose only, with little in the way of papules and pustules. This disorder does not respond well to any treatment, but intense antibiotic therapy is required coupled with a veto on alcohol and other vasodilators.
(4) **Lymphoedema.** This does not respond to antibiotics but the excess tissue may be removed by a plastic surgeon.

PERIORAL AND PERIORBITAL DERMATITIS

Definition
A papular eruption around the mouth or eyes secondary to the misuse of topical glucocorticosteroids.

> **Diagnostic features**
> • Red papules and erythema.
> • Around the mouth or eyes.
> • Secondary to topical steroids.
> • Responsive to oral antibiotics.

Aetiology
Perioral and orbital dermatitis is due to inappropriate treatment with topical steroids either mistakenly prescribed by a doctor or as a result of self-medication. Often the steroid is obtained from a well-meaning friend or had been prescribed for a totally unrelated condition. The initial disorder is either a mild seborrhoeic eczema or a mild acne around the nose and mouth or eye (Fig. 17.17).

Topical steroids are the treatment of choice for seborrhoeic eczema but only in the lowest strength as hydrocortisone. If a more potent steroid is used, perioral and periorbital dermatitis may result. If the

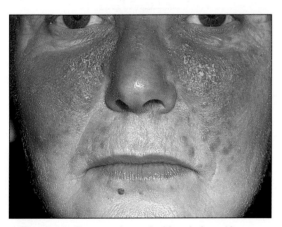

▲ **Fig. 17.16** *Rosacea mistreated with topical steroids. Although topical steroids initially calm rosacea, there is a 'rebound' vasodilatation and exacerbation of the papules and pustules.*

initial condition is acne, even the weakest steroid, hydrocortisone, is capable of causing the disorder. The acne is often misdiagnosed as eczema because it may be itchy and it is not always appreciated that acne may be itchy. The drug, particularly in cases of seborrhoeic eczema, seems to work at first, but each time the treatment is discontinued the condition flares (Fig. 17.18). Re-application of the steroid calms the rash so that many patients are led into believing that the steroid is controlling a progressive disease.

Topical steroids are potent acne-inducing agents, and *potent steroids should never be prescribed for acne or eczema of the face*. They can also cause permanent and disfiguring atrophy of the skin.

Clinical features
The history of the use of a steroid with deterioration or rebound on ceasing to use it is typical. The physical

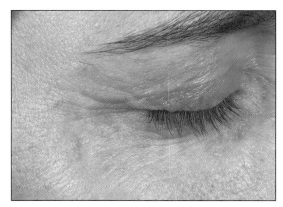

▲ **Fig. 17.17** *Periorbital dermatitis. Small red and often itchy papules occur around the eye. Steroids aggravate this.*

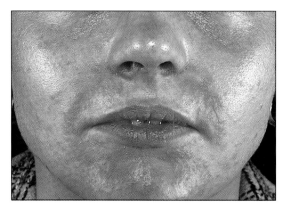

▲ **Fig. 17.18** *Perioral dermatitis. A perioral condition of erythema, papules and pustules results from the inappropriate use of steroids to treat either acne or seborrhoeic eczema.*

signs are of red papules, often on a background of erythema and scaling, involving the area of application of the drug, which is usually around the mouth or around an eye.

Management
Discontinuing the steroid and treatment with an antibiotic, usually oxytetracycline 250mg twice daily for a month, is successful. After an initial relapse (if the patient has been using the steroid up to the minute of the consultation), the condition begins to improve after 4 days and is very much better at 2 weeks. On stopping treatment the original condition often reveals itself. If it is seborrhoeic eczema, it should be treated with hydrocortisone as necessary or, if acne, with long-term antibiotics.

IDIOPATHIC LOCAL HYPERHIDROSIS

Definition
An over-production of sweat from the axillae, palms or soles.

Diagnostic features
- Inappropriate excess sweating.
- Axillae — ruins clothes.
- On palms and soles — disturbs function.

Aetiology
There are two distinct types of eccrine sweat glands, which respond either to heat or to emotion. Those responsible for heat adaptation and thermoregulation are distributed all over the body, except for the palms and soles (which are solely under the control of the emotions). The sweat glands in the axillae are under the control of both heat and emotion. Although hyperhidrosis occurs in disorders such as Graves' disease and acromegaly, its symptoms are usually secondary, not primary, presenting features. Idiopathic hyperhidrosis may be limited to the axillae or the extremities but occasionally both areas are affected. The condition becomes pathological, rather than a normal physiological response, when it interferes with function. It occurs most commonly in adolescents and young adults.

Clinical features
In pathological hyperhidrosis of the palms and soles the excess sweating is perfectly obvious and the sweat may be seen quite literally dripping onto the floor.

Those who suffer from axillary hyperhidrosis will show how the underarm portion of their blouses or shirts is stained and ruined within a few days of use.

Management
(1) Aluminium hexahydrate. Twenty per cent aluminium chloride hexahydrate in absolute anhydrous ethyl alcohol is useful for axillary hyperhidrosis, but disappointing for palmar or plantar disease.
(2) Iontophoresis. This is the introduction of an ionized substance through the skin by a direct current. It is useful for palmar/plantar hyperhidrosis. Initially various substances such as atropine, formaldehyde and anticholinergic drugs (for example glycopyrrhonium bromide) were introduced by this technique, but tap water alone is effective. Why the sweat glands shut down is unknown. It has been suggested that the sweat glands become blocked, or that there is some electrical gradient that controls the movement of sweat along the sweat duct, which is interfered with by iontophoresis. The method involves immersing one hand into a bowl of water with an electrode connected to a galvanic generator delivering direct current. A foot is placed in another bowl of water with an electrode to complete the circuit. The sweating ceases for many weeks and the treatment can be repeated. This treatment is usually carried out under hospital supervision, but there are units available for home use.
(3) Surgery. *(a) Sympathectomy:* as techniques for sympathectomy improve, this has become a much more effective and safe operation for hyperhidrosis of the palms. It is indicated only for those with severe disease, as there can be the disabling side-effect of permanent dryness, scaliness and fissuring of the palms, secondary to the total switching off of the sweat glands. *(b) Excision of axillary skin:* this is an excellent treatment for those disabled by axillary hyperhidrosis. The main sweat-producing area of axillary skin is excised. The procedure is uncomfortable post-operatively and secondary infection may occur. The resulting scars are unsightly but not usually disturbing to the patient.
(4) Oral anticholinergics. Although this would seem the logical treatment, the ocular and intestinal side-effects are such that they render the treatment difficult to comply with.
(5) Tranquillisers. Doses which induce drowsiness are relatively effective in reducing the emotional triggers, but the side-effects inhibit their usefulness.

HIDRADENITIS SUPPURATIVA

Definition
A chronic disorder of apocrine glands, which results in painful indolent papules and nodules that form sinuses and scars in the axillae and groins.

Diagnostic features
- Indolent painful papules and nodules, sinuses and scars.
- Axillae and groin.
- Often associated with acne.

Aetiology
The cause is unknown, although many patients also have acne conglobata. It commences after puberty and affects both sexes equally. There is occlusion of the apocrine glands. No primary pathogen has been found but exacerbations may be due to secondary infection or to the more androgenic progestogens in contraceptive pills.

Clinical features
Recurrent chronic suppurative papules and nodules result in sinuses and puckered scars (Fig. 17.19).

Management
Long-term antibiotic therapy as used in acne is helpful. Anti-androgens benefit females. 13-cis-retinoic acid has no effect. Intralesional steroids are worth trying. Local excision of lesions is often followed by recurrences. Wide excision and grafting is successful in some cases.

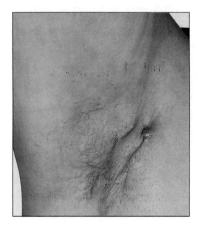

◄Fig. 17.19 *Hidradenitis suppurativa. Sinuses and puckered scarring result from indolent inflamed papules and nodules in the flexures.*

18 NAIL DISORDERS

INTRODUCTION

The nail consists of hard keratin which is formed from an invagination of the skin overlying the distal phalanx. It lies on a bed of epidermis to which it is firmly attached. It grows mainly from a matrix which is directly under the posterior nail fold and extends to the foremost portion of the lunular (half moon). The half moon is paler than the rest of the nail because keratinization is incomplete in this area, and possibly the connective tissue is packed more loosely. The cuticle is an extension of the stratum corneum of the skin, from the dorsal surface of the finger onto the nail plate. It plays an important role in sealing off the potential space between the roof of the nail fold and its floor. The nail acts as a protection to the under-lying distal phalanx, facilitates the picking up of small objects and contributes to the appreciation of fine touch.

Under normal circumstances, the fingernails take about 5 months to grow out, and the toenails 12-18 months, which is why the fingernails require cutting more frequently. Individual nails differ slightly in their growth rates, and those on the dominant hand grow fastest. Nail growth is accelerated in psoriasis, a disorder of epidermal proliferation, and decreased in severe illness or in ischaemic states.

The diagnosis of nail disorders is no more difficult than that of skin disorders, but the physical signs can be difficult to interpret. There is an understandable tendency to regard every abnormality as fungus and to treat accordingly, which is admirable in a sense because the fungal disorders are often the only ones which are treatable. However, it is always wise to take clippings and have the diagnosis of a fungal disorder established in the laboratory first, before commencing a potentially toxic and often protracted therapy.

INFECTIONS OF THE NAILS

Acute paronychia
Definition
An acute, usually staphylococcal infection of the lateral or posterior nail folds.

Diagnostic features
- Acute and painful.
- Erythema and swelling.
- Pus is often visible.

Aetiology
The organism, which is usually *Staphylococcus aureus* but sometimes *Streptococcus pyogenes*, gains entry to the posterior or lateral nail fold either through a minor injury (sometimes secondary to nail biting), or an already damaged nail. In the latter *Pseudomonas aeruginosa* is often involved. Sometimes the infection may develop deep under the nail plate.

Clinical features
The condition is acute in onset and painful. If it involves the nail folds, the infection may be quite superficial and the pus is evident (Fig. 18.1). Alternatively, it may be deeper and a red, tender swelling is present around the nail. If the infection is underneath the nail, the nail plate becomes loose and distorted, and may be lifted off to reveal purulent material.

Management
(1) **Broad spectrum antibiotics.** In the early stages of the infection, an antibiotic such as erythromycin 250mg four times daily for a week may be effective.

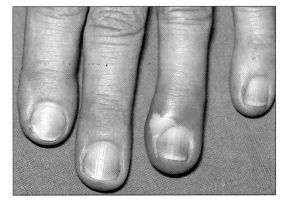

▲ **Fig. 18.1** *Acute paronychia. The condition is acute and painful. Pus is evident with surrounding inflammation.*

(2) **Surgery.** Pus from superficial infections can be released by incision, but may require surgical drainage if deeper. For infections underneath the nail, the nail may need to be removed.

Chronic paronychia
Definition
A chronic infection usually secondary to *Candida albicans* involving the posterior or lateral nail folds.

> **Diagnostic features**
> * Redness and swelling.
> * Occasional beads of pus.
> * Posterior and lateral nail folds.
> * Loss of cuticle.
> * Horizontal ridging of the nail.
> * Predominantly female.

Aetiology
The condition is common, affecting women far more than men and being most often seen in housewives. It is also encountered in anyone whose occupation requires continual immersion of the hands in water — nurses, bar staff, chefs, hairdressers, for example. It is important to understand the pathogenesis of this condition for it is more often mismanaged than misdiagnosed. Water is the cause, for it softens and eventually destroys the cuticle. The consequent damp and occluded microenvironment under the nail fold is ideal for the commensal and opportunistic organism *C. albicans*. Occasionally the patient also has diabetes mellitus or vaginal candidosis, both of which make the condition more likely. Often the patient is a keen manicurist and pushes her cuticles back too enthusiastically.

Clinical features
The index or middle finger is most commonly affected, although in neglected cases more than one fingernail is involved. The patient complains of a swelling around the nail which is not particularly uncomfortable unless an acute bacterial infection is superimposed. The patient often gives a history that a small bead of pus discharges from time to time. The physical signs are of a red, sometimes boggy, swelling of the posterior and lateral nail fold. The cuticle is absent and a gap is visible between the nail fold and the nail plate (Fig. 18.2). Later on the nail itself is affected by horizontal cross ridging, secondary to interference with nail growth, due to involvement of the nail matrix under the nail fold. In some cases the nail plate itself may become invaded by *C. albicans* (Fig. 18.3) or by *Pseudomonas pyocyanea*. The former gives it a brown and the latter a green colour.

Management
This is a challenging disorder to manage because cure depends on the doctor's powers of communication. The successful management ultimately lies in the patient's hands; failure to convince her of the significance of wet conditions will result in failure to cure the condition.

Many patients do not believe that it is possible to keep the skin dry if they are looking after a house, a husband and small children, but it is surprising how ingenious they can become if they are motivated. Plaster dressings must be forbidden, as they only increase the damp environment, and rubber gloves should be avoided because the skin will sweat under them and the nail will only be immersed in the

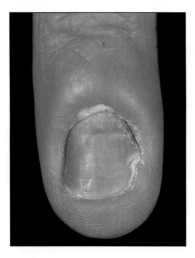

◀**Fig. 18.2**
Chronic paronychia. There is loss of the cuticle, oedema of the nail folds and horizontal ridging of the nail.

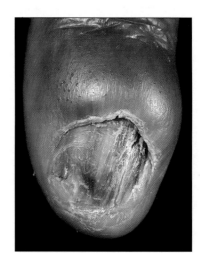

◀**Fig. 18.3**
Chronic paronychia. This lady was a domestic and continually had her hands in water. The cuticle is destroyed, the nail fold is bolstered and the nail is discoloured and dystrophic due to C. albicans.

patient's own saline. If gloves are to be worn, cotton-lined ones are to be preferred and they should not be worn for prolonged periods. Hand washing (including such social niceties as before a meal or after urination), preparation and cleaning of vegetables, laundry, washing up (other family members can do this) and manicuring should be disallowed. All this is essential to starve the microorganism of its ideal wet environment, and to allow the cuticle to reform.

Locally, the application of an anti-*Candida* preparation to the nail folds is all that is required. It should not be pushed up under the nail, because this will prohibit the reformation of the cuticle. The condition takes time to recover but if the patient is seen initially every fortnight, to ensure that the instructions are being adhered to, all will be well. Photographs or drawings are helpful to record progress.

If the nail plate is discoloured, clippings should be taken for mycology. If *Candida* is present in these clippings it is treatable with oral ketoconazole, 200mg daily, which may need to be taken for up to 4 months if severe. Ketoconazole is potentially hepatotoxic, so the drug should not be given unless the nail plate is proven by mycology to be involved.

Chronic paronychia is frequently mismanaged. It is important to emphasize that griseofulvin is ineffective against *Candida*, antibiotics are not appropriate unless bacterial sepsis has supervened, and surgical incision is not indicated.

Tinea unguium
Definition
An infection of the nail plate with a dermatophyte.

> #### Diagnostic features
> - Asymmetrical involvement of the toenails.
> - Unilateral hand involvement of fingernails.
> - Discolouration, thickening and destruction of the nail.
> - Begins at the lateral edges of the nails.

Aetiology
Trichophyton rubrum or *T. mentagrophytes* var. *interdigitale* are the most common causes of tinea unguium. However local species prevail in different countries. The condition usually begins in the skin of the feet as tinea pedis and is contracted in the same manner. There is subsequent infection of the toenails and occasionally it spreads to the skin of one hand and thence to the fingernails. It is unusual for fingernails to be infected without the toenails being involved but it can occur, particularly in children. The fungus

enters either from the lateral nail fold or from the nail bed. Many patients have a noticeably cool peripheral circulation.

Clinical features
Often the patient does not seek advice regarding the toenail changes until they are advanced. The sides of the nails are affected initially with a brown, white or yellow discolouration (Fig. 18.4). Subsequently the nail and its bed becomes thickened and the nail plate becomes crumbly, which is rather characteristic and can be observed when taking clippings for mycology. The nail bed becomes composed of a soft hyperkeratotic material which can be scraped out with a blunt scalpel. As invasion spreads, the whole nail and its bed becomes thickened, discoloured and distorted. The nail may separate from its bed (onycholysis), and may break away (Figs 18.5 & 18.6) altogether, causing complete destruction of the nail. It is an asymmetrical

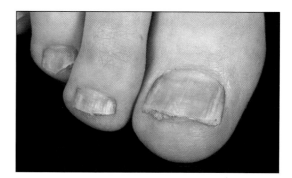

▲ **Fig. 18.4** *Tinea unguium. The nails are yellow and thickened with hyperkeratotic material underneath. The process commences at the sides of the nail as in the third toe.*

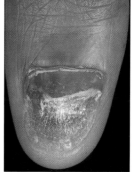 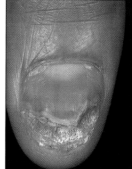

▲ **Figs 18.5 & 18.6** *Tinea unguium. The thumb nail is thickened and discoloured and the distal portion has broken off. Nail clippings were positive for* T. rubrum. *The nail is shown (Fig. 18.6) recovering after 2 months of griseofulvin.*

condition with variable degrees of involvement of the individual nails (Fig. 18.7) and this is a helpful physical sign. First the nails of one foot may be involved more than the other, and secondly the corresponding toe on the other foot may be either uninvolved or only affected to a limited degree. It is remarkable how several toenails may be extensively involved on one foot, and yet the others are relatively spared. It is even more extraordinary how several fingernails of one hand may be involved with complete sparing of those on the other. Indeed, one hand may be involved for many years before spread, if ever, occurs.

Diagnosis

It is important to take generous clippings of affected portions of the nail and of the subungual hyperkeratosis for mycology. It is not necessary to attempt to examine these oneself under direct microscopy, because the clippings need to be soaked in potash for some hours, and even then identification of the hyphae is not all that easy. Results of direct microscopy will be available quickly and results of the culture within 4 weeks. Although the fungus is usually visible under the microscope, it is not always easy to grow it on culture. Clippings are always worth repeating, if the tests are negative.

Management

Tinea of the nails responds to many months of systemic therapy with either griseofulvin or ketoconazole. *It is therefore imperative that the diagnosis is proven before commencing a treatment which might otherwise be fruitless.*

It is always worthwhile treating fingernail infections as they will clear within 6 months. It is more debatable whether toenail infection should be treated, for it is necessary to take griseofulvin or ketoconazole for 18 months to 2 years, and even then one cannot guarantee cure. It is probably reasonable to treat younger patients if they are likely to be conscientious in taking the tablets daily. They also appear to respond better than older groups, whose nails do not grow out as rapidly. These agents are fungistatic and do not therefore kill the fungus, but their presence in the newly forming nail is inimical to the fungus, so the patient recovers as the diseased nail grows out. Some advocate avulsion of the toenails to debulk the infection.

Topical agents have not been effective in the therapy of tinea of the nails. However, successful claims have been made for a new imidazole (tioconazole) in undecylenic acid, painted twice daily for several months. Certainly it seems to increase the chances of a cure if combined with a systemic agent.

Pseudomonas **infections**
Definition

A secondary infection of an abnormal nail (usually onycholysis or chronic paronychia) with *Pseudomonas pyocyanea*.

Diagnostic feature
- A green discolouration of the nail plate.

Aetiology

Pseudomonas pyocyanea is an ubiquitous pathogen, particularly associated with tap water. It is not surprising therefore that it will act as an opportunistic

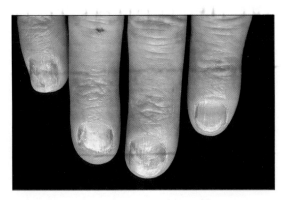

▲**Fig. 18.7** *Tinea unguium. The nails are affected to different degrees when dermatophytes affect the fingers; in adults it is usually due to* T. rubrum *and only one hand is affected although both feet are.*

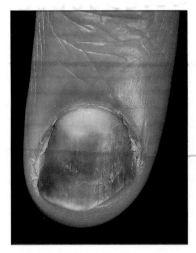

◀**Fig. 18.8** *Pseudomonas of the nail. This lady was a baker and her nails were continually wet. The green discolouration was due to P. pyocyanea. It responded to keeping the nail dry and painting with 15% sulphacetamide.*

pathogen in a diseased nail. It particularly colonizes onycholytic nails or those damaged by chronic parony-chia.

Clinical features

Pseudomonas pyocyanea imparts a green (Fig. 18.8), blue or black discolouration to the nail plate. It is a unique and easily identified phenomenon.

Management

Treatment is that of the primary condition. The superimposed *Pseudomonas* responds to 15% sulpha-cetamide in 50% spirit (30% sulphacetamide eye drops diluted by 50%) applied to the nail bed under-neath the nails.

PSORIASIS OF THE NAILS

Definition

Involvement of the nail secondary to psoriasis.

Diagnostic features

- Symmetry.
- Pitting.
- Onycholysis.
- Dystrophy.
- Psoriasis of the skin.

Aetiology

Nail changes are common in patients with psoriasis: probably most have them at some time, but the changes fluctuate in degree and may not be noticed.

Occasionally nail changes identical to those which occur in psoriasis occur in patients who have no evidence of cutaneous involvement, although the skin rash may appear years later. Sometimes gross changes occur with minimal psoriasis elsewhere, classically on the scalp and the genitalia.

Clinical features

There are three main groups of abnormality.

(1) Pitting. This is the commonest feature. The pits, which are usually minute, can occur in a random or uniform pattern across the nail plate (see Fig. 18.9) but may be arranged in lines. The lunula itself is often involved. The changes are frequently symmetrical. Pitting is thought to be due to parakeratosis (retention of nuclei in nail keratin) similar to that which occurs in the stratum corneum in psoriatic skin. These areas of parakeratosis are presumed to be weaker than the surrounding nail and they fall out leaving the pits behind. The parakeratosis is the result of the hyper-proliferation which occurs in psoriasis, which leads to an immature epithelium and hence nuclear remnants in horny tissue. Pitting is not specific to psoriasis, and identical changes occur in alopecia areata (see Fig. 20.13) and eczema.

(2) Onycholysis. This means a loosening of the nail away from the nail bed. It usually involves the free edge of the nail (Fig. 18.10) and a considerable gap is visible between the nail plate and its bed, but it can occur centrally. A characteristic feature which distin-guishes psoriatic onycholysis from other sorts is a yellow margin in between the white, separated, free edge and the pink, healthy nail. The onset of the condition may be quite sudden. The disorder is

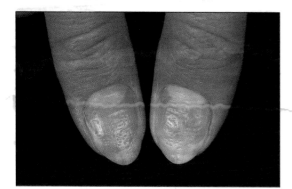

▲ **Fig. 18.9** *Pitting due to psoriasis. Small pits can occur in a random or uniform pattern sometimes producing lines.*

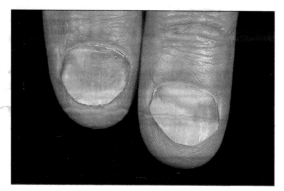

▲ **Fig. 18.10** *Onycholysis due to psoriasis. A yellow margin often separates the white separated free edge of the nail from the pink healthy nail.*

thought to be due to psoriasis involving the nail bed and this is sometimes actually visible underneath the lifted nail.

(3) Gross psoriatic nail dystrophy. This type is secondary to psoriasis underneath the posterior nail fold and lunular in the nail matrix. The nail lacks lustre, becomes opaque, and is thickened and discoloured. Symmetry (Fig. 18.11) distinguishes this type from fungal disorders, as all the nails are usually involved to some degree; but the situation is not static, with one nail recovering and then another deteriorating. Complete recovery is unusual. Patients with psoriatic arthropathy involving the distal joints often have this type of nail involvement, but nail changes frequently occur without arthropathy as well.

Management

It is always worthwhile taking clippings for mycological examination because occasionally patients with psoriasis also have fungal infections which are treatable, whereas psoriasis of the nails is not. Powerful topical steroids, in the form of scalp application applied under the nail,

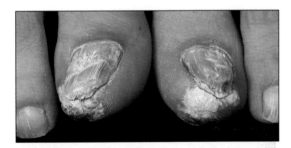

▲ **Fig. 18.11** *Gross psoriatic nail dystrophy. The nails are thickened, discoloured and distorted due to psoriasis in the nail matrix. The symmetry is striking, and in this patient the skin is also involved.*

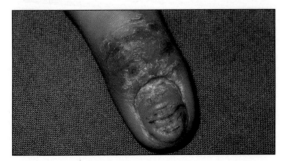

▲ **Fig. 18.12** *Eczema affecting the nails. Several horizontal ridges are present as well as active eczema, but this may have cleared by the time the patient presents.*

may be tried for onycholytic disorders. Matrix disorders do not respond to topical therapy but they do return to normality during systemic therapy, when this is given for extensive cutaneous disease. However, it must be questionable whether systemic treatment is justified for nail involvement only.

NAIL CHANGES ASSOCIATED WITH ECZEMA OF THE HANDS

Definition
Horizontal ridges in one or several nails secondary to eczema overlying the posterior nail fold.

Diagnostic features
- Horizontal depressions across one or more fingernails.
- Present or past eczema around posterior nail fold.

Aetiology
Eczema overlying the posterior nail fold disturbs the development of the' nail from the underlying nail matrix.

Clinical features
Usually several horizontal ridges are present across the nail (Fig. 18.12). Eczema of the fingers may be visible, or a past history of the disease may be obtained. One or more nails may be affected, depending on the degree of eczema. If the eczema has been severe the affected nail or nails may be temporarily shed.

Management
Treatment of the eczema on the skin stops the nail involvement. The ridging grows out over ensuing months.

ONYCHOLYSIS OF THE NAILS

Definition
Separation of the nail away from the nail bed.

Diagnostic features
- Opaque discolouration.
- Distal separation of the nail.
- Normal nail thickness.

Aetiology and clinical features

The nail may separate away from its bed as a result of psoriasis, eczema, tinea or poor peripheral circulation, but other manifestations of the condition are evident. The most common type, although known as *idiopathic onycholysis*, is most often due to trauma. A single nail, or sometimes more than one, is usually affected. It primarily occurs in females because women grow their nails long, and presumably the nail can be more easily detached by minor trauma from the bed upon which it lies. Secondary bacterial infection with *Pseudomonas* is not uncommon.

If all the fingernails (and often the toenails) are involved, a systemic effect is likely, usually phototoxic but occasionally due to thyrotoxicosis. Phototoxic onycholysis (Fig. 18.13) is a reaction between intense ultraviolet (UV) light exposure and a photosensitizing drug. These are most commonly tetracyclines, and especially the long-acting demethylchlortetracycline. A similar phenomenon was seen with the non-steroidal anti-inflammatory drug benoxaprofen (Opren). The widespread use of the photosensitizing chemicals 5- and 8-methoxypsoralens combined with UVA (PUVA) for the treatment of psoriasis and other skin diseases has led to an increase in iatrogenic photo-onycholysis.

Management

Idiopathic onycholysis often resolves spontaneously. Secondary infection is the commonest reason for the failure of the nail to reattach itself, coupled probably with further trauma. The nail should be kept clipped as short as possible to reduce further trauma, and the use of 15% sulphacetamide in 50% spirit is recommended as an anti-bacterial.

BEAU'S LINES

Definition

A horizontal depression occurring across the nail plate of all the nails.

> **Diagnostic features**
> - All the nails are affected.
> - A horizontal depression occurs across the nails.

Aetiology

The condition is common often in a minor degree which may not be noticed except by the fastidious. It is due to interruption in the growth of the nails occurring during an illness, whether it be influenza, an operation or even prolonged labour.

Clinical features

A horizontal trough across the nail plate is usually not noticed until it is halfway up the nail, that is at the level which corresponds to 2–3 months of nail growth after the precipitating episode. All the fingernails display the change (Fig. 18.14) and it is often possible to detect it in the toenails as well. The degree of change depends on the severity of the illness.

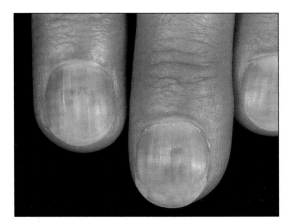

▲**Fig. 18.13** *Photo-onycholysis. All the nails are involved. The onycholysis resulted from an interaction between ultraviolet light and a photosensitizing drug. Haemorrhage can also be seen under the nail.*

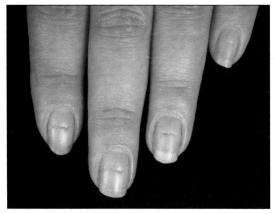

▲**Fig. 18.14** *Beau's lines. Horizontal troughs are visible across all the fingernails. They are usually not noticed until midway up the nail, about 3 months after an illness.*

Management

The deformity grows out and the patient can be reassured after suitable explanation.

LAMELLAR NAIL DYSTROPHY

Definition

A splitting of the nail plate into its component layers secondary to repeated wetting and drying out of the nails following frequent immersion in water.

Diagnostic features
- Most or all nails involved to some degree.
- Splitting of ends of fingernails into layers.

Aetiology

The condition is most common in women. It may occur in men but they rarely present for diagnosis. The normal nail consists of several layers of keratin. Frequent immersion of the hands and fingernails in water may soften the nail and the consequent drying damages the cells of the nail plate such that they do not adhere together properly. This permits the nail plate to separate into its component layers and these tend to split off distally (Fig. 18.15).

Clinical features

The tips of the fingernails are split into layers and an unmistakeable appearance results.

Management

Explanation and advice on reducing exposure to water coupled with protective measures is all that is required.

TRAUMA TO THE BIG TOENAIL

Definition

The big toenail, because of its prominence, is most vulnerable to external trauma or damage from ill-chosen footwear.

Diagnostic features
- Big toenail.
- Pin-point haemorrhage and brown or purple discolouration under nail (haematoma).
- Lateral growth, thickening and yellow colour (dystrophy).
- Granulation tissue at lateral border (ingrowing toenail).

Aetiology

The big toenail is most vulnerable because it is prominent and frequently injured, although the injury is often forgotten. Kicking a football, stubbing the toe accidentally, the wearing of shoes which are not large enough to accommodate the rapid growth of feet during childhood, high-heeled, pointed or open-toed shoes, allow minor trauma to lead ultimately to abnormal growth of the nail. The commonest abnormalities which result are haematoma, nail dystrophy and ingrowing toenails.

Clinical features

(1) **Haematoma.** The patient presents or the doctor refers because of an anxiety that the lesion may be a malignant melanoma. A red, brown or purple lesion (Fig. 18.16) is seen under the nail, often with pin-point haemorrhage. The discolouration will move up the nail as it grows.

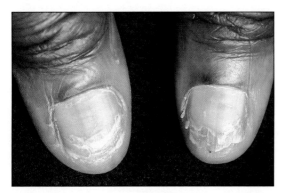

▲**Fig. 18.15** *Lamellar nail dystrophy. Frequent immersion in water causes the nail plate to separate into its component layers and these tend to split off distally.*

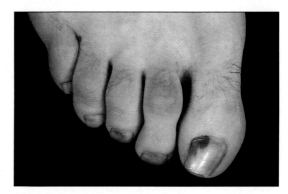

▲**Fig. 18.16** *Trauma to the big toenail. The big toenail is prominent and vulnerable to trauma. Haemorrhage may occur and ultimately the nail grows out laterally, as seen here.*

(2) Dystrophic nails. Chronic trivial trauma ultimately interferes with the growth of the prominent big toenails. The nail becomes discoloured and thickened and often grows out laterally (Fig. 18.16). In more severe cases the nail becomes grossly thickened, discoloured, excessively curved, hard and elongated, simulating a ram's horn (onychogryphosis). It was originally known as the ostler's nail, as it was usually seen in grooms who were frequently trampled on by horses.

(3) Ingrowing toenails. Discomfort and inflammation leading to granulation tissue (Fig. 18.17) result from small projections of the nail which cut into the lateral nail folds and sometimes detach and act as a foreign body.

Management

Patients with haematoma may be reassured. Dystrophic nails are often mistaken for a fungal disorder and treated as such, but as always it is wiser to take clippings for mycology before embarking on treatment. In a young healthy individual, it is reasonable to advise radical removal of the nail and its matrix. In the elderly, frequent chiropody is the best approach.

An ingrowing toenail usually results from ill-fitting footwear coupled with cutting the nail in a half-circle instead of straight across, which permits the nail to penetrate into the skin. Sometimes it results from a chronic tinea infection, which so distorts the nail bed that the nail grows abnormally into the skin. Rectification of these factors, use of potassium permanganate soaks as an antiseptic and insertion of a cottonwool plug under the edge of the nail to allow it to grow out straight are helpful measures. Granulation tissue should be destroyed by cautery. If this fails, the nail fold should be excised under a digital nerve block. Sometimes the nail has to be avulsed.

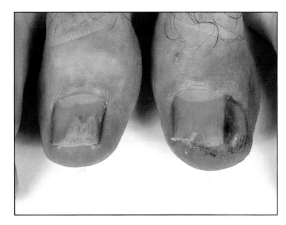

▲ **Fig. 18.17** *Ingrowing toenail. Heaped up granulation tissue occurs at the side of the big toe. Tinea is present here but ill-fitting shoes and poor nail cutting are the major cause.*

INTRODUCTION

In the skin, melanocytes are found in the basal cell layer of the epidermis and are responsible for producing the pigment known as melanin. They occur in a ratio of approximately one melanocyte to five basal cells. Since they do not stain with haematoxylin and eosin, they appear as clear cells in routine sections. They also occur in the retina, brain and mesentery.

Melanocytes are derived from melanoblasts which migrate from the neural crest (an ectodermal structure) during fetal development. If melanoblasts fail to migrate from the neural crest or fail to differentiate into melanocytes, a condition known as *piebaldism* (white forelock of hair with white patches on the skin) results. If they are arrested deep in the dermis on the way to the epidermis a blue naevus (see Fig. 7.12) or mongolian blue spot (see Fig. 7.13) results.

Caucasians have the same number of melanocytes as Negroes but have fewer and smaller melanosomes. Melanosomes are pigment-containing electron-dense granules produced within the melanocyte during the process of manufacturing melanin (melanogenesis); they are present in the dendrites of melanocytes and are ingested by neighbouring keratinocytes. These melanin granules partially surround the nucleus of the keratinocyte and protect it from ultraviolet light. Each melanocyte serves several keratinocytes. Melanosome abnormalities may occur, so that giant melanosomes are found in the café au lait patches of neurofibromatosis and in certain birth marks such as naevus spilus (see Fig. 1.7).

Melanocytes are largely protective against ultraviolet irradiation. Each individual has a constitutional amount of melanin which is capable of increasing either as a result of ultraviolet irradiation or of the increased production of certain hormones, in particular melanocyte stimulating hormone (MSH) and adrenocorticotrophic hormone (ACTH). Increases in

CAUSES OF INCREASED PRODUCTION OF MSH AND ACTH
adrenal failure
pituitary adenoma causing Cushing's syndrome
Nelson's syndrome (functioning pituitary tumour after bilateral adrenalectomy)
ectopic ACTH syndrome

▲ **Fig. 19.1** *Causes of increased production of MSH and ACTH.*

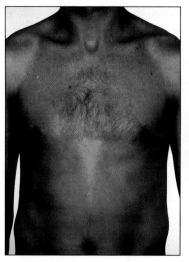
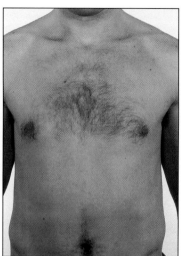

◄ **Figs 19.2 & 19.3** *Generalized hyperpigmentation. The cause of generalized hyperpigmentation must be investigated. This patient was suffering from adrenal failure and his anterior pituitary was over producing ACTH and MSH. The skin colour returned to normal (Fig. 19.3) with steroid replacement.*

MSH and ACTH production occur as a result of a pituitary tumour, an ectopic ACTH syndrome or a failure of the adrenal response (Figs 19.1–19.3). Conversely their production is decreased in hypopituitarism, which accounts for the pallor of the skin in this condition. In renal failure hyperpigmentation results from decreased degradation of MSH. Oestrogens also increase pigmentation such that pregnant women become temporarily generally more pigmented and their nipples, linea alba, axillae and genitalia become permanently pigmented.

Melanin is produced from phenylalanine, an essential amino acid, under the influence of the enzyme tyrosinase. The steps are illustrated in Figure 19.4. If the enzyme phenylalanine hydroxylase is deficient, tyrosine is not formed and phenylalanine accumulates leading to *phenylketonuria*, a condition of fair skin and hair due to impaired melanin synthesis and of mental retardation if the disorder is not promptly treated by a low phenylalanine diet. If tyrosinase is absent or nonfunctioning, *albinism* results, with varying degrees of white skin, blonde hair and photophobia. Squamous cell carcinoma is common in albinos, particularly those living in sunny climates.

Melanocytes may malfunction as a result of certain pathological states. Thus they may proliferate in a benign manner under the influence of ultraviolet light, as in solar lentigines or in certain genetic disorders such as the *Peutz Jegher syndrome*, a condition of pigmented macules of the mouth and extremities associated with intestinal polyps. They may proliferate in a malignant manner, as in malignant melanoma. Melanocytes may be destroyed as part of an autoimmune process, as in vitiligo, or following inflammatory conditions that disrupt the basal layer of the epidermis, such as lichen planus and discoid lupus erythematosus. Disorders of pigmentation are classified in Figure 19.5.

HYPERPIGMENTATION

The more common causes of generalized hyperpigmentation of the skin are summarized in Figure 19.6. The commonest skin disorders which result in localized hyperpigmentation are discussed below.

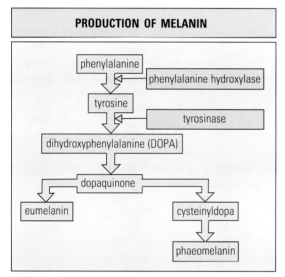

PRODUCTION OF MELANIN

▲ **Fig. 19.4** *Production of melanin.*

CLASSIFICATION OF PIGMENTARY DISORDERS

failure of melanocytes to arrive in the epidermis, e.g. blue naevus

enzymatic disorders of melanin synthesis, e.g. phenylketonuria and albinism

hormonal disorders affecting melanogenesis, e.g. Addison's disease

loss of melanocytes, e.g. vitiligo

proliferation of melanocytes, e.g. benign (lentigo), malignant (melanoma)

post-inflammatory disorders of pigmentation, e.g. lichen planus

▲ **Fig. 19.5** *Classification of pigmentary disorders.*

CAUSES OF GENERALIZED HYPERPIGMENTATION

hormonal (Fig. 19.1)

chronic infection, e.g. tuberculosis

neoplasia, especially with cachexia, e.g. carcinoma of the bronchus

lymphoma

vitamin B_{12} deficiency

liver disease especially primary biliary cirrhosis and haemochromatosis

malabsorption and nutritional deficiency

drugs, e.g. chlorpromazine, busulphan, cyclophosphamide, amiodarone, arsenic

▲ **Fig. 19.6** *Causes of generalized hyperpigmentation.*

Melasma (chloasma)
Definition
A patchy increased pigmentation of the face.

> **Diagnostic features**
> - Forehead, cheeks, nose and around the mouth.
> - Patchy hyperpigmentation.
> - Precipitated by pregnancy or oral contraceptives.
> - Worsened by sunlight.
> - Mostly female.

Aetiology
The condition is common. Many women observe it whilst pregnant, and for the majority the condition fades after delivery. Some acquire it whilst taking oral contraceptives but it does not always fade on their cessation. All sufferers find that it is increased with exposure to ultraviolet (UV) light, and in those for whom there is no obvious hormonal explanation it may be the final result of years of sun exposure. It is not confined to women and indeed is common in Mediterranean, Middle Eastern and Asian men but not in Anglo Saxon men. Almost certainly excess ultraviolet irradiation is the most important factor in affected males. MSH levels are quite normal in patients with melasma.

Clinical features
The pigmentation is light brown or darker, depending on recent solar exposure. It is ill-defined and usually symmetrical and patchily distributed on the forehead,

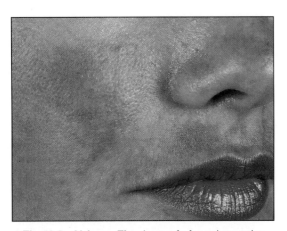

▲ **Fig. 19.7** *Melasma. There is a patchy hyperpigmentation on the cheeks and upper lip. Although it may be precipitated by pregnancy or oral contraceptives, sunlight makes it worse.*

cheeks (Fig. 19.7), over the nose, on the upper lip (often simulating a moustache), chin and neck. The prognosis for recovery varies greatly.

Management
Explanation and solar protection are most important as the condition is impossible to treat at present.

Fair-skinned individuals have the best prognosis and many recover completely after pregnancy or stopping the contraceptive pill. They must however be advised to use a sunscreen on the face in the sun, to ensure that the pigmentation does not return and remain indefinitely.

In darker skinned individuals, the condition can be remarkably persistent. They too should be advised to protect the skin obsessionally with high protection sunscreens which have not only UVB but also UVA protection.

Depigmenting agents, based on 2% hydroquinone (which inhibits the conversion of tyrosine to melanin) and available over the counter in proprietary preparations, are disappointingly ineffective. Dermatologists have advocated preparations containing hydroquinone (2%), retinoic acid (0.05%) in hydrocortisone (1% cream; to counteract the irritant effect of the retinoic acid), but this is not effective either. Higher concentrations of hydroquinone (4–6%) can be tried, but an exogenous ochronosis may occur. Monobenzylether of hydroquinone is quite effective but it has two major disadvantages: it damages melanocytes permanently such that an unacceptable depigmentation may result, and contact sensitization is common.

Ochronosis
Definition
A hyperpigmentation with papules occurring on the face which in localized ochronosis is secondary to the prolonged use of hydroquinone-containing skin-lightening creams, and in generalized ochronosis is inherited.

> **Diagnostic features**
> - Hyperpigmented patches and papules.
> - Cheeks, temples, ears.
> - Dark urine, arthritis (inherited alkaptonuria).
> - Use of hydroquinone skin lighteners (localized ochronosis).

Aetiology
Generalized ochronosis is a rare inborn error of metabolism, occurring as a result of an enzyme deficiency

(homogentisic acid oxidase) which leads to an accumulation of homogentisic acid. As a result a melanin-like pigment is deposited in connective tissues, cartilage and skin. It is inherited as an autosomal recessive, is characterized by dark urine, arthritis and a distinctive cutaneous pigmentation and is known as *alkaptonuria*. It may also occur as an acquired disorder secondary to certain drugs (for example phenol and mepacrine) which inhibit sulphydryl groups in the enzyme.

Localized ochronosis has become commonplace amongst Negroes who use high concentrations (6–8%) of hydroquinone to lighten the skin. A hyperpigmentation occurs on prominent parts of the face. Occasionally ochronosis of the cartilage of the ear occurs.

Clinical features

Pigmented papules are present on a background of hyperpigmentation particularly over bony prominences such as the cheeks (Fig. 19.8) and lateral to the eyes. The skin in between the papules is often quite normal when stretched. In alkaptonuria, skin directly over cartilage (pinna and ribs) and tendons (backs of hands) also becomes pigmented.

Management

A skin biopsy is helpful in the diagnosis because the ochronotic fibres may be demonstrated in the dermis.

Management of both conditions is difficult. The pigmentation of localized ochronosis shows little tendency to fade and patients often revert to using the preparation again. There is no specific treatment for alkaptonuria.

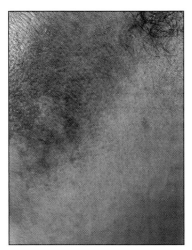

◄**Fig. 19.8**
Localized ochronosis. Localized hyperpigmentation over bony prominences such as the cheeks occurs secondary to the use of skin-lightening creams containing hydroquinone.

POST-INFLAMMATORY HYPERPIGMENTATION

Hyperpigmentation may follow any skin disorder but particularly one which affects the basal cell layer of the epidermis. Thus lichen planus (see Fig. 6.10) and lupus erythematosus are always followed by post-inflammatory hyperpigmentation because the basal cell layer is destroyed and melanin is deposited in the dermis (pigmentary incontinence). Although macrophages ingest the pigment, they may take a long time to clear it, particularly in coloured races. Other diseases such as acne, pityriasis rosea or eczema produce barely any discernible pigmentation in the Caucasian but may produce long-lasting hyperpigmentation in coloured races (see Figs 17.7 & 6.4). The pigmentary changes are quite untreatable, so it is necessary to prevent the inflammation as much as possible, by treating the initial condition.

The identification of the cause of the hyperpigmentation depends upon knowing the history of the preceding condition and observing the configuration and distribution of the pigmentation. For example in a fixed drug eruption (see Fig. 15.36) the condition keeps recurring in the same place. In pityriasis versicolor (see Fig. 12.9) the pigmented macules are found on the trunk.

HYPOPIGMENTATION

Introduction

Generalized hypopigmentation occurs in hypopituitarism but is seldom noticed by the patient. Localized loss of pigmentation is a common complaint. Partial loss is known as hypopigmentation and complete loss as depigmentation, of which vitiligo is the best example.

Vitiligo
Definition
An acquired destruction of melanocytes resulting in white patches on the skin.

> **Diagnostic features**
> - Usually symmetrical.
> - Sharply defined patches.
> - Totally white (depigmented).

Aetiology

The disorder is common (possibly with an incidence of 1%), affects both sexes and in about a third of cases has a family history. All races are affected. It occurs at any age from infancy to old age, but most commonly in the third decade. It is thought to be an autoimmune disorder in that it is associated with known autoimmune conditions such as thyroiditis, diabetes mellitus, pernicious anaemia, alopecia areata and adrenal insufficiency. Antibodies to pigmented human melanocytes have been demonstrated in the blood. As vitiligo sometimes occurs in a segmental distribution, it is possible that a neurochemical mediator which destroys melanocytes is responsible. Chemicals may be implicated since it is known that those used in the rubber industry, such as monobenzylether of hydroquinone, can cause depigmentation in factory workers. Pathologically there is an absence of melanocytes and melanin in the epidermis.

Clinical features

The patches are usually completely depigmented and appear totally white (Fig. 19.9). There is no other cutaneous change. They are well-defined and may have a hyperpigmented margin. They have convex borders which are oval or round and of varying sizes. They are usually symmetrical but occasionally segmental. They occur particularly on the face (Fig. 19.10), in the axillae and groins, around the areolae and orifices, and on the genitalia, backs of the hands, feet, elbows, knees and ankles. Hair growing within vitiliginous patches may appear white (Fig. 19.10). Universal involvement may occasionally occur. Lesions are usually asymptomatic but some patients note a premonitory itch. The patches are liable to sunburn but surprisingly are not particularly liable to malignant change. Vitiligo is barely perceptible in the fair-skinned in winter, but tanning of surrounding normal skin heightens its contrast with vitiligo and may reveal it for the first time. The condition may be precipitated by trauma (Koebner phenomenon).

Spontaneous repigmentation occurs tantalizingly in a minority, particularly around the hair follicle orifices, but rarely with satisfactory total repigmentation.

Management

The disorder may be devastating in coloured races. The condition is so noticeable that the patient may be socially ostracized and have no marriage prospects. It is extremely difficult to treat; the prognosis is given in Figure 19.11. Management consists of:

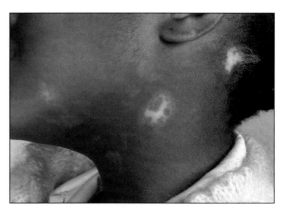

▲**Fig. 19.10** *Vitiligo. Repigmentation sometimes occurs on the face in coloured individuals. Hair affected by vitiligo grows out white.*

PROGNOSIS FOR VITILIGO	
Fair	face, neck, chest, upper arm and legs
	coloured races
Bad	widespread
	mucosae, fingers, toes, palms (Lip Tip syndrome)
	Caucasians

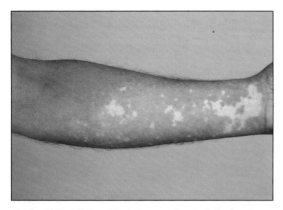

▲**Fig. 19.9** *Vitiligo. The lesions are sharply defined and totally white. They are usually symmetrical and are much more obvious in a coloured or tanned skin.*

▲**Fig. 19.11** *Prognosis for vitiligo.*

(1) Photoprotection. High protection factor sun-screens which block UVB and UVA are mandatory to prevent contrasting tanning of the surrounding normal skin and burning of the affected skin. They should be applied every day and sun exposure strictly avoided.
(2) Topical glucocorticosteroids. Very potent topical steroids are indicated for those areas which potentially may recover, such as the face. However, they must be adequately supervised and risk of facial steroid side-effects explained (although these are unusual if the ointment is applied accurately to the areas of vitiligo).
(3) Camouflage. Camouflage with sunscreen-containing make-up (Covermark, Keromask) is helpful, especially if the guidance of a camouflage instructor is available. Dihydroxyacetone may be used to stain the vitiligo a more acceptable colour.
(4) Psoralens. Photochemotherapy (PUVA) using psoralens topically or systemically has been tried, although phototoxicity (burning and blistering) is common with the former. Treatment is extremely prolonged, requiring anywhere between 100 and 300 treatments. Those in whom disease affects the face and neck have a 50% chance of repigmenting (increasing to 80% with over 200 treatments), although for general vitiligo (excluding mucosal or fingers) there is only a 28% chance (increasing to 80% with over 200 treatments). These figures come from North America and not all centres have been so fortunate.

In the Middle East and India, patients are instruct-ed to take the 8-methoxypsoralen or trimethylpsoralen 2 hours before exposure to the midday sun. The patient exposes the affected skin for increasing periods each day. Treatment has to be continued for months and often years.
(5) Monobenzylether of hydroquinone. This treat-ment is rarely used. It causes permanent loss of pigment and should be used only for depigmenting residual normal skin in patients with near universal vitiligo. It is hazardous because contact and irritant dermatitis may occur in addition to unwanted pig-mentary effects.

POST-INFLAMMATORY HYPOPIGMENTATION

The concept of loss of pigmentation secondary to inflammation is similar to that of hyperpigmentation. The history and distribution of the problem aids diagnosis. The loss of pigmentation is incomplete and therefore an off-white colour is seen, unlike the chalk white colour seen in vitiligo. The common causes of post-inflammatory hypopigmentation are:
(1) Pityriasis alba (see below).
(2) Pityriasis versicolor (see Fig. 12.11).
(3) Hypopigmented eczema (see Fig. 3.29).
(4) Leprosy.
(5) Sarcoidosis.

Pityriasis alba
Definition
Patches of hypopigmentation limited to the face of coloured children or adolescents.

> **Diagnostic features**
> * Patches.
> * Hypopigmentation.
> * Cheeks.
> * Children and adolescents.
> * Coloured races.

Aetiology
The condition is common but the cause is unknown. It is thought to be post-inflammatory in origin, pos-sibly due to a preceding eczema but this is never visible, and the children are not atopic and the condition does not respond to topical steroids.

Clinical features
The lesions are quite flat with no surface changes of inflammation or scaling. There are patches of hypo-pigmentation limited to the face and especially the cheeks (Fig. 19.12). It is confined to coloured races.

Management
There is no effective treatment but the disorder clears after a number of years.

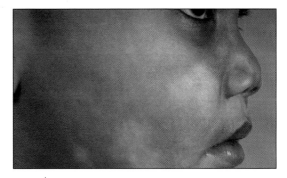

▲**Fig. 19.12** *Pityriasis alba. A patchy hypopigmentation on the cheeks is common in coloured children and adolescents. Although thought to be secondary to eczema, this is rarely observed. It eventually recovers.*

INTRODUCTION

Hair structure

Hair is composed of keratin, which is a protein made by mitotically active cells at the base of the hair follicle. The follicle is an invagination of the epidermis and the bulb at its base encloses a highly vascular area of dermis. Any influence that interferes with mitosis or compromises the blood supply will affect the hair.

The hair shaft consists of several layers. The principle one is the cortex, which in terminal hair has a central medulla. Surrounding the cortex is a cuticle and an outer and inner root sheath. Since the hair is keratinous, it may be invaded by fungi. Structural abnormalities, either genetically determined or induced by trauma, may occur and result in increased fragility of the hair shaft and shortened hair; most are too uncommon to be discussed here.

Hair types

(1) **Lanugo hair.** This is present *in utero* and is shed during the eighth month, so it will therefore only be visible in premature babies. It is soft, fine, unmedullated and usually unpigmented.

(2) **Vellous hair.** This is the fine, downy hair which covers the entire cutaneous surface other than the palms, soles and parts of the genitalia. It is capable of being transformed into terminal hair by androgens.

(3) **Terminal hair.** This is the usual, medullated hair of the scalp, eyebrows and eyelashes which is thicker and more pigmented than vellous hair. At puberty it develops in the axillae and pubic area of both sexes and also in the beard area and body in the male. It may also occur in these latter areas in the female, when it constitutes a problem known as *hirsutism* (Fig. 20.1), which may or may not be part of a more general problem known as *virilism*. *Hypertrichosis*, on the other hand, is a term used to describe growth of terminal hair in an area which is not normally hairy, for example on the forehead in porphyria.

Hair colour

Hair colour is dependent on which type of melanin is formed. Thus eumelanin is present in brown or black hair, and phaeomelanin (a product of dopaquinone and cysteine) in blonde or red hair (Fig. 19.4). As the amount of melanin in the hair shaft decreases with age, greying (*canities*) occurs. This may occur prematurely and is an inherited predisposition. Greying also occurs in pernicious anaemia and thyroiditis. In

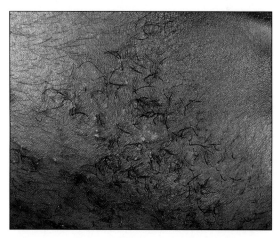

▲ **Fig. 20.1** *Hirsutism. Hirsutism is growth of coarse terminal hairs in sites normally reserved for males. It is frequently a racial characteristic but occasionally is a sign of virilism.*

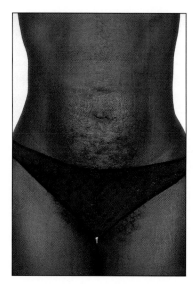

◄ **Fig. 20.2**
Male escutcheon in a female. The upper triangle of pubic hair growth towards the umbilicus is under the influence of testosterone only and is therefore absent in normal females.

certain forms of albinism and phenylketonuria the hair is white or blonde. In copper deficiency, as in *Menkes' kinky hair syndrome*, the hair colour is light because copper is required by tyrosinase for the production of melanin. Severe protein malnutrition and iron deficiency also lighten hair.

Hormonal influences on hair growth

Secondary sexual hair growth results from the change of vellous to terminal hair. This is under the direct control of androgens at puberty. Pubic and axillary hairs develop first, followed by facial and body hair.

PHYSICAL SIGNS OF VIRILISM
thickened coarse skin
enlarged pores and oiliness
acne
temporal recession and male pattern thinning
hirsutism
masculinized genitalia
clitoromegaly in females
hypertrophy of the penis and increased folding of
scrotal skin in boys
hyperpigmentation of sexual zones in children
male musculature
accelerated growth of long bones
premature closure of epiphyses
loss of subcutaneous fat around shoulders and girdle
deepening of the voice
oligo- or amenorrhoea
infertility

▲ **Fig. 20.3** *Physical signs of virilism.*

CAUSES OF HIRSUTISM	
increased production of ovarian androgens	polycystic ovaries ovarian tumours
increased production of adrenal androgens	adrenal tumour or hyperplasia hyperpituitarism
defects in steroid metabolism	adrenogenital syndrome
ovarian failure	post-menopausal post-oophorectomy
androgenic drugs	testosterone danazol systemic steroids

▲ **Fig. 20.4** *Causes of hirsutism.*

Androgens are secreted as testosterone by the Leydig cells of the testis in the male and as weak androgenic steroids, androstenedione and dehydroxyepiandrosterone, by the ovaries in females and by the adrenals in both sexes. Pubic and axillary hair are extremely sensitive to these androgens and are maximally developed in both sexes. The upper triangle of pubic hair which grows towards the umbilicus is under the control of testosterone alone, which explains why males have hair in this area and females do not. It is known as the male escutcheon (Fig. 20.2). The lower triangle of pubic hair is under the control of both adrenal and testicular androgens.

Testosterone is a powerful androgen and, after the completion of puberty, males are maximally virilized by it so that no further hair growth can occur in the male, even in the presence of an adrenal tumour secreting androgen. Thus virilization is a term which is only applicable to a prepubertal child or a female; its signs are given in Figure 20.3, and its causes in Figure 20.4, but further discussion of it is without the scope of this book.

Hormonal causes of decreased hair growth include adrenal failure and hypopituitarism (Fig. 20.5). The former is more evident in females than males because in males testicular androgen metabolism is not impaired. In hypopituitarism, axillary hair growth diminishes first, followed by pubic hair growth and then beard growth, resulting in decreased shaving in males. There may be generalized thinning of scalp hair. The skin is also thin and fine, with decreased sebum, sweat and pigment production.

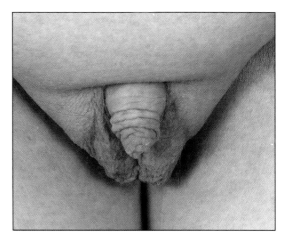

▲ **Fig. 20.5** *Hypopituitarism. Hypopituitarism results in adrenal and testicular failure so that secondary sexual hair growth fails.*

CONSTITUTIONAL HIRSUTISM

Definition
The growth of terminal hair on areas of the body on which it is not wanted by the patient, usually female.

> **Diagnostic features**
> - Excess undesired terminal hair.
> - No gross endocrine abnormalities.
> - Females.

Aetiology
Once known causes of hirsutism and virilism have been excluded, the vast majority of patients are labelled as having constitutional hirsutism. This is largely racial, being rare in the Japanese and Chinese and much more common in Mediterranean, Middle Eastern, Indian and Negro races — although it is fair to say that most women develop some degree of hirsutism as they grow older, particularly after the menopause once the protective influence of oestrogens has been reduced. Racial hirsutism may be accepted as normal in the patient's own country but Western culture decrees that it is unnatural and the patient regards it as unacceptable. The growth of the hair is thought to be due to increased sensitivity of the hair follicle to dihydrotestosterone produced from testosterone by 5-alpha-reductase; a similar explanation as is provided for acne and male pattern alopecia. Circulating levels of testosterone are usually normal (albeit sometimes at the higher end of the range) or alternatively sex hormone binding globulin levels are low so that free serum androgen levels are raised even though total levels are normal. Although males may be hirsute, and often bald as well, this is not considered a disease because it is socially acceptable.

Clinical features
The disorder is the growth of terminal hairs on the upper lip especially at the edges, producing a moustache, the chin and sideburns, down the cheeks, around the areolae of the breasts, sternum, limbs and lower abdomen producing a male escutcheon.

Management
The patient requires investigation if there is any clinical suspicion of virilism (Fig. 20.3) which may lead to elucidation of the cause. The basic tests are listed in Figure 20.6.

Management is highly unsatisfactory, and this exacerbates the psychological distress to the patient.

The traditional methods are:

(1) Plucking. This is satisfactory for minimal involvement.

(2) Shaving. This is highly unsatisfactory and completely unacceptable to many patients, being final proof, to them, that they are not female.

(3) Electrolysis. This is very satisfactory for limited disease. A fine wire is passed down the hair follicle and the bulb is cauterized and destroyed. It must be performed skilfully, otherwise scarring occurs. It is time-consuming and expensive but in skilled hands is permanent.

(4) Bleaching. Hydrogen peroxide, 10–20 vol. plus enough ammonia to turn litmus paper blue, is used to bleach melanin and also alter keratin. There are various proprietary preparations.

(5) Depilatories. These consist of strontium or barium sulphide 20% in a suitable vehicle or thioglycollic acid. They are widely available commercially.

(6) Waxing. This is very commonly used especially for the legs.

(7) Anti-androgens. These remain the hope for the future. Unfortunately, they are not effective topically at this time, but oral cyproterone acetate is a useful treatment. It is available in the UK as 2mg combined with $30\mu g$ of ethinyloestradiol (Dianette), and thus has a contraceptive as well as a therapeutic effect. Usually larger doses are required and it is reasonable to prescribe 50–100mg of cyproterone acetate on days 5–15 of the cycle, in addition to the Dianette. The effect is not seen for 6 or 9 months, but there is some benefit in some patients. The drawbacks are that the condition returns on cessation of treatment and the long-term hazards of the cyproterone acetate are not known.

BASIC TESTS TO INVESTIGATE HIRSUTISM

full blood count
plasma testosterone
plasma cortisol at 9 a.m. and midnight
24-hour urinary 17-hydroxy- and ketocorticosteroids
dehydroepiandrosterone sulphate levels
prolactin levels
luteinizing hormone/follicle stimulating hormone
    levels (LH/FSH)
ovarian scan
X-rays of the pituitary fossa

▲**Fig. 20.6** *Basic tests which should be used in investigating hirsutism.*

TELOGEN AND ANAGEN EFFLUVIUM

Introduction: the hair cycle

Human hair grows in an asynchronous manner, unlike animal hair which falls out synchronously in the form of a moult. 'Moulting' only occurs in humans as part of a pathological state. There are three phases of hair growth. *Anagen* is the active and longest phase, lasting up to 4 or 5 years, which explains why hair will only grow to a certain length, usually to the waist or buttocks, but not down to the ground. The majority of the hair is in anagen at any one time. Following anagen, cell division ceases in the hair bulb and involution (*catagen*) occurs. The hair follicle regresses and the hair shaft becomes shortened and club shaped. Catagen lasts a few weeks and is followed by *telogen* during which hair is shed for about 3 months. The hair cell cycle is one of the most active in the body and is very susceptible to external influences. Three recognizable clinical states occur.

Anagen effluvium
Definition
Acute, diffuse loss of scalp hair.

Diagnostic features
- Sudden onset.
- Diffuse loss of hair.
- Obvious immediate cause, usually a drug.

Aetiology
Drugs used in cancer chemotherapy are now probably the most common causes of acute hair loss that results from mitotic arrest of the cells of the hair bulb. The hair falls out within a few days. Other agents are listed in Figure 20.7. X-Rays used to be used therapeutically to induce epilation of hairs infected with ringworm, until this became unnecessary with the advent of griseofulvin.

Clinical features
The hair fall is acute and often extreme necessitating the wearing of a wig.

Management
The patient will recover but clearly requires to be forewarned of the occurrence.

Telogen effluvium
Definition
An acute, diffuse hair loss occurring 3–4 months after a medical event.

Diagnostic features
- Sudden onset.
- Diffuse loss of hair.
- Medical event 3 months previously.

Aetiology
Surgical shock, haemorrhage (including occasionally blood donation), high fever, crash dieting and psychological illness are common causes of hair loss. Women notice the complaint much more frequently than men. During the illness, anagen hairs are prematurely precipitated into catagen. Nothing untoward happens during this time, but as the hairs reach the telogen phase, new anagen hairs develop and displace the telogen hairs, causing them to fall abruptly and alarmingly.

DRUGS THAT MAY CAUSE ACUTE HAIR LOSS
cytotoxics especially cyclophosphamide
anticoagulants
thyroid antagonists
excess vitamin A and other retinoids
thallium salts
X-rays

▲ **Fig. 20.7** *Drugs that may cause acute hair loss.*

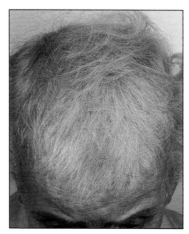

◄ **Fig. 20.8** *Telogen effluvium. Anagen hair may be prematurely precipitated into a resting phase (catagen) during an illness. Some weeks later the telogen phase begins and hair is shed quite profusely for about 3 months.*

A similar occurrence may occur after childbirth, particularly if it is a complicated birth. The explanation in this case is slightly different. During pregnancy hair grows luxuriantly because anagen hairs which should have passed into the catagen phase during this time do not do so and continue to grow until after parturition. Then all the hairs which should have gone into catagen during pregnancy do so, and 3 months later fall out precipitously in a similar manner to that described above.

A number of drugs are recorded as causing telogen effluvium, in particular thyroid antagonists (thiouracil or carbimazole), anticoagulants (heparin and coumarins), and hypervitaminosis A.

Clinical features
The patient does not associate her hair loss with the illness because of the time interval. The hair loss is often profuse (Fig. 20.8). The patient notices that it comes out 'in handfuls', especially after being brushed or washed, and that the pillow case is covered in hairs in the morning. On examination, hairs can easily be removed and the scalp is clearly visible. The nails may also be affected and horizontal Beau's lines (Fig. 18.14) may be found.

Management
The patient can be reassured that recovery will take place spontaneously within 3–4 months.

DIFFUSE HAIR LOSS

Introduction
Diffuse insidious loss of hair is a common complaint, particularly in females. The commonest cause is

CAUSES OF DIFFUSE HAIR LOSS
malnutrition: marasmus and kwashiorkor, malabsorption, iron deficiency, zinc deficiency, prolonged inadequate parenteral nutrition endocrine: myxoedema, hyperthyroidism, hypopituitarism, hypoparathyroidism syphilis lupus erythematosus drugs male pattern alopecia

▲**Fig. 20.9** *Causes of diffuse hair loss.*

androgenetic alopecia. Occasionally the hair loss is due to an associated illness and the main causes are listed in Figure 20.9.

Male pattern alopecia (androgenetic alopecia)
Definition
Loss of hair to a varying degree with retention of parietal and occipital hair, usually genetically inherited.

Diagnostic features
- Uniform symmetrical thinning or total loss of hair.
- Frontal and temporal regions.
- Crown of head.
- Normal parietal and occipital hair.
- Autosomal dominance.

Aetiology
The disorder is very common in males but also occurs in females, although to a lesser degree because of the protective influence of oestrogens. The propensity is inherited, and there is frequently a family history of hair loss or baldness. Similar abnormalities of androgen metabolism to those found in hirsutism occur. Males castrated prior to puberty never go bald, even in the presence of a strong family history.

Clinical features
Pubertal male fronto-temporal recession is normal, but this may be followed by frontal thinning (type I), some loss on the crown (type II) and various degrees of hair loss thereafter, leading to total baldness apart from the sides and back of the scalp. Eighty per cent of males will have developed at least type I baldness by the seventh decade. Some 15% eventually go completely bald and 1–2% are completely bald by the age of 30.

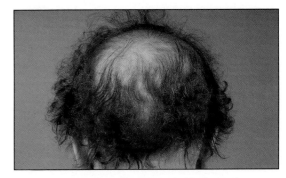

▲**Fig. 20.10** *Male pattern (androgenetic) alopecia in a female. This is inherited and becomes more evident after the menopause as the protective effects of oestrogens fail.*

In females the picture is less obvious and less rapid in progress. The hair is fine and the loss is diffuse across the vertex (Fig. 20.10). Twenty-five per cent of women have type I loss by the age of 40, the condition being much more common than generally appreciated.

Management

All men know that there is no treatment for baldness but this does not stop them from seeking it. Women regard thinning of the hair as quite abnormal and do not appreciate the rôle of heredity. Treatment in women is unsatisfactory, but at least hormonal therapy with cyproterone acetate may be considered. Wigs are only popular with some patients as are hair transplants, although the latter are commonplace in the US. Plugs of hair taken from the occipital and parietal areas are used to replace the bald areas but the technique requires expertise and patience. The hairs fall out some weeks later but then regrow, although it may be 2–3 years before the hair begins to look 'normal'.

HAIR LOSS WITHOUT PHYSICAL SIGNS

Definition

A complaint of diffuse hair loss without any objective evidence for it.

Aetiology

The complaint is usually psychosomatic and indicative of depression since there is nothing abnormal to find on examination.

Clinical features

The patient is always female and complains of considerable loss of hair, such that she finds it on her pillow or on her comb. Examination usually reveals a magnificent head of hair and the physician can find nothing wrong. It is particularly common in young women from Middle Eastern countries where abundant hair is particularly desirable.

Management

Reassurance may be all that is required and the patient may be told that the hair is falling out but is being replaced at the same rate, so that all is in balance and no permanent alopecia will occur. Often, however, there is an underlying depression.

SKIN DISORDERS AFFECTING THE HAIR AND SCALP

Introduction

Tinea, psoriasis, dandruff and seborrhoeic eczema have been dealt with elsewhere. Other disorders are described here.

Alopecia areata
Definition

A loss of hair with no appreciable abnormality of the underlying skin, ranging in severity from localized patches to universal involvement. Spontaneous recovery occurs in uncomplicated cases.

Diagnostic features
- Alopecia.
- Single or more round patches.
- Occasionally extensive or universal.
- No abnormality visible on the skin.

Aetiology

The disorder is common and affects both sexes equally. It is currently believed to be an autoimmune disorder because many patients have a personal or family history of other autoimmune disorders, such as Hashimoto's thyroiditis and diabetes mellitus, as well as organ-specific antibodies. Vitiligo is associated with 4% of cases and there is a positive family history of alopecia in 10% of cases of vitiligo. Histologically there is a lymphocytic infiltrate around the hair follicles which supports the autoimmune theory but, unlike other autoimmune disorders, there is no permanent destruction of the target organ and the hair may regrow. The condition is much more common in Down's Syndrome (6% incidence at any one time) and a majority of these cases have alopecia universalis. A number of patients have associated atopic eczema and this is associated with a poor prognosis.

Clinical features

The condition is most common before the age of 40 but can occur at any time. There are a wide range of patterns associated with it so that although a single patch of hair loss is most usual there may be several patches, or indeed the whole scalp (*totalis*) or body (*universalis*) may be involved. The eyelashes, eyebrows and beard area (Fig. 2.2) may be involved separately or in combination with scalp hair loss.

Similarly, the secondary sexual hairs may be involved. Whichever area is affected, there is a round patch of complete hair loss with no visible change in the skin (Fig. 20.11).

The majority of patients recover without any treatment within 9 months, especially those who have one or two patches and have never been afflicted before, but a number of other factors must be considered. Features of a poor, guarded prognosis are:

- Several patches.
- Ophthiasis (occipital hair loss).
- Loss of eyebrows and eyelashes.
- Early onset.
- Alopecia totalis/universalis.
- Associated atopic disease.
- Previous attack.

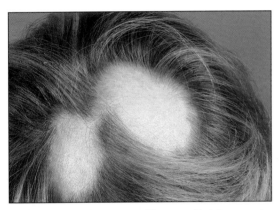

▲ **Fig. 20.11** *Alopecia areata. The areas of hair loss are quite round with no scalp abnormality. The recovering hair is depigmented initially.*

The onset of the disease in childhood causes the most concern. The patches may recover, but recurrent attacks and alopecia totalis or even universalis are a common outcome. Widespread involvement (Fig. 20.12) is also serious prognostically, with only a third or less of those with alopecia universalis recovering. The distribution is important: ophthiasis is always associated with a poor prognosis.

The features to be assessed in determining recovery are the presence or absence of exclamation mark hairs and the type of regrowth. Exclamation mark hairs are a few millimetres long. The stump appears normal but the proximal portion nearest the scalp is thin and depigmented. Exclamation mark hairs indicate continued activity of the disease and that the hair loss may deteriorate. As patients recover, fine white hairs appear and subsequently these become pigmented and return to their normal colour. The nails are involved in the minority of cases: pits, often found in longitudinal lines (Fig. 20.13), which are slightly larger than those seen in psoriasis occur.

Occasionally a patient complains that he has gone 'white overnight' (Figs 20.14 & 20.15). This occurs in an adult who normally has a mixture of white and black hairs: the black hairs are preferentially shed and the white hairs remain, producing this somewhat startling effect.

Management

If the alopecia is minimal, reassurance that it will regrow may be all that is necessary. The results of specific treatment are always difficult to assess because the majority of cases resolve spontaneously, but they include:

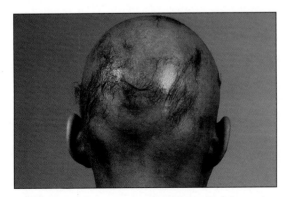

▲ **Fig. 20.12** *Alopecia areata. The degrees of hair loss varies. Occipital hair loss (ophthiasis), total scalp hair loss (totalis) and total body hair loss (universalis) are associated with a poor prognosis.*

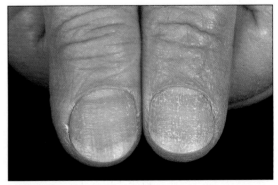

▲ **Fig. 20.13** *Nail pitting in alopecia areata. In alopecia areata the pitting occurs in a linear arrangement.*

(1) Steroids. The standard treatment is topical steroids or intralesional triamcinolone. Systemic steroids are effective and have been used for alopecia universalis, but the hair usually falls out at the cessation of treatment and the risks involved in therapy are unacceptable. Intralesional steroids certainly produce a rather convincing picture of hairs growing in the site of the injections but subcutaneous atrophy is a potential side-effect, particularly in the beard area (Fig. 2.8) where they should be avoided. Topical potent glucocorticosteroids applied each night for 3 months are probably the treatment of choice if any treatment is indicated.

(2) Irritants and sensitizers. Dithranol (Anthralin), which is the standard treatment for psoriasis, is a potent irritant of the skin, and some success has been claimed for applications of this drug to areas of alopecia. Dinitrochlorobenzene (DNCB) is a potent contact allergen, producing a contact dermatitis after the patient has been primed. The dermatitis is unpleasant, being acute and weeping, often with regional lymphadenopathy. Primin (which is the sensitizer in primula obconica) and poison ivy, which is the commonest cause of plant dermatitis in North America, have been tried. Diphencyprone is presently enjoying a vogue, since DNCB is considered to be a potential carcinogen to the skin. All these remedies are unpleasant and should probably only be used by a dermatologist. The results of these therapies vary.

(3) Ultraviolet light. Irradiation with ultraviolet B (UVB) in order to cause erythema is a time-honoured treatment. In recent times, psoralens and UV (PUVA) have been used in extreme cases with variable results.

Pityriasis amantacea
Definition
A distinctive morphological entity of thick scales attached to the hair shaft, sometimes secondary to seborrhoeic dermatitis or psoriasis.

Diagnostic features
- Thick scales attached to the lower hair shaft.
- Does not respond to topical steroids.
- Must be treated with tar-containing preparations.
- Hair will fall out but always regrows.

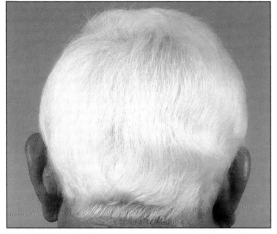

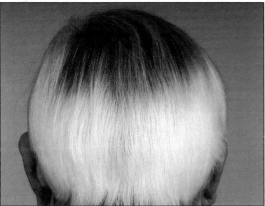

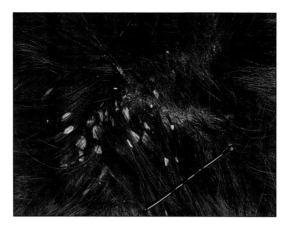

▲ **Figs 20.14 & 20.15** *Alopecia areata. A patient may 'go white overnight'. This is due to retention of his white hairs and preferential loss of pigmented hairs, which may be visible as the patient recovers (Fig. 20.15).*

▲**Fig. 20.16** *Pityriasis amantacea. Thick scales are attached to the lowest parts of the hair shaft, rather like tiles overlapping on a roof.*

Aetiology

The condition is common in children and young adults. The cause is quite unknown but in some cases the condition is a manifestation of psoriasis or seborrhoeic eczema.

Clinical features

There is a considerable build-up on the scalp of scales which appear to be attached to the lower part of the hair shaft, rather like tiles overlapping on a roof (Fig. 20.16). There may be evidence of psoriasis or seborrhoeic dermatitis elsewhere on the body, but usually there is none. For many patients it is a single episode which does not recur, but in those in which it does an underlying psoriasis or seborrhoeic dermatitis should be suspected.

Management

The condition does not respond to topical steroids and has to be treated with tar-containing remedies such as ung. cocois co. The latter is very effective, but the patient must be warned that many of the affected hairs will fall out; however, this hair loss is temporary and replacement occurs.

Trichotillomania
Definition

A rather fanciful name to describe a condition of self-induced hair loss.

Diagnostic features
- Asymmetrical hair loss.
- Side affected corresponds to dominant hand.
- Broken hairs of unequal length.
- Scalp is normal.

Aetiology

This is a disorder primarily of children. It does not usually represent any deep emotional trauma but is a habit tic rather like nail-biting. It results from the child fiddling, twisting and pulling at the hairs, causing them to fall out or break off. It tends to be a temporary behaviour pattern. It does occur, though less commonly, in adults when a varying degree of depression and unhappiness is usually present, or psychosis, in which case the prognosis is poor.

Clinical features

There are one or more asymmetrical patches of hair loss. The hairs are broken off at various lengths above the surface, without any inflammatory changes in the scalp (Fig. 20.17).

Management

Once it is recognized that the condition is self-induced, it is necessary to assess the degree of emotional disturbance and treat accordingly.

Traction alopecia
Definition

A localized hair loss usually secondary to an unsuitable method of hair styling.

Diagnostic features
- Patchy hair loss.
- Fractured hairs.
- No scalp abnormality.
- Female.
- Plaits or ponytail.

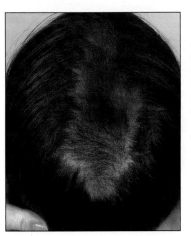

◀ **Fig. 20.17**
Trichotillomania. Asymmetrical loss of hair secondary to pulling and twisting is a common temporary habit in children. The broken hairs are of uneven lengths.

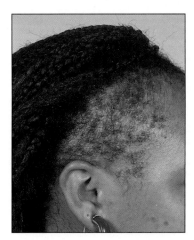

◀ **Fig. 20.18**
Traction alopecia. This patient has frontal marginal alopecia secondary to her hair being pulled back too tightly, which causes undue traction on the hair follicles.

Aetiology

Any manner of trauma may damage the hair. The infant rubbing the occiput on the cot can cause temporary damage. Over-zealous massage of the scalp, permanent waves or straightening hair with hot combs may damage the hair. The frontal marginal alopecia (Fig. 20.18) caused by the hair being pulled back too tightly in a ponytail over a long period of time is fairly obvious. Negroes frequently plait their hair; if this is done incorrectly and too much traction is exerted on the hair and its follicle, the hair becomes thin, barely attached and eventually breaks away.

Clinical features

The patient, usually female and frequently a child, often presents with a patchy hair loss. The style causing it may have been abandoned because the cause of the problem was suspected, but surprisingly it may not even then be accepted as the correct diagnosis.

Management

The cause needs to be carefully explained, but in a number of cases the condition is recognized too late or the patient may be unwilling to abandon this traditional style and regrettably the hair loss is often permanent.

Scarring alopecia (cicatricial alopecia)
Definition

A permanent loss of hair on the scalp secondary to a disorder which results in destruction of the hair follicle.

Diagnostic features
- Hair loss.
- Tethered, smooth, shiny, atrophic and scarred skin.
- Scalp.
- Other manifestations of underlying cause.

Aetiology

Any disorder which causes destruction and scarring of the hair follicle may result in a permanent loss of hair. Commoner causes include discoid lupus erythematosus, lichen planus, favus (a fungal disorder of the scalp which is rare in this country but common in the Middle East) and X-irradiation of the scalp for ringworm in the past. The term *pseudopelade* is given to the condition when the aetiology is unknown.

Clinical features

The hairless skin on the scalp becomes tethered to the underlying subcutaneous tissue, so that it is not possible to pick it up and pinch the skin. The most common cause of scarring alopecia in the West is discoid lupus erythematosus (Fig. 20.19).

Management

Once scarring has occurred there is no more that can be done as far as treatment is concerned. If the diagnosis is made early in the inflammatory stage of treatable conditions such as lichen planus, discoid lupus erythematosus or favus, the scarring may be prevented by the appropriate therapy.

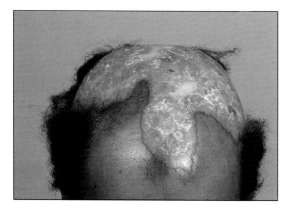

▲ **Fig. 20.19** *Scarring alopecia. Discoid lupus erythematosus may result in well-defined red patches with tenacious scales surrounded by hyperpigmentation and permanent scarring and hair loss.*

21 BLISTERING DISORDERS OF THE SKIN

INTRODUCTION

Blisters are a common cutaneous physical sign and are usually due to benign causes such as insect bites (Fig. 13.4) or a burn (Fig. 21.1). Impetigo (Fig. 10.1) starts as a blister and confusion has been caused by calling impetigo in the new-born 'pemphigus neonatorum', but as this has absolutely nothing whatsoever to do with primary blistering diseases such as pemphigus the term should be abandoned. Erythema multiforme can sometimes be bullous in appearance (Fig. 15.8) and formerly was confused clinically with bullous pemphigoid. The whole subject has however been clarified by the technique of immunofluorescence such that the disorders described in this chapter are characterized by the abnormal deposition of antibodies between the epithelial cells (pemphigus), at the basement membrane (pemphigoid) or in the dermal papillae (dermatitis herpetiformis). These disorders are admittedly rare, so they are only discussed briefly, but they do represent an area of intense immunological research and may be serious if not diagnosed and treated.

BULLOUS PEMPHIGOID

Definition
A serious condition of spontaneous blistering characterized by itchy tense blisters due to an autoimmune process affecting the dermo-epidermal junction.

Diagnostic features
- Usually itchy.
- Elderly.
- Tense blisters, with erythema.
- Symmetrical.
- On the limbs and trunk.

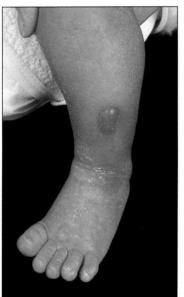

◀**Fig. 21.1** *Burn. Blisters are a common physical sign and are more likely to be due to insect bites, impetigo or, in this case, to a cup of tea which the infant has upset over his leg.*

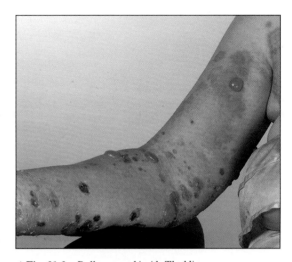

▲**Fig. 21.2** *Bullous pemphigoid. The blisters occur spontaneously in a widespread manner first on the limbs and subsequently on the trunk.*

Aetiology

The condition is relatively common in the elderly, affecting both sexes equally and all races. It is considered to be an autoimmune process as it is often seen in patients suffering from other such disorders, for example myasthenia gravis, pernicious anaemia, rheumatoid arthritis, systemic lupus erythematosus and Hashimoto's thyroiditis. More specifically, circulating IgG antibodies to the basement membrane zone of the dermo-epidermal junction have been demonstrated in the sera by indirect immunofluorescence. A clear green band of fluorescence is visible as a result of the interaction of the labelled antibody with the antigenic lamina lucida of the basement membrane. Complement (C3) deposition is also present. It has been suggested that bullous pemphigoid may be a manifestation of co-existent malignant disease, but it is more probable that elderly patients are simply more likely to develop malignant disease.

Clinical features

The condition is usually intensely itchy and the patient presents with blisters which are symmetrical in distribution, often beginning on the inner thighs, then spreading down the legs and involving the arms (Fig. 21.2) and ultimately the trunk. These blisters are full of clear fluid initially and are tense (Fig. 1.12) and are quite firm to feel. They start as tiny vesicles (Fig. 21.3) but rapidly enlarge and coalesce to form bullae. They are usually but not always surrounded by erythema. The blisters eventually become haemorrhagic and break leaving behind denuded, eroded skin often covered with scabs. The lesions may become secondarily infected and the clear blister fluid becomes purulent and yellow crusts form. With prompt treatment the lesions heal without scarring. Occasionally, in the early stages of the disease, no frank blisters are seen and the lesions are of a more urticarial nature but are much more persistent than ordinary urticaria. Ultimately frank blisters appear.

An identical clinical and pathological eruption occurs extremely rarely in pregnancy, commencing in the second trimester and recurring with successive pregnancies and occasionally with each period. It has previously been known as herpes gestationis but is better termed *pemphigoid gestationis*. Generally mucous membranes are not involved in straightforward bullous pemphigoid, but are involved in a rare variant known as *benign mucous membrane pemphigoid*.

Diagnosis

It is essential that a skin biopsy is taken for routine histopathology and more particularly for immunofluorescence to confirm the diagnosis (Fig. 21.4). The pathology shows that the entire epidermis makes up the roof of the blister which explains why the intact vesicles or blisters are so firm and do not break easily. There are usually many eosinophils within the blisters and surrounding the dermal blood vessels. The blister is subepidermal in location.

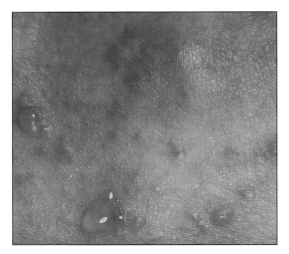

▲ **Fig. 21.3** *Bullous pemphigoid. The blisters are firm, tense and itchy. They gradually become haemorrhagic and break after a few days to form erosions and scabs.*

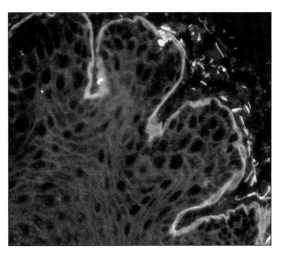

▲ **Fig. 21.4** *Bullous pemphigoid: immunofluorescence. IgG antibodies and complement (C3) may be demonstrated as a green band of fluorescence at the basement membrane which separates the epidermis from the dermis.*

The techniques of direct and indirect immuno-fluorescence are illustrated in Figure 21.5. They involve the raising of antibodies to human immuno-globulin by injecting it into an animal. These antibodies are labelled with a fluorescein marker which can then be incubated either with the patient's skin (direct immunofluorescence) or with the patient's serum and a foreign substrate, such as monkey oesophagus (indirect immunofluorescence). In the direct test, if antibody is present in the skin, it will be recognized by the fluorescein-labelled antibody which will be deposited as a pale green fluorescence. In the indirect test, if antibodies are present in the serum, the anti-human antibody will label them with fluorescein and be deposited at their target site on the foreign substrate, which will fluoresce.

Management

The condition is more benign than pemphigus. However the patients are elderly and are at risk from infection of the skin, urinary tract and lungs and from secondary septicaemia. Infection must be diagnosed, investigated and treated promptly. Patients feel generally unwell and often take to their beds and they may develop deep venous thrombosis and pulmonary embolism. The disease may compromise coexisting disorders, especially once the patient has been started on systemic steroids, which are the treatment of choice, often coupled with other immunosuppressive therapy, in particular azathioprine.

Most patients require 40mg of prednisolone daily to gain control. This is best commenced in hospital. The steroid dosage may be reduced once the blistering process has stopped (this usually takes 10 days) by 5mg every fifth day, although maintenance is required often for several months at a dose of 12.5mg daily. Once the patient has been maintained free of disease for 3 months it is reasonable to reduce to 10mg daily and then by 1mg each week provided no fresh blisters occur. Azathioprine starting at 50mg daily and then increasing up to 2mg/kg is thought to have a steroid-sparing effect.

Potent topical steroids are usually of limited value in this disease although in the rare localized variants of bullous pemphigoid they are the treatment of choice. The old-fashioned remedy of potassium permanganate added to the daily bath is of great value.

PEMPHIGUS

Definition

A serious autoimmune disorder affecting interepidermal cell cohesion resulting in flaccid blisters and painful erosions of the skin and mucous membranes.

Diagnostic features
- Flaccid easily broken blisters.
- Painful erosions.
- Face, trunk, flexures.
- Mucous membranes especially the mouth.
- Positive Nikolsky sign.

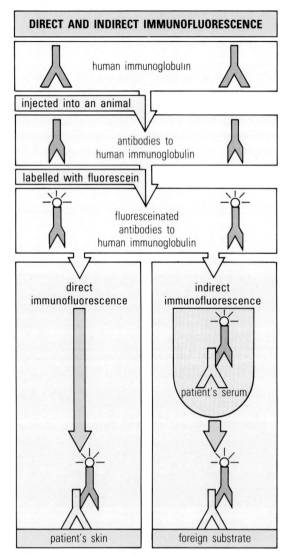

DIRECT AND INDIRECT IMMUNOFLUORESCENCE

human immunoglobulin

injected into an animal

antibodies to human immunoglobulin

labelled with fluorescein

fluoresceinated antibodies to human immunoglobulin

direct immunofluorescence

indirect immunofluorescence

patient's serum

patient's skin

foreign substrate

▲ **Fig. 21.5** *Direct and indirect immunofluorescence.*

Aetiology

Pemphigus is a very rare autoimmune disorder which is most common in Jews. It commences in the fourth or fifth decade. The antibodies are directed against the intercellular cement substance and can be demonstrated by direct or indirect immunofluorescence. Fragile blisters result within the epidermis (Fig. 21.6). If the split is low in the epidermis (suprabasal) erosions are the prominent physical sign (*pemphigus vulgaris*), but if it is more superficial crusts are more pronounced (*pemphigus foliaceus*) and the disorder is less severe. Pemphigus may be induced by certain drugs, in particular penicillamine and captopril.

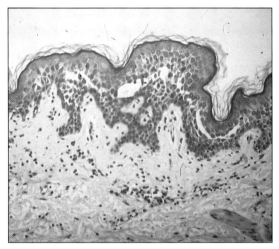

▲ **Fig. 21.6** *Pemphigus vulgaris. The epidermal cells separate from one another and a split is visible within the epidermis which results in a fragile blister.*

Clinical features

The blisters are flaccid and break easily to leave erosions behind, in contrast to the tense and firm blisters of pemphigoid. The erosions (Fig. 21.7) in pemphigus heal slowly, usually with crusting and subsequently pigmentation. They are painful and extensive. The mucous membranes are involved and are often the presenting feature in the mouth (Fig. 21.8) or genitalia. Because epidermal cell cohesion is damaged the upper layer of the epidermis may be made to slide over the lower by the examining finger (Nikolsky's sign). The disease was lethal in many patients before the advent of systemic steroids. The complications are similar to those of a patient with extensive burns with loss of fluid, infection both of the skin and other organs and septicaemia and toxaemia being prominent.

Diagnosis

The diagnosis may be confirmed by a skin biopsy. The histology shows clefting within the epidermis and the epidermal cells are separated away from one another, an appearance known as acantholysis. Acantholysis may also be demonstrated with exfoliative cytology. However diagnosis by immunofluorescence is definitive and deposits of IgG and C3 are visible between the epidermal cells. Indirect immunofluorescence is helpful in management in that the disease activity can be monitored by the antibody titre.

Management

Patients require specialist care, usually in hospital, in order to gain control of the disease. High doses of

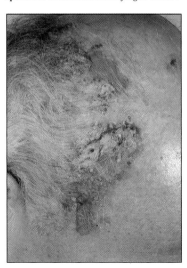

◀**Fig. 21.7** *Pemphigus vulgaris. The blisters are flaccid and break easily to form painful erosions and crusts which have little tendency to heal without therapy.*

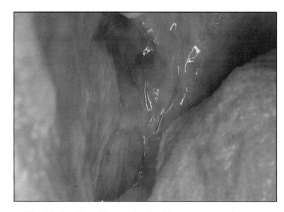

▲ **Fig. 21.8** *Pemphigus vulgaris. The mucous membranes are involved. The blisters break so easily that erosions are the most obvious abnormality. The condition often presents in the mouth or genitalia.*

systemic steroids (120mg of prednisolone) are required initially. Other immunosuppressants such as cyclophosphamide or azathioprine are often incorporated into treatment for their steroid sparing effect. Gold is also effective in less severe cases.

DERMATITIS HERPETIFORMIS

Definition
A very pruritic condition of grouped vesicles localized to certain areas of the skin, associated with a gluten-sensitive enteropathy.

> **Diagnostic features**
> - Excoriated papules and vesicles.
> - Grouped, symmetrical.
> - Intensely itchy.
> - Elbows, knees, buttocks, shoulders and scalp.
> - Rapidly alleviated by dapsone.

Aetiology
The condition is rare but has been the subject of intense investigation since the discovery that it is associated with a gluten-sensitive enteropathy identical on jejunal biopsy to that of coeliac disease but without overt symptoms of malabsorption. This enteropathy is relevant for it is possible to produce a remission of the disease if gluten is excluded from the diet for several months. The rash will return, however, if gluten is reintroduced into the diet.

Dermatitis herpetiformis mainly begins in early adult life.

All patients can be demonstrated, by immunofluorescence, to have deposits of IgA in the dermal papillae or along the basement membrane in their normal skin.

Clinical features
The condition is very itchy and the skin lesions start as vesicles or urticarial papules which the patient usually describes as blisters, which occur symmetrically in a grouped (herpetiform) manner just below the elbows (Fig. 21.9) and knees, on the buttocks, on the front and back of the shoulders and on the scalp. It has little tendency to remit. The patient is otherwise well.

Management
The itching ceases within a few hours of taking dapsone 50mg twice daily but recurs on stopping the drug. If a patient can tolerate a gluten-free diet the disorder will remit within a few months (sometimes longer), but will recur if the diet is abandoned. The gluten-free diet is unpleasant and many patients compromise with a partial diet and low doses of dapsone.

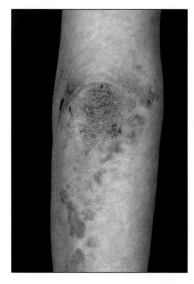

◀**Fig. 21.9** *Dermatitis herpetiformis. The intensely itchy vesicles are usually broken by scratching, and symmetrical, grouped, excoriated papules are seen on the elbows, knees, buttocks and in the scalp.*

PSYCHOLOGICAL DISORDERS OF THE SKIN

Many patients with symptoms referable to the skin have psychological problems. They may present in various manners.

APPROPRIATE REACTIONS

It is natural that a patient should be anxious or depressed regarding a disfiguring condition such as acne or psoriasis. He or she may feel embarrassed or even 'leprous' and have difficulty in making satisfactory relationships. The patient may be withdrawn and introverted or aggressive as a result. The degree of involvement of the skin is no guide to the degree of unhappiness. Mild psoriasis may be devastating to one patient whereas severe disease may be borne with good humour and tolerance by another, but most would give a lot to be free of it. Clearly sympathy, understanding, compassion and a desire to help are important, but they are not always forthcoming from doctors more accustomed to serious medical disorders.

OVERCONCERN REGARDING MINOR BLEMISHES

Symptoms involving the skin are common presentations of anxiety and depression. In particular, patients complain or are anxious about minor blemishes, particularly skin tags, haemangiomata, seborrhoeic warts, etc. (see chapter 8). If these patients were happy the lesions would merit no concern, but in the distressed they assume a disproportionate importance. The patients are usually middle-aged and are either depressed because of marital failure or anxious because of excessive pressure and stress at work.

LACK OF ABNORMAL PHYSICAL SIGNS

Alternatively, affective disorders may present as complaints for which no abnormal physical signs may be found on examination. This is sometimes known as *dermatological non-disease*. It includes a group who are suffering from *dysmorphophobia*, a rare and serious disorder in which the patient, usually female, is convinced that there is something wrong with her face. The condition is not amenable to reason and is thus a delusion. It is very difficult to treat and may end in suicide. Much more commonly, however, patients have less severe forms which are amenable to psychological treatment but are sometimes perplexing to practitioners who are taken in by the patient and believe that there must be something wrong with the skin, even though there is nothing abnormal to see. The common symptom complexes are referable to:

(1) **The scalp.** The patient may complain of excessive itching or burning of the scalp or, in females in particular, of excessive hair loss. In the former, the scalp appears quite normal on examination. In the latter, there may be abundant or acceptable amounts of hair and no adequate explanation, such as telogen effluvium, for the 'loss'. Depression and unhappiness in personal relationships are usually the explanation.

(2) **The face.** Burning is the most usual symptom — an unusual one in skin disorders — and should alert the practitioner. Complaints regarding redness of the face are common too, even when there is none to be seen.

(3) **The genitals.** In males the patient becomes preoccupied with the penis and scrotum. He describes irritation of the scrotum and redness of the glans or corona, particularly during an erection, and may find intercourse painful. He tends to examine his penis regularly and conscientiously and describes the abnormality in a painstaking manner (*penile preoccupation*). The condition is invariably diagnosed and treated as thrush and yet there are no real abnormal physical signs apart from possibly minimal erythema. The patient usually receives a multiplicity of topical remedies but none are effective because the patient requires counselling. Marital disharmony, sexual inexperience, stress and depression are the most common causes.

In females the complaint is usually of symptoms referable to the vulva without any abnormality on examination. In previous generations itching (*pruritus vulvae*) was the symptom, but for some reason this has been replaced by burning (*vulvodynia*). The discomfort may interfere with walking and sitting and certainly precludes sexual intercourse. The condition is often persistent and extremely difficult to treat, the patient consulting many doctors unsuccessfully and being reluctant to accept psychiatric help.

(4) The eyelids. The patient, usually female, complains of irritation of the eyelids. This *itchy eyelid syndrome* has usually baffled several doctors, including ophthalmologists, who can find nothing wrong but suspect an allergic cause. It is the lack of abnormal physical signs on examination of the skin of the eyelids that should alert the practitioner (Fig. 22.1). It possibly represents a suppression of the need to weep to display the pent-up unhappiness. Often the patient will readily recount her problems to the enquiring family practitioner if challenged.

(5) The mouth. *Glossodynia* is quite a common symptom of depression. The patient complains of burning or soreness in the mouth, particularly of the tip of the tongue, and may describe abnormalities such as

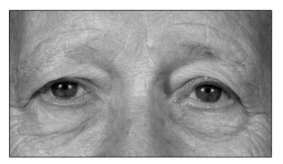

▲**Fig. 22.1** *Itchy eyelid syndrome. This man complained bitterly of irritation of his eyelids. The ophthalmologist and the dermatologist could find no abnormality. The condition was psychosomatic.*

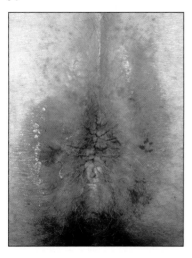

◀**Fig. 22.2** *Dermatitis medicamentosa. This man had suffered from pruritus ani for many years. There was never any abnormality on examination until he developed a contact dermatitis to one of his medicaments.*

blisters or ulcers, but there is never anything to see. The patient is usually diagnosed as having thrush or an allergy to dentures, but treatment is of no avail as the psychological nature of the condition requires recognition. It may respond well to counselling, and low-dose antidepressants such as amitriptyline 25mg at night.

(6) The anus. *Pruritus ani* is a common disorder, especially in males. Although many explanations are given for the intense irritation, for example anal sphincter dysfunction, anal tags, fissures, haemorrhoids, faecal soiling and thus 'allergy' to bacterial endopeptidases, a psychological disorder is more probable. There are no abnormal physical signs on examination and the condition is remarkably chronic and resistant to all manner of therapies. Certainly by the time the patient consults a dermatologist he will bring an accurate list (most unusual for other skin conditions) of numerous medications he has tried unsuccessfully. He is usually introspective, obsessional and mildly hypochondriacal, and will describe the malady in intimate detail. It does not respond well to psychological measures and it is best to tell him that many are similarly affected, that it is an oversensitivity of the cutaneous nerve endings and to continue to use whichever cream suits him best. It is wise, however, to avoid medicaments containing antibiotics, anaesthetics and other potential allergens because dermatitis medicamentosa (Fig. 22.2) may result.

PHOBIAS

The other variety of psychological skin disorder with no physical abnormality is the phobia. Venereophobia manifests itself in different ways depending on the diseases that are in the news at the time. Syphilis was the standard until it was superceded by herpes genitalis in the 1970s, now replaced by the acquired immune deficiency syndrome (AIDS). Clearly the patient may have good reason to fear these disorders, but in true venereophobia the patient is not at risk at all but just severely depressed and this should be recognized. The condition does not respond to reassurance but does respond to treatment of the depression.

A rare and bizarre phobia is parasitophobia, better known as *delusional parasitosis*. It is a true delusion quite unamenable to reason and should be recognized and treated as such. The patient has usually consulted several doctors, called in pest control agencies, had innumerable therapies for infestations and brings along the evidence (bits of dust and skin, but not parasites) for the doctor to see. There are no abnormalities on the skin, other than occasional scratch marks, and certainly no parasites. It is not easy to treat but if the patient will take the neuroleptic drug, pimozide, starting at 2mg and gradually increasing, the delusion may cease and the patient may acquire insight into the condition, and an underlying depression is revealed, which should be treated.

SKIN DISORDERS WITH A PSYCHOLOGICAL COMPONENT

Some disorders have a varying degree of psychological abnormality. Lichen simplex (chapter 3) probably results from scratching or rubbing of the skin secondary to a minor affective disorder, but it persists until treated with topical steroids because the condition induced is eczematous and therefore pruritic in its own right. Acne excoriée des jeunes filles (chapter 17) may commence as a minor degree of acne, but ultima-

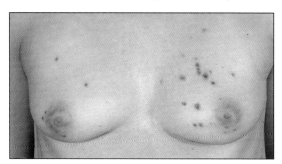

▲ **Fig. 22.3** *Neurotic excoriations. Discrete excoriations (scratch marks) were limited to the breasts in this patient. She admitted that they were self-induced and willingly accepted psychiatric help.*

tely the acne is non-existant and the abnormality has become a self-perpetuating and self-induced neurotic disorder. Trichotillomania (chapter 20) is a nervous habit tic for the most part, similar to biting the nails. Neurotic excoriations and habit tics are described below.

Neurotic excoriations
Definition
An itchy condition characterized by scratching or picking at healthy skin where the underlying cause is anxiety.

Diagnostic features
- Itching.
- Excoriations and sometimes hyperpigmentation and scarring.
- Localized excoriated thickening of the skin.
- No other skin abnormality.
- No systemic disturbance.

Aetiology
Generalized excoriation is more common in women and is a demonstration of unhappiness. Localized picking at the skin is a mild form of neurosis.

Clinical features
The patient complains of irritation of the skin. The condition may be generalized, in which case examination reveals excoriations at various stages of development, either fresh or healing, with post-inflammatory hyperpigmentation and scarring. Frequently the limbs are involved. Sometimes the lesions are localized excoriations (Fig. 22.3) or consist of thickened areas of skin (Fig. 22.4), often induced on the back of the hand by continually picking at it. The thumbnail (Fig. 22.5) may be affected in a similar way. These are forms of habit tic.

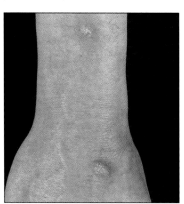

◀ **Fig. 22.4**
Habitual picking at the skin. These two thickened nodules were the result of continuous picking at the skin. This habit tic is a manifestation of anxiety.

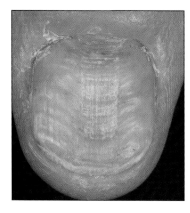

◀ **Fig. 22.5**
Habitual picking at the nail. A ridge along the length of the thumbnail has resulted from the continuous running of the index fingernail along it.

Management

Once a skin disorder or systemic explanation for the itching has been ruled out, recognition and elucidation of the root of the psychological problem and its treatment is important. The lesions themselves may be treated with, for example, medicated bandages if the limbs are involved, or topical steroids under occlusion, such that the patient cannot scratch the skin.

Prurigo
Definition

A chronic disorder characterized by intense generalized itching and widespread excoriations.

> **Diagnostic features**
> * Generalized irritation.
> * Excoriations.
> * Often excoriated nodules.
> * Limbs and upper back.

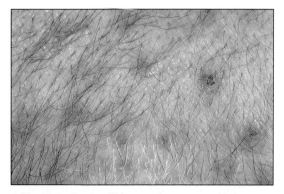

▲ **Fig. 22.6** *Prurigo. This term refers to a general irritation of the skin for which no explanation can be found. Only scratch marks are found on examination of the skin.*

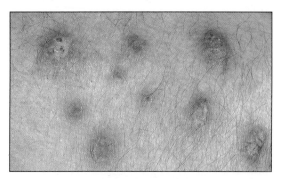

▲ **Fig. 22.7** *Nodular prurigo. This disorder is a variant of prurigo where the degree of scratching of the skin results in excoriated nodules.*

Aetiology

The cause is quite unknown. Emotional factors are suspected but not proven, but it is convenient to discuss the condition here. It occurs in both sexes but more commonly in middle-aged women. The term prurigo is used when there is no cutaneous or systemic explanation for the itching. (Confusingly, atopic eczema where excoriations predominate is known as Besnier's prurigo, and the itch of pregnancy which starts at the end of the second trimester and persists until just after delivery is known as 'prurigo of pregnancy', but these are unrelated.) Biopsy reveals non-specific inflammation initially, but in nodular cases gross thickening of the epidermis and hyperkeratosis is notable with a moderately dense mixed inflammatory infiltrate in the dermis.

Clinical features

The lesions are small excoriated papules (Fig. 22.6), usually on the extensor aspects of the limbs, upper trunk and buttocks. The condition is chronic over many years and may lead eventually to nodule formation (Fig. 22.7).

Management

Topical steroids are of limited value but antihistamines are helpful, especially hydroxyzine hydrochloride. Nodular prurigo may be treated with intralesional steroids, and ultraviolet light and PUVA are helpful in extensive nodular cases. Psychological remedies have a variable success. Occlusive bandaging is very helpful, especially to the limbs.

Dermatitis artefacta
Definition

A mutilation of the skin induced, but not admitted to, by the patient.

> **Diagnostic features**
> * Bizarre lesions.
> * Linear or geometric in configuration.
> * Do not conform to a recognized skin disorder.

Aetiology

The condition is rare and only included here for the sake of completeness. Any number of ingenious methods are used to induce the lesions. In many patients the condition is a psychosis which is completely denied by the patient and is very difficult to treat. In others it is a 'cri de coeur' which responds well to counselling.

Clinical features

The lesions are bizarre in appearance and do not conform to the configuration and distribution of any recognized pattern of dermatological disease. Linear (Fig. 22.8) and geometric shaped lesions are present. Gross mutilation may occur.

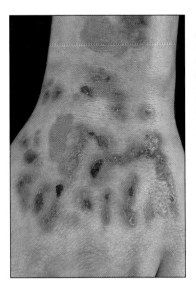

◀**Fig. 22.8**
Dermatitis artefacta. Linear excoriations were present on the back of this young woman's hand with no cutaneous abnormalities elsewhere. The lesions were self-induced.

Management

Confrontation with the patient is disastrous because patients do not accept psychiatric referral. The condition requires the greatest skill on the part of the physician who recognizes the condition, with the building up of an understanding. Hospitalization, skilled nursing and psychotropic drugs may all be helpful.

EXACERBATIONS OF SKIN DISORDERS BY EMOTIONAL FACTORS

Clearly psoriasis is not a psychiatric disorder. Its cause is at present obscure. However, many patients observe that their psoriasis will deteriorate after a shock or when they are highly stressed. Other conditions which are affected in this manner are atopic eczema, alopecia areata, pompholyx, seborrhoeic eczema, herpes simplex and dermographism and chronic urticaria. It is always worth enquiring about the patient's personal life because simple counselling may frequently help the patient cope with this exacerbation of their disorder whilst it is being treated with standard topical remedies.

CUTANEOUS SIGNS OF SYSTEMIC DISEASE

INTRODUCTION

The disorders described in this chapter are not common but the recognition of their physical signs is important because this may aid the diagnosis of an underlying systemic disease. The principal cutaneous signs only of these conditions are described and depicted here and the reader is referred to a general medical text for a full description of the disorders.

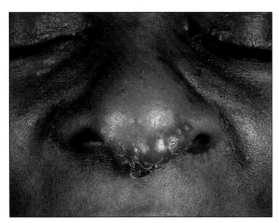

▲ **Fig. 23.1** *Sarcoidosis. Brown papules or nodules particularly around the nose are characteristic of sarcoidosis in Negroes.*

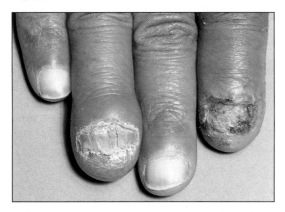

▲ **Fig. 23.2** *Sarcoidosis. Granulomatous infiltration of the skin and subcutaneous tissues occurs in the phalanges with the destruction of the nails. Erosions and cysts are usually found on X-ray.*

GRANULOMATOUS DISEASE

Leprosy and tuberculosis are discussed in chapter 10.

Sarcoidosis
Sarcoidosis is a multi-system disease of unknown aetiology characterized by non-caseating granulomatous infiltrations which may present in the skin as
(1) Erythema nodosum (Figs 15.11 & 15.12).
(2) Granulomatous infiltrations. Red-brown or purple, smooth-surfaced papules, plaques and nodules may occur anywhere on the body. Annular configurations are common (Fig. 1.27). Skin biopsy helps to establish the diagnosis. Because the pathology is confined to the dermis and subcutaneous tissues and the epidermis is not involved the lesions are never scaly.
(3) Granulomatous invasion of old scars.
(4) Sarcoidosis in the Negro. Brown-red papules around the nose (Fig. 23.1) and on the cheeks are characteristic.
(5) Sarcoidosis of the distal phalanges. Infiltration of the skin (Fig. 23.2) and destruction of the nails occur in association with erosions and cysts in the distal phalanges.
(6) Lupus pernio. In rare cases diffuse purple plaques occur on the nose and cheeks.

ENDOCRINE DISORDERS

Diabetes mellitus
Although boils are always mentioned as an indication for testing for glycosuria, candidosis and dermatophyte infections are much more commonly associated with diabetes. Two conditions which are associated with diabetes mellitus more than might be expected by chance are:
(1) Granuloma annulare. The lesions are ring-shaped (Fig. 23.3). The margin is seen to be composed of individual red papules, especially on the fingers (Fig. 23.4) and over the knuckles but also on the elbows, limbs and ankles. Although frequently mistaken for ringworm, there is no scaling since there is no epidermal involvement but a granulomatous infiltration of the dermis, the cause of which is obscure. It is by

no means always associated with diabetes. It is more common in children and young adults. It may respond to intralesional steroids or disappear spontaneously. (2) **Necrobiosis lipoidica.** These lesions occur classically on the shins as well-defined yellowish plaques with a waxy consistency, dilated small blood vessels on the surface (telangiectasia) and a violaceous margin (Fig. 23.5). They occasionally ulcerate.

Thyroid disease

Generalized pruritus and diffuse hair loss are occasionally presenting features of hyper- or hypothyroidism. The cutaneous signs of myxoedema are a dry and somewhat yellow skin. The hair lacks lustre, is coarse and may fall out. Purpura may occur. The features are coarse and there is oedema around the eyes (Fig. 23.6) which returns to normal with treatment (Fig. 23.7). A specific skin eruption is pretibial myxoedema.

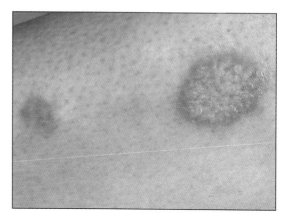

▲ **Fig. 23.5** *Necrobiosis lipoidica. Well-defined, yellow, telangiectatic plaques with a purple margin occur on the fronts of the shins. A significant proportion of patients have diabetes mellitus.*

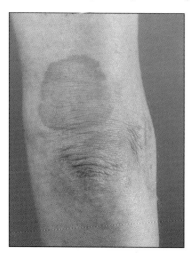

◄**Fig. 23.3** *Granuloma annulare. The lesions are ring-shaped but unlike ringworm, for which they are often mistaken, they have no surface change. The elbows are a typical site.*

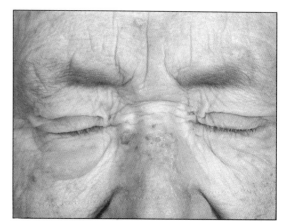

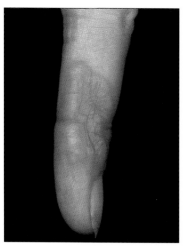

◄**Fig. 23.4** *Granuloma annulare. Individual discrete, flat-topped papules make up the border of the annular lesions. The digits and knuckles are commonly affected.*

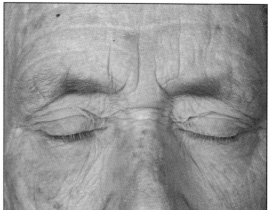

▲ **Figs 23.6 & 23.7** *Myxoedema. The skin is coarse, dry and somewhat yellow. The hair lacks lustre and falls out. There is oedema around the eyes which returns to normal (Fig. 23.7) with therapy.*

Pretibial myxoedema

Well-defined nodules occur on the shins (Fig. 23.8), often with patulous follicular orifices and hypertrichosis. There is mucinous infiltration of the dermis. Pretibial myxoedema occurs in thyrotoxic patients with high long-acting thyroid stimulating hormone (LATS) levels.

Cushing's syndrome

The buffalo hump, puffy telangiectatic face and obese trunk with slender, wasted limbs are a familiar picture due to iatrogenic Cushing's syndrome. Purple striae and atrophic skin which heals poorly are occasional modes of presentation (Fig. 23.9) of the disease. If an adrenal adenoma is the cause rather than adrenal hyperplasia secondary to a pituitary tumour, acne, hirsutism and virilism may be present.

Addison's disease

An insidious hyperpigmentation is characteristic (Figs 19.2 & 19.3).

METABOLIC DISORDERS

Porphyria

The porphyrias are a rare group of, usually inherited, inborn errors of the metabolism of haem, which result in the accumulation of porphyrin precursors, some of which are photosensitizers. The cutaneous physical signs are of:

- Vesicles, blisters and erosions (Fig. 23.10).
- Fragility of the skin.
- Hypertrichosis.
- Premature ageing of the skin.
- Scarring and scleroderma.
- In light exposed areas.

Hyperlipidaemia

Disorders of lipid metabolism may present in the skin as:

(1) **Xanthelasma.** These are yellow plaques which occur around the eyes (Fig. 23.11). They are common in normolipidaemic subjects.

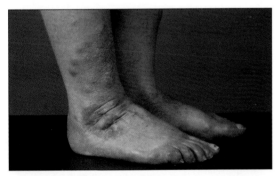

▲**Fig. 23.8** *Pretibial myxoedema. Well-defined nodules occur on the fronts of the shins with patulous follicular orifices and hypertrichosis in thyrotoxic patients with high LATS levels.*

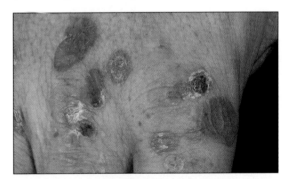

▲**Fig. 23.10** *Porphyria cutanea tarda. Fragility of the skin in light-exposed areas with blisters and erosions are characteristic. The backs of the hands are particularly affected.*

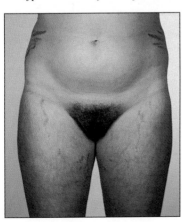

◄**Fig. 23.9** *Cushing's disease. This young woman presented with purple striae on her thighs and on her waist. The skin on the thighs is noticeably atrophic.*

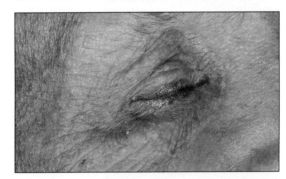

▲**Fig. 23.11** *Xanthelasmata. Diffuse yellow plaques occur around the eyes in primary and secondary (in this case due to multiple myeloma) hyperlipidaemia.*

(2) **Xanthomata.** These are yellow papules or nodules (Fig. 1.23) which appear quite suddenly in an eruptive manner, principally on the buttocks, elbows and knees.

(3) **Plane xanthomata.** Yellow deposits occur in the palmar creases and are rather typical of type III hyperlipidaemia.

COLLAGEN VASCULAR DISORDERS

Lupus erythematosus

Lupus erythematosus is a spectrum which varies from a potentially fatal, multi-system disorder (SLE) characterized by various immunological irregularities (most specifically antibodies to nuclear material and DNA) to a chronic discoid form (DLE) which is confined to the skin. The cutaneous signs may be precipitated by sunlight and cold. They consist of:
(1) a diffuse blotchy erythema (SLE) or
(2) well-defined, red, discoid lesions with an adherent scale with follicular plugging and sometimes scarring (DLE) (Fig. 23.12).
They occur on:
(1) sunlight-exposed sites (Fig. 23.13) and
(2) areas exposed to cold — ears, nose and fingers, so-called chilblain lupus (Fig. 16.16).
Hair loss — diffuse in active SLE or localized due to scarring DLE (Fig. 20.19) — may be present.

Dermatomyositis

This is a rare skin disease associated with a polymyositis which may occur in childhood or adult life. In a significant proportion of the latter it is associated with an underlying carcinoma. The major skin changes are:

(1) **A mauve ('heliotrope') discolouration** sometimes with oedema around the eyes (Fig. 23.14) is almost diagnostic. This may also occur on the cheeks, back of the neck, elbows and knees.

(2) **Purple papules** occur over the knuckles and around the nail folds (Fig. 23.15).

(3) **Cuticular splinter haemorrhages** (see Fig. 23.16).

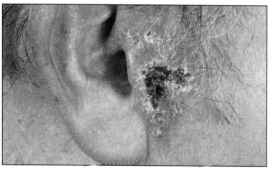

▲ **Fig. 23.12** *Discoid lupus erythematosus. A well-defined red plaque with adherent scale and scarring is present. The sideburn is often involved.*

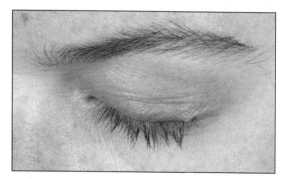

▲ **Fig. 23.14** *Dermatomyositis. A mauve discolouration around the eyes is characteristic. The cheeks, neck, elbows, knees and fingers are similarly discoloured.*

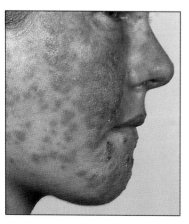

◀ **Fig. 23.13** *Systemic lupus erythematosus. A diffuse erythema is present on the cheeks, nose and ears. This exacerbation of her disease was initiated by sunbathing.*

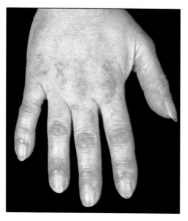

◀ **Fig. 23.15** *Dermatomyositis. Purple papules occur symmetrically over all the knuckles. This lady had proximal myositis and an associated carcinoma of the breast.*

Scleroderma

Scleroderma may occur as part of a systemic process (progressive systemic sclerosis) or as a localized abnormality confined to the skin (morphoea and lichen sclerosus et atrophicus).

Systemic sclerosis

This is a rare disease in which atrophy and sclerosis of the peripheral skin follows Raynaud's phenomenon and is associated with multi-systemic vasculitis. The predominant skin changes are:

(1) **Raynaud's phenomenon** (Fig. 23.17).

(2) **Sclerosis, deformity and dysfunction.** The skin overlying the subcutaneous tissue becomes tethered so that it feels hard (sclerotic) and cannot be pinched. There is loss of the normal skin creases and tapering of the fingers due to atrophy of their pulps.

(3) **Ischaemia.** Digital ischaemia leads to cutaneous infarction with ulceration and gangrene.

(4) **Facial changes.** Matt-like telangiectasia and sclerosis causing a beak-like appearance of the nose and a shrunken mouth with radiating furrows (Fig. 23.18).

(5) **Calcinosis** in the fingers and subcutaneous tissues.

(6) **Hirsutism.**

(7) **Hyperpigmentation.**

Localized scleroderma (morphoea)

Although occasionally patients with systemic sclerosis have patches of localized scleroderma, the likelihood of a patient with morphoea developing systemic disease is practically nil. The lesion is usually a single, well-defined plaque with a smooth, shiny surface which is impossible to pinch (Fig. 23.19). There is loss of hair and the margin is lilac in colour. The plaque may occur anywhere on the body but particularly on the trunk, thighs, eyes and upper arms. The cause is unknown but the disorder may disappear.

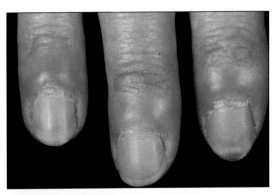

▲ **Fig. 23.16** *Dermatomyositis. Cuticular splinter haemorrhages occur with nail fold oedema and mauve discolouration.*

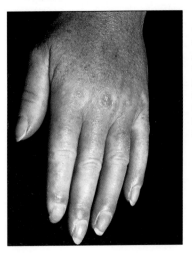

◀ **Fig. 23.17** *Scleroderma. The condition frequently presents as Raynaud's phenomenon. The skin goes white with cold. Later the fingers become tapered.*

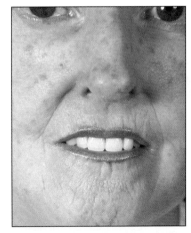

◀ **Fig. 23.18** *Scleroderma. The skin is tethered. Furrows radiate out from the mouth. The nose is pinched and the mouth is contracted. Mat-like telangiectasia is prominent.*

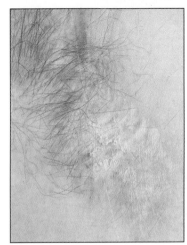

◀ **Fig. 23.19** *Morphoea (localized scleroderma). The lesion is a well-defined plaque with a smooth shiny sclerotic surface with loss of hair with a lilac or brown margin.*

Lichen sclerosus et atrophicus

Scleroderma-like changes may occur around the vulva and anus and on the glans penis (then often known as *balanitis xerotica obliterans*). The cause is not known. Occasionally extra-mucosal lesions (Fig. 1.20) occur, particularly on the wrists, neck and shoulders.

In the female the lesions consist of shiny, white, smooth-surfaced papules which coalesce and occur in a symmetrical manner around the vulva and anus (Fig. 23.20). These sclerotic papules become atrophic and telangiectasia and purpura may occur. The architecture of the labia and introitus become shrunken and obliterated. Very occasionally malignant change may occur.

An identical condition occurs on the foreskin of the glans penis (Fig. 23.21). The atrophy frequently leads to meatal stenosis and phimosis.

MALIGNANCY AND THE SKIN

As a general rule it is unusual for a patient with cancer to present with skin abnormalities, although generalized pruritis, hyperpigmentation, clubbing of the nails and cutaneous deposits are common enough during the course of the illness. Dermatomyositis and *acanthosis nigricans* are very rare disorders but are associated with malignancy. *Pseudoacanthosis nigricans* is a very common benign disorder in the obese Mediterranean or Arab: the physical signs are identical to those of true acanthosis nigricans. A velvety thickening and pigmentation of the skin occurs in the flexures (Fig. 23.22) often with skin tags.

Carcinoma of the breast may present as Paget's disease (Fig. 23.23).

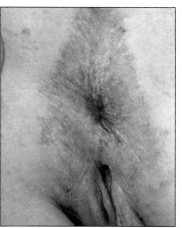

◀ **Fig. 23.20** *Lichen sclerosus et atrophicus. Symmetrical shiny white smooth-surfaced papules occur initially and are followed by atrophy, telangiectasia and purpura of the skin around the vulva and anus.*

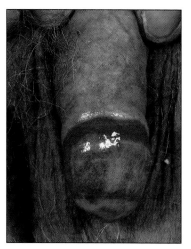

◀ **Fig. 23.21** *Balanitis xerotica obliterans. White sclerotic papules are visible on the glans and tip of the penis. Haemorrhage occurs readily into the atrophic areas.*

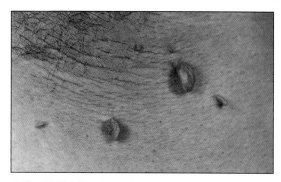

▲ **Fig. 23.22** *Pseudoacanthosis nigricans. Hyperpigmentated velvety thickening of the skin with exaggerated skin creases and skin tags occur in flexural areas in the obese. An identical picture occurs in association with a carcinoma.*

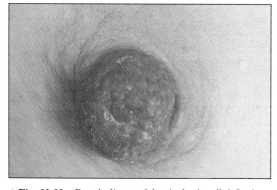

▲ **Fig. 23.23** *Paget's disease of the nipple. A well-defined red thickening of the nipple is present. Biopsy showed pagetoid cells (large cells with pale-staining granular cytoplasm and prominent nuclei and nucleoli) in the epidermis.*

Paget's disease

This occurs most frequently in the nipple as a result of the invasion of the skin by cells from an intraduct carcinoma of the breast. The nipple and then areola become reddened and indurated with scaling and crusting (see Fig. 23.23). The condition can also occur around the anus and genitalia secondary to a prostatic or gastrointestinal malignancy.

LYMPHOMA AND THE SKIN

Lymphomas present comparatively commonly in the skin. The skin may be the predominant organ affected, with spread to lymph nodes and elsewhere occurring latterly if at all (mycosis fungoides), or be involved from secondary deposits of non-Hodgkin's lymphoma.

Mycosis fungoides

Mycosis fungoides is a disorder of the thymus-derived lymphocytes which infiltrate the dermis and epidermis, producing large patches and plaques on the skin. In most patients it is a chronic disorder and the patients come to no harm, but in a minority it progresses to produce tumours and involve lymph nodes and other organs. Occasionally the entire cutaneous surface is involved (Fig. 23.24) and there is intense pruritus, erythroderma, loss of hair and hyperkeratosis of the palms and soles. Skin biopsy reveals an identical histology to that of mycosis fungoides but there may be circulating abnormal T cells as well as lymphadenopathy and the condition is known as the *Sezary syndrome* (Fig. 23.25). The salient changes are as follows.

Early stage disease
- Well-defined patches and/or plaques.
- Colour variation from pink to deep red.
- Asymmetrical.
- Bizarre shapes.
- Poikiloderma (atrophy, pigmentation and telangiectasia of the skin).

Late stage disease
- Tumours.
- Erythroderma (Sezary syndrome).
- Lymphadenopathy.

Hodgkin's and non-Hodgkin's lymphoma

These disorders may present in the skin as a generalized pruritus, acquired ichthyosis or infection secondary to immunosuppression, for example generalized

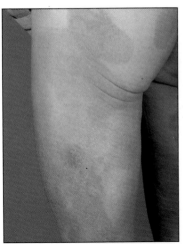

◀ **Fig. 23.24** *Mycosis fungoides. Well-defined patches and plaques occur in the early stages with sharply angulated edges and varying shades of pink and red.*

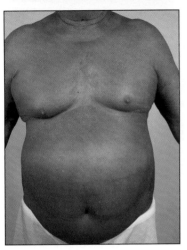

◀ **Fig. 23.25** *Sezary syndrome. The whole skin is red (erythrodermic) and intensely itchy. The skin, lymph nodes and bone marrow are infiltrated by large 'mycosis' cells with cerebriform hyperchromatic nuclei. The syndrome is a T cell leukaemic variant of mycosis fungoides.*

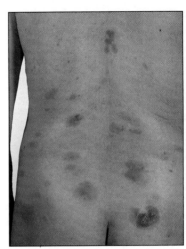

◀ **Fig. 23.26** *Non-Hodgkin's lymphoma. Purple papules, nodules and tumours are extensively distributed in the skin. The diagnosis can be made by skin biopsy.*

herpes zoster. Very occasionally mycosis fungoides may be followed by Hodgkin's disease. More frequently non-Hodgkin's lymphoma may be accompanied by or present with cutaneous deposits which are purple papules, plaques or tumours (Fig. 23.26) with no surface change. The diagnosis may be made by a skin biopsy.

MISCELLANEOUS CONDITIONS

Pyoderma gangrenosum

This is a rare disorder which evolves from a sterile pustule or boil-like lesion into an ulcer with a characteristic blue oedematous margin (Fig. 23.27). It is most commonly associated with inflammatory bowel disease, rheumatoid arthritis, Behçet's syndrome or plasma cell abnormalities such as multiple myeloma.

Reiter's disease

This is a disorder characterized by a non-suppurative polyarthritis, iritis and psoriasiform mucocutaneous lesions occurring in young adult males with the HLA-27 antigen. It follows either a dysenteric episode or a non-specific urethritis. The psoriasiform eruption is classically seen on the penis and palms and soles, where it is referred to as *keratoderma blenorrhagicum* (Fig. 23.28) since the skin may be grossly thickened.

Behçet's syndrome

This is a condition of oro-genital ulceration associated with recurrent uveitis, arthralgias and systemic (in particular, central nervous system) involvement. The skin lesions may be summarized as:

- Recurrent deep and painful oro-genital ulceration (Figs 23.29 & 23.30).
- Erythema nodosum.
- Sterile pustules, especially at venepuncture sites.
- Sterile pyodermas (see Fig. 23.31).

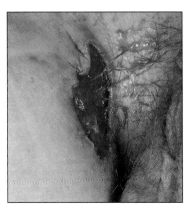

◀**Fig. 23.27** *Pyoderma gangrenosum. The ulcer has an indurated purple margin. This lady had associated rheumatoid arthritis.*

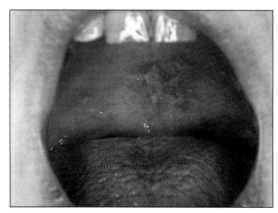

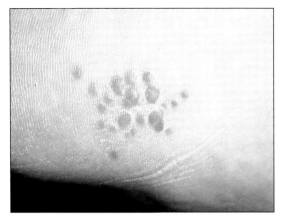

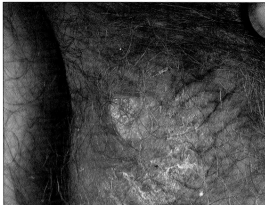

▲**Fig. 23.28** *Reiter's syndrome. Conical hyperkeratotic lesions present on the soles or palms are known as keratoderma blenorrhagicum. In other cases the lesions are more psoriasiform.*

▲**Figs 23.29 & 23.30** *Behçet's syndrome. Oral (Fig. 23.29) and genital ulceration (Fig. 23.30), iritis, arthritis, pyodermas and sometimes CNS involvement are characteristic.*

Generalized pruritis

Itching is a very common symptom. If it is due to a skin disorder (Fig. 23.32), physical signs of that skin disorder, for example burrows in scabies, will be found. In generalized pruritis due to an underlying medical or psychological disorder there will be either no abnormal physical signs or solely scratch marks (excoriations) and their consequences (post-inflammatory pigmentation and scarring) (Figs 23.33 & 23.34).

A full medical history and examination and investigation are required. The common causes of generalized pruritis are given in Figure 23.35. If no systemic abnormality is discovered on further investigation the pruritis may be psychosomatic, as in neurotic excoriations, or be termed prurigo (chapter 22).

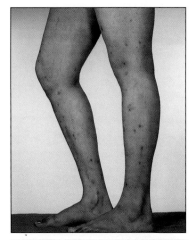

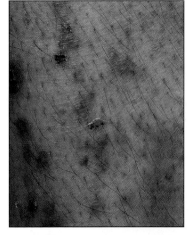

◀**Figs 23.33 & 23.34** *Generalized pruritis. The complaint is of irritation of the skin but on examination only excoriations and post-inflammatory pigmentation (Fig. 23.34) are found on the limbs. In this case the itching was due to iron deficiency anaemia.*

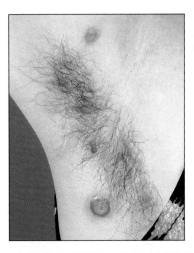

◀**Fig. 23.31** *Behcet's syndrome. Sterile pyodermas are sometimes present.*

PRURITIC SKIN DISORDERS
eczema
lichen planus
scabies
pediculosis
urticaria
insect bites
polymorphic light eruptions
drug eruptions
dermatitis herpetiformis
bullous pemphigoid

▲**Fig. 23.32** *Pruritic skin disorders.*

COMMON CAUSES OF GENERALIZED PRURITIS	
Haematological	iron deficiency anaemia polycythaemia rubra vera paraproteinaemia
Hepatic disease	primary biliary cirrhosis extra hepatic obstruction cholestasis of pregnancy cholestatic drugs
Renal disease	chronic renal failure
Malignancy	lymphoma, leukaemia abdominal cancer
Endocrine	hyperthyroidism diabetes mellitus
Drugs	opiates and derivatives aspirin
Psychological	

▲**Fig. 23.35** *Common causes of generalized pruritis.*

PREGNANCY

There are certain changes in pregnancy which are almost physiological. Thus spider naevi, palmar erythema, a generalized pigmentation coupled with a local pigmentation of the areolae, linea alba and genitalia are commonplace. Chloasma (Fig. 19.7) may occur. Moles and skin tags may increase in number and size. Striae are common. Hair growth is more luxuriant because anagen is prolonged in pregnancy. A compensatory precipitation of hair into telogen occurs at delivery so that a telogen effluvium three months later is normal. Prurigo gravidarum is the most common specific skin disorder. The others are rare. Their distinguishing features are summarized in Figure 23.36.

Prurigo gravidarum

This is very common and the skin appears quite normal apart from excoriations (Fig. 23.37). It is at its peak in the last month before delivery but can start as early as the third month. The condition is thought to be due to cholestasis induced by oestrogens, and in a minority the liver function tests are abnormal and jaundice may occur. This condition recurs in subsequent pregnancies.

Polymorphic eruption of pregnancy (pruritic urticarial papules and plaques of pregnancy, PUPPP)

This is an extremely pruritic condition of the last trimester of pregnancy (usually of primigravidae) which begins in the abdominal striae and consists of erythematous or urticarial papules or plaques (Figs 23.38 & 23.39) without excoriations. It clears with delivery or shortly thereafter and does not recur.

◀**Fig. 23.36** *Distinguishing features of pregnancy eruptions.*

DISTINGUISHING FEATURES OF PREGNANCY ERUPTIONS			
	Signs	Trimester	Subsequent
Prurigo gravidarum	Excoriations	Any time but especially late third	Yes
PUPPP	Urticarial papules, plaques	Late third	No
Pemphigoid gestationis	Urticarial lesions, blisters	Any time	Yes

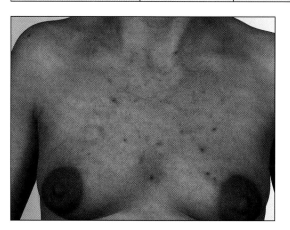

▲**Fig. 23.37** *Prurigo gravidarum. Only scratch marks are evident. It is most frequent in the last trimester and is recurrent. Occasionally cholestatic changes occur.*

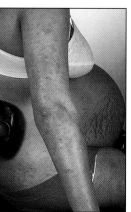 

▲**Figs 23.38 & 23.39** *Pruritic urticarial papules and plaques of pregnancy (PUPPP). There are urticarial papules and plaques (Fig. 23.39) which are intensely itchy. It begins in the abdominal striae in the last trimester in primigravidae and recovers with delivery.*

Pemphigoid (herpes) gestationis

This condition is virtually identical to bullous pemphigoid. It may occur at any time during pregnancy, and recurs in subsequent pregnancies and may be exacerbated post partum, premenstrually or with oral contraceptives. The lesions (Figs 23.40 & 23.41) are initially urticarial but subsequently become bullous. It is intensely pruritic and usually requires systemic steroids.

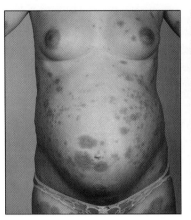 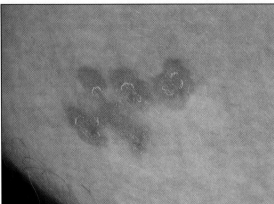

◀ **Figs 23.40 & 23.41** *Pemphigoid (herpes) gestationis. Intensely itchy urticarial and blistering lesions (Fig. 23.41) occur which are identical clinically to bullous pemphigoid.*

GLOSSARY OF TOPICAL THERAPIES

INTRODUCTION

The convention is to use generic and chemical names in medical textbooks. These are sometimes cumbersome for dermatological medicaments, especially in the case of glucocorticosteroids, so that product names are often used in common parlance. The purpose of this glossary is to give the British and North American proprietary names of these chemicals (the latter are given in parentheses). It is not all-inclusive and inevitably new products will be marketed and others withdrawn over the next few years. Systemic agents are not included because their generic names are generally well known.

BATH ADDITIVES AND EMOLLIENTS

British National Formulary
Aqueous cream (30% emulsifying ointment, 1% phenoxyethanol in water).

Emulsifying ointment (30% emulsifying wax, 50% white soft paraffin, 20% liquid paraffin).

Proprietary preparations
based on liquid paraffin: Alcoderm, Oilatum, Keri, Hydromol, Emulsiderm.
with lanolin: Alpha Keri (UK, US).
with white soft paraffin: Unguentum Merck, Diprobase, Ultrabase (Acidmantle creme, Nutraderm, Cetaphil, Eucerin, US).
based on soya oil: Balneum.
based on colloidal oat fraction: Aveeno.
based on urea: Aquadrate.
with lactic acid: Calmurid.

DITHRANOL (UK) ANTHRALIN (US)

British National Formulary
Available as ointment and in Lassar's paste (zinc and salicylic acid).

Proprietary preparations
alone: Dithrocream, Anthranol, Exolan, Antraderm (Anthraderm, Drithocreme, Lasan, US).
+ *urea*: Psoradrate.
+ *salicylic acid*: Dithrolan.
+ *tar*: Psorin.

Caution – Dithranol may burn the skin, particularly in higher concentrations.

TAR

British National Formulary
Available as coal tar and salicylic acid ointment, coal tar paste, zinc and coal tar paste and coal tar bath solution.

Proprietary preparations
Tar alone
shampoos: Alphosyl, Baltar, Gelcotar, Polytar, Genisol, Clinitar, T gel, Ionil T (UK and US) (Denorex, Pentrax, Zetar, Sebutone, US).
bath preparations: Polytar, Psoriderm, Balneum + Tar bath oil (Balnetar, Zetar, US).
creams, lotions and/or gels: Carbodome, Alphosyl, Clinitar, Psoriderm, Gelcotar, Psorigel (Estar, Fototar, Sebutone, US).
medicated bandages (zinc and coal tar): Coltapaste, Tarband.

Tar and hydrocortisone creams
Alphosyl HC, Tarcortin, Carbocort.

Tar and salicylic acid
Gelcosal, Pragmatar.

Ichthammol
Ichthammol is a mild form of tar from wood shale.

British National Formulary
Available as ointment and zinc and ichthammol cream.

Proprietary bandages (zinc and ichthammol)
Ichthaband, Icthopaste.

Non-tar medicated bandages
zinc paste: Zincaband, Viscopaste.
zinc paste and calamine: Calaband.
zinc paste, calamine and clioquinol: Quinoband.
hydrocortisone and silicone: Cortacream.

TOPICAL GLUCOCORTICOSTEROIDS

The classification system used by Polano has been
adopted in this textbook (i.e. class I are weakest,
class IV are strongest) because class V steroids may
become available whereas weaker ones will not
because they would be ineffective. Others
confusingly classify the steroids the other way
around, so that class I are the strongest, but this
leaves no room for the inclusion of stronger steroids
at a later date.

Class I (weakest)

Hydrocortisone
Alone
Cobadex, Dioderm, Efcortelan, Hydrocortistab,
Hydrocortisyl (Hytone, Cortdome, Cortril, Penecort,
Lacticare, Synacort, Texacort, US).

+ urea
Sential.

+ antibacterials
neomycin, bacitracin and polymyxin B:
   Corticosporin (US).
tetracycline: Terracortril.
framycetin: Framycort.
fucidin: Fucidin H.
gentamycin: Genticin HC.
clioquinol: Barquinol HC, Vioform HC (US
equivalent Vytone = hydrocortisone + iodoquinol).

+ Nystatin
+ benzalkonium chloride: Timodine.
+ chlorhexidine: Nystaform HC.
+ neomycin: Gregoderm.

+ Imidazoles
Canesten HC, Daktacort, Econacort.

Other class I steroids
alclometasone dipropionate: Modrasone (Aclovate US).

Class II
desoxymethasone: Stiedex.
flucortolone: Ultradil and Ultralanum.
hydrocortisone + urea: Calmurid HC, Alphaderm.
clobetasone butyrate: Eumovate.
   + nystatin and oxytetracycline: Trimovate.
flurandrenolone: Haelan.
   + clioquinol: Haelan C.

Class III
hydrocortisone butyrate: Locoid (UK and US).
beclomethasone dipropionate: Propaderm.
   + aureomycin: Propaderm A.
betamethasone dipropionate: Diprosone (UK and
US) (Diprolene, Maxivate, Alphatrex, US).
   + clotrimazole: Lotriderm (Lotrisone US).
   + salicylic acid: Diprosalic.
betamethasone valerate: Betnovate (Betatrex,
Valisone, US).
   (Also available in dilutions of 1/4.)
   + clioquinol: Betnovate C.
   + neomycin: Betnovate N.
   + fucidin: Fucibet.
diflorasone diacetate: Florone, Maxiflor, Psoreon (US).
fluocinolone acetonide: Synalar (UK and US).
   (Dilutions of 1/10 and 1/4 available.)
   + clioquinol: Synalar C.
   + neomycin: Synalar N (Neosynalar US).
fluocinonide: Metosyn (Lidex US).
desonide: Tridesilon (Desowen US).
triamcinolone acetonide: Adcortyl, Ledercort
(Kenalog, Aristocort A, US).
   + graneodin and neomycin: Adcortyl with
      graneodin (UK).
   + tetracycline: Aureocort.
   + nystatin: Nystadermal (Mycolog II, Mytrex F,
      US).
   + nystatin, gramicidin and neomycin:
      Triadcortyl.

For oral lesions
triamcinolone: Adcortyl in orabase (Kenalog in
orabase, US).

For intralesional use
triamcinolone hexacetonide 5mg/ml: Lederspan
(Aristospan US).
triamcinolone acetonide 10mg/ml: Adcortyl (Kenalog US).

Class IV (most potent)
halcinonide: Halciderm.
diflucortolone valerate 0.3%: Nerisone forte.
fluocinolone acetonide 0.2%: Synalar HP (US).
clobetasol propionate: Dermovate (Temovate US).
  + neomycin and nystatin: Dermovate NN.

ANTIBACTERIALS

framycetin: Framygen, Soframycin.
mupirocin: Bactroban (UK and US).
neomycin: Myciguent.
  + bacitracin: Cicatrin.
  + bacitracin + polymyxin: Polybactrin, Tribiotic.
  + gramicidin: Graneodin.
  + chlorhexidine: Naseptin.
nitrofurazone: Furacin (UK and US).
polymyxin B sulphate: Polyfax.
silver sulphadiazine: Flamazine.
chlortetracycline hydrochloride: Aureomycin.
tetracycline hydrochloride: Achromycin (UK and US).
fusidic acid: Fucidin.
gentamycin: Cidomycin, Genticin, Garamycin (all US).

ANTIFUNGALS

Anti-candida
amphotericin: Fungilin (Fungizone US).
nystatin: Nystan, Multilind (Mycostatin, Nilstar, US).
natamycin: Pimafucin.

**Candida, tinea and pityriasis versicolor
(Broad spectrum imidazoles)**
clotrimazole: Canesten (Lotrimin, Mycelex, US).
econazole: Ecostatin, Pevaryl, Spectrazole (UK, US).
miconazole: Daktarin, Dermonistat (Monistat, Micatin, US).
ketoconazole: Nizoral (UK and US).
sulconazole: Exelderm.

Tinea and candida nail plate infection:
tioconazole: Trosyl nail solution.

Tinea
undecenoates: Phytocil, Tineafax (Breezee US).
tolnaftate: Timoped.

Tinea and candida
nystatin and tolnaftate: Tinaderm-M.

Pityriasis versicolor
Selenium sulphide shampoo: Lenium, Selsun, (Exsel US).

ANTIVIRAL PREPARATIONS
(Herpes simplex and Zoster)

acyclovir: Zovirax (UK and US).
idoxuridine: Herpid, Iduridin, Virudox.

PARASITICIDAL PREPARATIONS

Insect bites
crotamiton: Eurax (UK and US).
  + hydrocortisone: Eurax HC.

Pediculosis
carbaryl: Carylderm, Clinicide, Derbac, Suleo-C.
permethryn: Nix (US).
malathion: Derbac-M, Prioderm, Suleo-M.

Scabies
lindane = gamma benzene hexachloride: Lorexane, Quellada (Kwell, Scabene, US).
benzyl benzoate: Ascabiol.

Caution – Benzyl benzoate irritates the skin and is best avoided. Crotamiton is inadequate as a scabicide.

PREPARATIONS FOR WARTS
AND CALLUSES

salicylic acid: Salatac gel (UK), Verrugon, Compound W (UK and US), (Occlusal, Wart off, Trans-plantar, Duoplant, US).
salicylic acid and lactic acid: Cuplex, Salactol, Duofilm (UK and US) (Viranol, Salactic film, US).
salicylic acid and podophyllum resin: Posalfilin (Cantharone plus, US).
formaldehyde: Veracur.
glutaraldehyde: Glutarol, Verucasep.

Podophyllum resin
British National Formulary
podophyllin paint compound.

Proprietary preparations
podophyllotoxin: Warticon (Pod-ben 25 US).

TREATMENT FOR ACNE

Topical antibiotics
clindamycin: Dalacin T (Cleocin T US).
tetracycline: Topicycline (UK and US).
benzoyl peroxide: Acetoxyl, Acnegel, Acnidazil, Benoxyl, Nericur, Benzagel (UK and US), Panoxyl (UK and US) (Theraderm, Desquam X, Persagel, US).
+ sulphur: Benoxyl with sulphur
+ quinolines: Quinoderm.
+ quinolone + hydrocortisone: Quinoderm HC.
chloramphenicol with hydrocortisone acetate: Actinac.
erythromycin: Stiemycin (Erymax, Eryderm, Erycette, US).
+ benzoyl peroxide: Benzamycin, T Stat (both US).

Vitamin A derivatives
tretinoin: Retin A (UK and US).

Keratolytics
British National Formulary: salicylic acid and sulphur; sulphur lotion and cream.
Proprietary preparations: resorcinol and sulphur – Eskamel.

Abrasives
aluminium oxide: Brasivol.
polyethylene granules: Ionax.

SUNSCREENS

There are a multitude of commercially available sunscreens. Virtually all block UVB (e.g. para amino benzoic acid (PABA) and ethylhexyl-*p*-methoxycinnamate). Some have an additional effect against UVA (e.g. oxybenzone and mexenone). Butyl-methoxydibenzoylmethane is effective against UVA only. Titanium dioxide is an opaque reflectant which blocks all wavelengths but is not cosmetically very acceptable. The sun protection factor (SPF) indicates how much longer one may remain in the sun without burning. PABA occasionally causes allergic reactions.

Oxybenzone, padimate: Coppertone supershade 15.
Ethylhexyl-*p*-methoxycinnamate, oxybenzone, padimate: Coppertone ultrashade 23, Piz Buin 12.
Ethylhexyl *p*-methoxycinnamate, zinc oxide: Roc Total Sunblock.
Ethylhexyl-*p*-methoxycinnamate, butyl methoxydibenzoylmethane: Piz Buin 24.
Aminobenzoic acid, padimate: Spectraban 15.
Mexenone, ethyl *p*-methoxycinnamate: Uvistat 10.
Octyldimethyl PABA, oxybenzone: Pre-Sun (US).

ANTIPERSPIRANTS

aluminium chloride: Anhydrol forte, Driclor, Hyperdrol (Drysol US).

TOPICAL CYTOSTATICS

5 fluorouracil: Efudix (Fluroplex US).

INDEX